Cardiovascular MRI in Practice

Cardiovascular MRI in Practice

A Teaching File Approach

By

John D. Grizzard, MD
Assistant Professor, Department of Radiology, Director, Non-invasive Cardiovascular Imaging, VCU Medical Center, Richmond, VA, USA

Robert M. Judd, PhD
Associate Professor, Department of Medicine and Radiology, Co-Director, Duke Cardiovascular Magnetic Resonance Center, Duke University Medical Center, Durham, NC, USA

Raymond J. Kim, MD
Associate Professor, Department of Medicine and Radiology, Co-Director, Duke Cardiovascular Magnetic Resonance Center, Duke University Medical Center, Durham, NC, USA

Springer

John D. Grizzard, MD
Assistant Professor, Department of Radiology, Director, Non-invasive Cardiovascular Imaging, VCU Medical Center, Richmond, VA, USA

Robert M. Judd, PhD
Associate Professor, Department of Medicine and Radiology, Co-Director, Duke Cardiovascular Magnetic Resonance Center, Duke University Medical Center, Durham, NC, USA

Raymond J. Kim, MD
Associate Professor, Department of Medicine and Radiology, Co-Director, Duke Cardiovascular Magnetic Resonance Center, Duke University Medical Center, Durham, NC, USA

ISBN 978-1-84800-089-6 ISBN 978-1-84800-090-2 (eBook)
DOI 10.1007/978-1-84800-090-2

Additional material to this book can be downloaded from http://extras.springer.com

Library of Congress Control Number: 2008921382

Printed on acid-free paper

9 8 7 6 5 4 3 2 1

springer.com

To my three sons– Patrick, Michael, and Kevin– with love. And to Louisa for her encouragement.

– JDG

To my immediate family—Sue, Matt, Kevin, and Elizabeth, and to the grandfather I never met, Herbert Alvin Judd, who left a wife and four children when he died of heart disease at the age of 46.

–RMJ

To Enn-ling, Alison, and 'Kiwi'—my treasures.

–RJK

And to those patients whose heart or vascular disease is portrayed herein with the hope that this endeavor may ultimately prove helpful to other patients and the physicians involved in their care.

–JDG, RMJ, RJK

Preface

Cardiovascular MR imaging has become a robust, clinically useful modality, and the rapid pace of innovation and important information it conveys have attracted many students whose goal is to become adept practitioners. In turn, many excellent textbooks have been written to aid this process. These books are necessary and useful in helping the student learn the underlying pulse sequences used in CMR, as well as the imaging findings in a variety of disorders. However, one of the difficulties inherent in learning CMR from a book is that the printed format is not the ideal medium to display the dynamic imaging that comprises a typical CMR case. For instance, it may be difficult to perceive focal areas of wall motion abnormality on serial static pictures, but these abnormalities are often easily seen on cine loops. One might say that trying to learn CMR solely from a standard textbook with illustrations is like trying to learn to drive by looking at snapshots obtained through the windshield of a moving car. The learner needs to see the cardiac motion and decide if it is normal or abnormal; he or she needs to be in the driver's seat. An additional limitation of the available textbooks on CMR is that while they often have superb illustrations of abnormal findings, these images have been preselected. In transitioning to the "real world," the challenge is for the student to be able to find the pathology. Therefore, ideally the student should make an initial attempt at deciding what is normal and abnormal in a given scan, as it is our experience that it is not uncommon for patients to leave the CMR facility with a diagnosis that differs importantly from the original indication for the scan. To do this successfully, the student needs to see the entire scan, with the mistakes and inconclusive images included, rather than attempt to become proficient in CMR based solely on preselected images that simply support the final diagnosis.

This book represents a new and different way of learning CMR. The entire project is encoded on a single (dual-layer) DVD as a series of Web pages that can be displayed offline in any Web browser (e.g. Internet Explorer, Firefox, Safari). Unlike previous CMR textbooks, which typically contain a few preselected views for each case, the DVD contains the *entire scan* for each of the 150 clinical cases (a total of 88,535 CMR images). Within each case, all the necessary tools to make the diagnosis are presented in exactly the same format as they are used every day at leading CMR clinical centers, including side-by-side movies, image magnification, single stepping, and even measurement tools (measurements require an internet connection). This format provides the student of CMR with the unprecedented opportunity to review all of the data and attempt to reach their own conclusion and then reference an expert opinion simply by clicking on the "Case Discussion" Web link.

The cases comprising this Teaching File demonstrate the utility of CMR for the entire spectrum of cardiovascular pathology. Straightforward "bread-and-butter" cases are presented, along with more unusual entities. The first few cases are designed to introduce the reader to the display format and to the techniques used in CMR, including the mechanics and nuances of image acquisition. The cases that then follow can be sorted by category (congenital heart disease, cardiomyopathies, etc.) if desired, but are otherwise presented in a random format to allow readers to test themselves in interpreting "unknowns." In the initial presentation of the images, the history is withheld, but clicking the "history" button at the top of the page will reveal it.

Through this presentation of unknown cases, the reader can encounter the unfiltered "raw data" of real patient scans, can formulate their own opinion, and then can obtain immediate feedback by reading the discussion. In addition, references are attached to virtually every case. Since the cases are viewed using a standard web browser, if one is connected to the Internet, clicking on the associated links will take one directly to the abstract in PubMed. From there, one can do additional reading as desired.

The print portion of this project, which accompanies the DVD, is organized into two sections: Part I is an overview of CMR imaging, with an introduction to current techniques and applications. Part II is comprised of the Case Discussions that explain each case. Part III reviews scan planning and standard protocols. The printed material is thus available for offline reading, but is also reproduced on the DVD. This duplication is done to take advantage of the Web page format of the DVD, which allows the creation of links between related subjects. Since the DVD contents are displayed in a browser window, links from the Case Discussions to the Overview allow easy navigation from cases to didactic material and back to cases, facilitating the learning process (when using the DVD).

It is our hope that this assemblage of CMR cases will be helpful to those cardiologists and radiologists in training who are interested in learning CMR, particularly those training at facilities where they may not have an abundance of cases. We are biased of course, but we believe that CMR is one of the most exciting fields in medicine. We hope that the introduction to its various implementations as contained in this Teaching File will stimulate in the reader a broad and sustained interest.

John D. Grizzard, MD
Robert M. Judd, PhD
Raymond J. Kim, MD

Acknowledgments

This work would not have been possible without the hard work and expertise of a multitude of individuals. First among these is Tarik Koc, who did much of the laborious work of HTML coding involved in making the DVD an effective teaching tool, with links between sections and cases. Thanks also go to the many current and former cardiology fellows, radiology house staff, and technologists both at Duke and VCU who performed scans and suggested cases for inclusion.

We would also like to point out that the sections of this book relating to myocardial delayed contrast enhancement reflect knowledge gained from U.S. National Institutes of Health projects R01-HL064726 and R01-HL063268.

John D. Grizzard, MD
Robert M. Judd, PhD
Raymond J. Kim, MD

Contents

How to Use the DVD and the Book Together

As opposed to many book-DVD combinations, in the instance of this endeavor, the DVD is the "heart" of the project, while the printed material is supplementary. To get started, simply insert the DVD into your computer and navigate to and open the folder containing the Book. Then, click the "Getting_Started.html" icon and the Teaching File will load in a browser window. The reader will note that the home page for the project has a "window-frame" appearance wherein the navigation placemarks (Book, Cases, Training, etc.) are present along the left margin of the screen, while the central "pane" shows the case images, or the book text, etc. Selecting "Cases" will result in the display of a drop-down menu allowing choice "by number" of the cases in 20 case increments. However, the cases can also be sorted by category. Clicking on "The Book" will take one to the title page of the Book. Choosing the "Table of Contents" drop-down menu will take the reader to an interactive Table of Contents that has links to the various sections and chapters of the Book.

The Webpax® interface used for the presentation of the cases provides a user-friendly format for the display of cardiovascular images. This unique interface allows visualization of cardiac motion at the patient's native heart rate (assuming sufficient computer resources) as present during the scan. These images can be viewed using any standard web browser, although the authors' prefer Firefox® (http://www.mozilla.com/en-US/firefox/) since this browser appears to more faithfully follow W3C web standards. Multiple looping images can be viewed simultaneously, facilitating comparison of the various segments. Clicking on any given image will result in the image being magnified. In addition, a scroll bar will then become evident, which provides the reader the ability to rapidly move back and forth through the stack of images. If two or more "magnified" views are desired, one can open multiple browser windows, each with their own view. The thumbnail images are presented as animated GIFs, and right clicking on the image and "saving as" will allow one to save the image. Alternatively, if one has an Apple computer, one can simply drag the image and drop it onto the desktop or directly onto a PowerPoint slide. Many tools, including the ability to download the magnified views as AVI or animated GIF files, have been disabled for offline viewing, however, if an internet connection is available these tools will be available during online viewing. For AVI files, the reader can select the play speed or frame rate, but the default (for cine images) is the patient's native heart rate.

The majority of cases are displayed in a standardized format, wherein the short-axis cine views are presented in the top row, arranged from base to apex as one proceeds from left to right. In the case of a stress / rest perfusion study, the stress images are presented in the first three or four images of the second row, and are arranged so that they are directly below the corresponding cine image acquired at the same location. The rest perfusion images are displayed in the third row, again at exactly the same image locations. Finally, the delayed-enhancement images (again spatially matched to the cine and perfusion images) are displayed in the fourth row. This arrangement facilitates the comparison of wall motion with stress and rest perfusion and viability. In cases performed without perfusion imaging, the display arrangement may demonstrate some variability, but the essential images necessary for diagnosis will be available.

Each case has an associated discussion that reviews the imaging findings and reveals the diagnosis. In addition, references are attached to virtually every case. Since the cases are viewed using a standard web browser, if one is connected to the Internet, clicking on the associated links will take one directly to the abstract in PubMed. From there, one can do additional reading as desired.

It is suggested that the reader initially attempt evaluation of the images alone, before turning to the discussion. It is our hope that the discussions will suggest to the reader a systematic approach to the evaluation of CMR images. The abundance of information presented in a typical CMR case can be overwhelming at times, and only through the application of a consistent reading format will one be assured of detecting all the important findings in a given case. In general, the approach used in the Teaching File follows this sequence: 1) LV–Cavity size, wall thickness, global and regional wall motion (using the 17-segment model). 2) RV–Cavity size, wall thickness, global and regional wall motion. 3) Valves–Mitral, aortic, tricuspid, pulmonic; evaluate for morphology and thickening, regurgitation, and stenosis. 4) Atria –Size, emptying, masses/ thrombi (left atrial appendage in particular). 5) Perfusion images (if performed)–Compare stress/rest images if both performed in order to exclude artifact. Evaluate for defects; compare to analogous regions on cine and delayed-enhancement images. 6) Delayed-enhancement imaging–Compare to perfusion and cine images at same spatial locations. If hyperenhancement is present, determine if it is in a CAD or Non-CAD pattern. Determine the transmural extent of hyperenhancement (infarction for patients with CAD) using the 17-segment model and a 5-point scale for each segment. Evaluate long-inversion-time images for thrombi. 7) Global overview–Evaluate pericardium for thickening, fluid; mediastinum and lungs for masses, etc.

MR angiographic images are also presented, and the utility of MRA for imaging a variety of vascular territories will be discussed. Because of the variety of body regions examined, it is difficult to suggest a single reading technique. A few caveats, however, are offered: 1) When possible, think physiologically when evaluating an MRA study, and not simply anatomically. For instance, looking for associated collaterals that would be expected in cases of chronic occlusion facilitates the correct characterization of an abrupt vessel-cutoff as being due to a stent artifact rather than an occlusion. 2) These studies encompass a lot of anatomy, and attention to extra-vascular structures is important to avoid missing significant pathology.

The Overview of Cardiovascular MR Imaging included with the Teaching File is not designed as a comprehensive textbook, but rather is intended to serve as a quick reference to the current techniques and principles used in everyday CMR imaging. It can be read prior to attempting to tackle the Teaching File cases, or may simply be referred to on an "as-needed" basis, depending on one's experience and training. The scanning protocols used by the authors for a variety of indications are included in the Appendix, along with a glossary of acronyms to help the reader decode the "alphabet soup" of abbreviations found in CMR.

John D. Grizzard, MD
Robert M. Judd, PhD
Raymond J. Kim, MD

Part I
Techniques and Applications

1
Overview

Introduction

Over the last several years, cardiovascular magnetic resonance (CMR) has undergone rapid evolution, and tremendous advances in pulse sequence design, scanner hardware, and coil technology have resulted in progressive expansion of the clinical applications.[1–4] In particular, new pulse sequences have leveraged the inherently superior soft tissue contrast provided by MR so that it now provides the reference standard for in vivo viability imaging.[5] Additionally, the pattern and distribution of scar as demonstrated by CMR often provides useful information regarding the specific etiology of various cardiac disorders.[6, 7] Similarly, for imaging cardiac structure and function, pulse sequence and hardware developments have resulted in improvement in image quality with simultaneous acceleration of image acquisitions, resulting in shorter but better examinations. Improved coil design now allows the use of parallel imaging technology, resulting in further reductions in acquisition times.[8, 9] These improvements have led to the recognition of CMR as the reference standard for the assessment of regional and global systolic function,[10, 11] the detection of myocardial infarction and viability,[12, 13] and the evaluation of pericardial disease and cardiac masses.[14, 15] In some centers, CMR is emerging as the test of choice for the detection of ischemic heart disease, as well as for the initial work-up of patients presenting with heart failure.[16, 17]

As CMR moves from a research tool into the clinical mainstream, there has been a gradual recognition of the need for standardized imaging protocols. This process is ongoing, but the Society of Cardiovascular Magnetic Resonance has formulated initial guidelines for imaging modules that can be combined as needed for a variety of different examinations. The cases presented in the Teaching File in Part II were acquired using protocols similar to these guidelines, and our versions of these guidelines are listed in the appendix. This chapter provides a brief overview of the common techniques used in CMR. The subsequent chapters then outline the standard cardiac examination, discuss specific applications for the assessment of a variety of cardiac disorders, and provide some suggestions on how to optimally use this Teaching File. Several of the individual Teaching File cases will also review the techniques of image acquisition, and the parameters used for given sequences.

CMR Techniques

A unique characteristic of MR imaging is that a variety of information can be obtained simply by selecting different software sequences to probe the tissue characteristics of the organ in question. Multiple pulse sequences are available for cardiac MR imaging and can provide morphologic, cine, perfusion, viability, and velocity-encoded flow images. Also, certain image sequences may be utilized to produce cine images wherein multiple phases at the same slice location are obtained, or the same sequence may be run as a multislice acquisition where single phases at multiple locations are obtained. Although the physics underlying these pulse sequences are beyond the scope of this overview, a brief consideration of pulse sequences and the resulting images is presented to provide background for the Teaching File cases.

Morphologic Imaging Using Dark-Blood Sequences

This was the initial application of MR imaging for evaluating the heart. Initial implementations used spin-echo techniques, and subsequently fast spin-echo acquisitions were developed that resulted in decreased imaging time. For the most part, morphologic black blood imaging is now performed with single-shot double inversion fast spin-echo techniques (Double-IR FSE, and HASTE or half-Fourier acquisition turbo spin-echo). These result in still-frame images and are usually acquired in the standard orthogonal imaging planes (axial, sagittal, or coronal) (Figure 1.1) (Case 66, series 2 and 4). The TR is typically set at 90% of the R-R interval, and adjusted to null the signal from blood. The images are acquired at every other heartbeat, and are quite useful for rapid morphologic imaging. A fat-saturation prepulse can also be applied. The rapidity of acquisition is such that breath holding is not required. These produce excellent depiction of the overall myocardial structure, as well as the relationships of the great vessels. They also provide excellent depiction of the walls of the great vessels and myocardium.

Occasionally, segmented fast spin-echo images are acquired when higher spatial resolution and/or

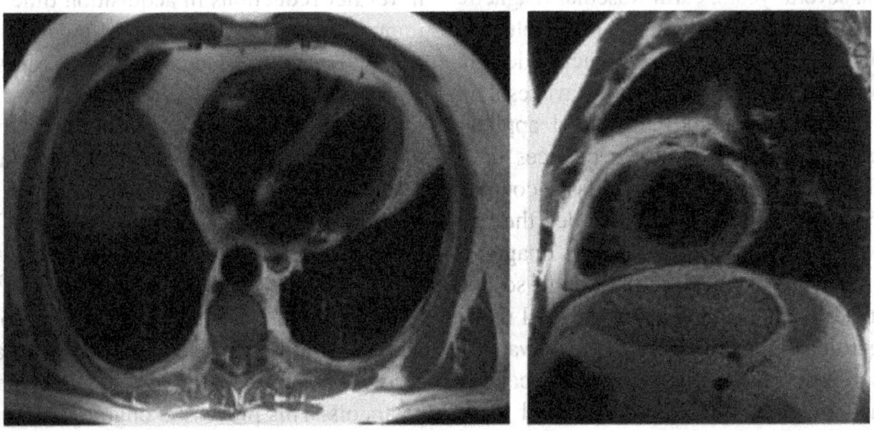

A B

FIGURE 1.1. Axial (A) and sagittal (B) half-Fourier acquisition single-shot turbo spin-echo (HASTE) images

improved T1- or T2-weighting is desired, such as when characterizing cardiac masses. These acquisitions take approximately 7 to 10 seconds per image and require breath holding. They can be performed either with or without fat saturation.

Morphologic Imaging Using Bright-Blood Sequences

Bright blood imaging was usually performed with gradient-recalled echo pulse sequences, which resulted in bright intracavitary signal due to the inflow of moving blood. However, slow flow could result in poor depiction of the interface between the blood pool and myocardium.

Steady state free precession (SSFP) sequences have resulted in significant improvement in bright blood imaging. With these sequences, image contrast is not as dependent on inflow effects, but rather on the different physical characteristics of tissues. Specifically, signal intensity is dependent on the T2/T1 ratio of the tissue being imaged[18] (not including effects from prepulses), and this results in bright signal for intracavitary blood, and a relatively dark appearance for myocardium. Images can be rapidly acquired typically in less than 300–400 ms per image. These sequences do not require breath holding and are similar to HASTE sequences in that they are a form of single-shot imaging. For cardiovascular structures, one image is typically acquired each heartbeat (at the same cardiac phase), and a stack of 30 images can be acquired in approximately 30 seconds (Figure 1.2) (Case 66, series 3 and 5) SSFP sequences are very useful in the evaluation of disorders producing intraluminal abnormalities. For example, they can be used for the evaluation of aortic dissection and for localization of the pulmonary veins prior to MR angiography.

Cine Imaging

The same steady state free precession (SSFP) technique used to produce bright blood static images may be adapted for cine acquisition. In this instance, multiple images are obtained at a single slice location in rapid succession during different phases of the cardiac cycle and can be displayed as a continuous movie loop.[19, 20] Cine imaging allows evaluation of ventricular wall motion abnormalities, dynamic changes in wall thickness, and measurement of chamber sizes. It also allows assessment of valvular morphology and function (Figure 1.3) (Case 66, series 33).

The standard cine sequence is a segmented, retrospectively gated acquisition, in which the data is acquired throughout the cardiac cycle and is "time stamped" to allow assignment to the proper cardiac phase. The segmented acquisition indicates that data from several heart beats is combined to yield the image. As such, irregularities in

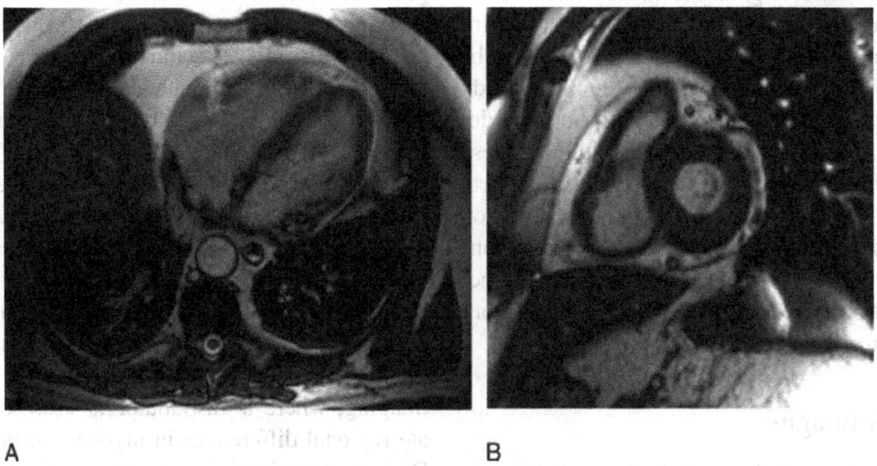

FIGURE 1.2. Axial (**A**) and sagittal (**B**) steady-state free precession (SSFP) images

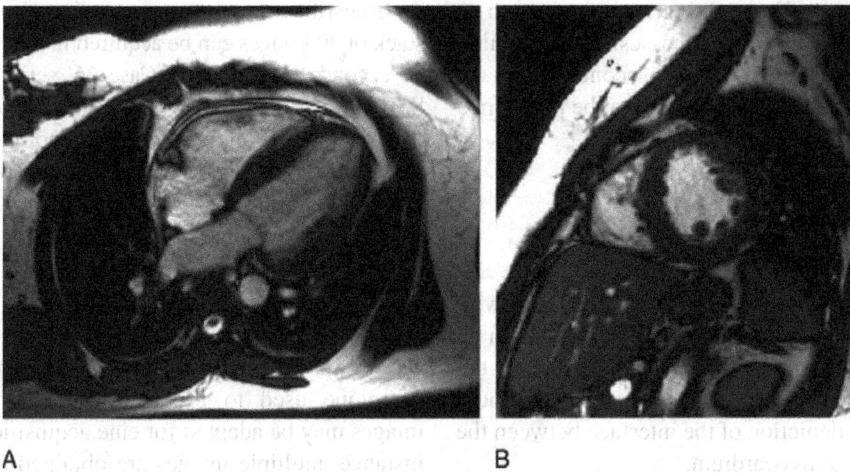

FIGURE 1.3. Four-chamber (**A**) and short-axis (**B**) cine images using SSFP

the patient's heart rate and rhythm may degrade image quality.

In cases of arrhythmia, prospectively triggered acquisitions may be helpful. Since changes in heart rate predominately affect the length of diastole rather than systole, this strategy by beginning with the R wave and acquiring a predetermined length of time (usually up to early or mid diastole), can remove some of the artifacts that result from irregular cycle lengths. Unfortunately, prospectively triggered acquisitions often result in the loss of the terminal phase of diastole, and correspondingly, measurements of ventricular ejection fraction and chamber volumes from these acquisitions may be slightly imprecise. If gating is unsuccessful, or the arrhythmia is severe, or the patient cannot breath-hold adequately, real-time cine acquisitions may be necessary. These acquisitions also employ steady state free precession sequences, albeit in a single-shot rather then segmented fashion. Although these acquisitions have lower spatial and temporal resolution, they may provide sufficient information for diagnosis. In addition, real-time cine acquisitions can be helpful in the detection of dynamic processes, as they can be acquired during inspiratory and expiratory maneuvers.

Perfusion Imaging

These sequences are designed to demonstrate contrast media passage through the myocardium in a manner that reliably reflects myocardial blood flow. It is desirable to have multiple slices during each heartbeat in order to ensure sufficient ventricular coverage, with high temporal resolution.[12, 21, 22] The sequences used by different manufacturers differ, but the general strategy is to utilize a saturation prepulse to accentuate T1-weighting, and thus accurately depict the passage of a T1 shortening contrast agent such as gadolinium.[23] These sequences are very gradient intensive, such that only high performance magnets are capable of executing these sequences with adequate temporal and spatial resolution. In the implementation used throughout this teaching file, a saturation recovery gradient-recalled echo sequence has been used. Each slice takes approximately 160 ms to acquire (120 ms for image acquisition, 40 ms to allow partial recovery of magnetization) and therefore 4 slices require a total of 640 ms. Given that the R-R interval is approximately 640 ms when the heart rate is 94 beats per minute, 4 slices can be obtained in most patients unless tachycardia is present.

Perfusion imaging is most often used for the detection of obstructive coronary artery disease, where it is performed with pharmacological vasodilation (e.g. adenosine). The underlying principle is similar to that in nuclear perfusion imaging, where a vasodilator is used to accentuate regional differences in myocardial blood flow. During adenosine infusion, myocardial blood flow increases approximately 4-fold downstream of

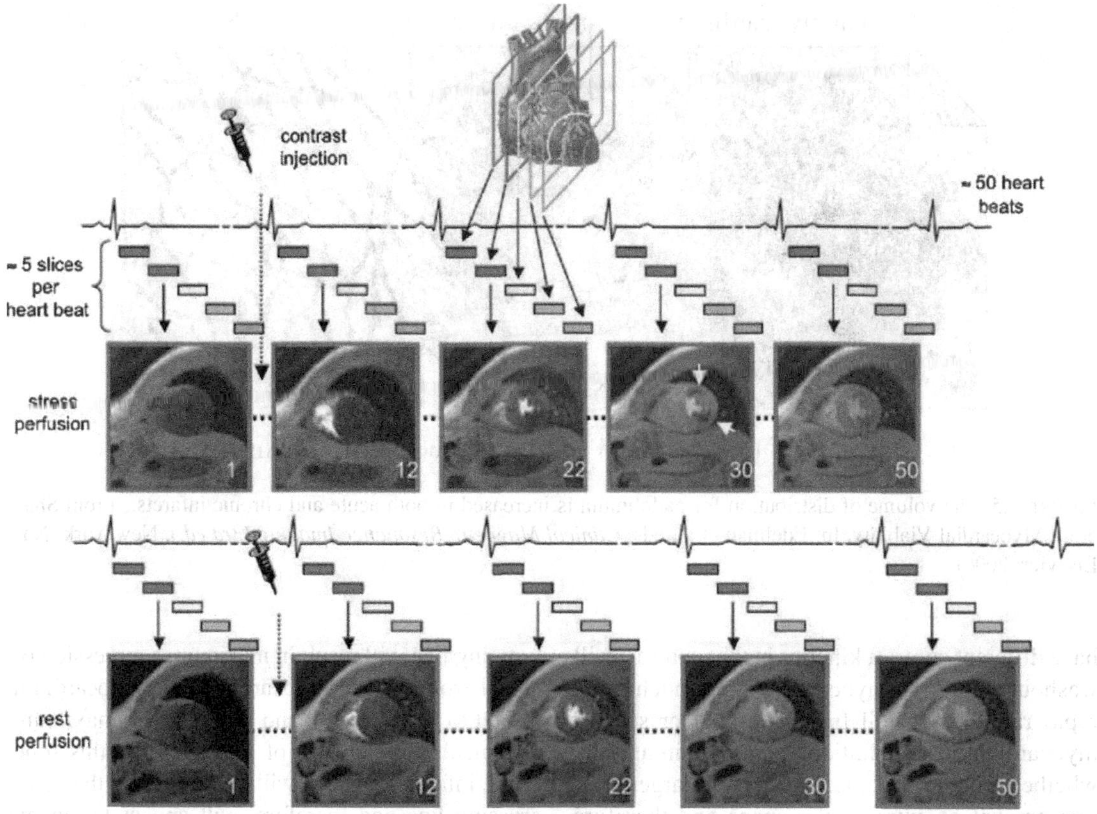

FIGURE 1.4. First-pass perfusion MR image acquisition. Images are acquired serially at multiple slice locations (usually four to five short-axis views for left ventricular coverage) every heartbeat to depict the passage of a compact contrast bolus as it transits the heart. Example images of one slice location are shown at several representative timepoints: before arrival of contrast (frame 1); contrast in RV cavity (frame 12); contrast in LV cavity (frame 22); peak contrast in LV myocardium (frame 30), showing normal perfusion in the septum *(open arrowhead)* and abnormal perfusion in both the anterior and inferolateral walls *(solid arrowheads)*; and the contrast wash-out phase (frame 50)

normal coronary arteries, but does not increase (or increases minimally) downstream of severely diseased arteries because the arteriolar beds are already maximally vasodilated (Figure 1.4) (Case 25, series 21.3). However, there are some differences as compared with nuclear perfusion imaging, MR perfusion imaging is a first pass imaging study that directly images the passage of contrast, and therefore is performed using an abbreviated adenosine protocol (~3 minutes). Also, MR perfusion imaging has higher spatial resolution than nuclear techniques, and can depict a perfusion defect that is only subendocardial. MR perfusion imaging has the additional advantage of providing a more linear depiction of myocardial blood flow in response to vasodilatation, without the plateau phenomenon seen with nuclear agents.[24] Although research studies often emphasize analysis of the upslope curves and other complex post-processing of the perfusion data, recent reports using visual analysis demonstrated comparable sensitivity and specificity.[25,26] This is the approach used throughout this Teaching File.

Perfusion imaging can also be used in the evaluation of suspected intracardiac shunts, as well as in the characterization of cardiac masses.

Viability Imaging

It is important to note that normal myocardium as well as infarcted and scarred myocardium will demonstrate contrast enhancement. However, they

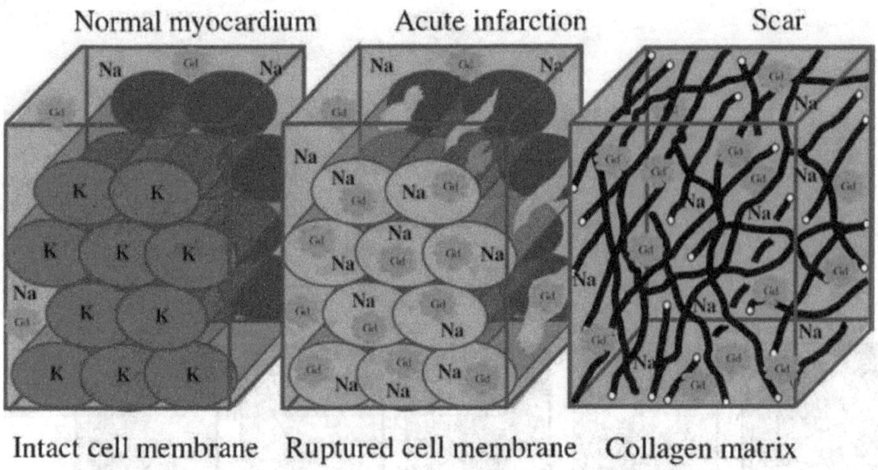

FIGURE 1.5. The volume of distribution for gadolinium is increased in both acute and chronic infarcts. (From Shah et al, Myocardial Viability. In: Edelman et al, eds. *Clinical Magnetic Resonance Imaging (3rd ed.)*. New York, NY: Elsevier; 2006)

have different contrast kinetics in that contrast will washout of normal myocardium at a much more rapid rate than it will from infarcted or scarred myocardium.[27] In addition, areas of infarction, whether acute or chronic, will have a larger relative amount of extracellular space and therefore a greater volume of distribution for gadolinium contrast than will normal myocardium (Figure 1.5) Accordingly, areas of prior infarction will have higher concentrations of contrast on delayed images (5 to 10 minutes after intravenous administration).[28] The delayed-enhancement sequences used for infarct detection are designed to maximize the differential signal intensity between normal myocardium and infarcted myocardium.[29]

The standard delayed-enhancement imaging sequence incorporates a segmented gradient echo read-out and an inversion prepulse to produce heavy T1-weighting.[30] The inversion pulse serves to flip the magnetization 180 degrees. The recovery of magnetization back to baseline by areas that have a higher gadolinium concentration will be more rapid (as they have a lower T1 value) than those with a lower concentration of gadolinium such as normal myocardium. Therefore, the increased concentration of gadolinium in an area of scar will be reflected by more rapid return above the zero-crossing line and back to baseline longitudinal magnetization (Figure 1.6) The time after the inversion pulse at which normal myocardium is at the zero-crossing line will result in maximum suppression of signal from normal myocardium (the myocardium is said to be "nulled"), and will result in maximum conspicuity of the area of infarction. At this time point, infarcted regions will be well above the zero-crossing line and therefore, will appear bright on these images (Figure 1.7) (Case 3, series 50).

The standard delayed-enhancement sequences are segmented acquisitions, acquired at every other heartbeat in order to allow normal myocardial regions to recover longitudinal magnetization before the next inversion pulse is applied. Therefore, they are constructed from the data of multiple heartbeats. They typically take approximately 8 to 12 seconds to acquire. For patients with significant arrhythmia, or difficulty with breath holding, single-shot delayed-enhancement images using an SSFP inversion recovery sequence can provide a reasonable alternative in a fraction of the imaging time.[31, 32] These images are slightly lower in contrast to noise ratio, and have a mildly reduced sensitivity for the detection of infarction, but provide a satisfactory option in these circumstances (Case 3, series 30).

Single-shot delayed-enhancement imaging may also be obtained with a long inversion time (550 to 600ms). These are quite useful in the detection of thrombi.[15] On these images, thrombi will appear dark in contrast to normal myocardium and infarcted myocardium, which will be grey and bright in image intensity, respectively (Figure 1.8) (Case 11, series 39).

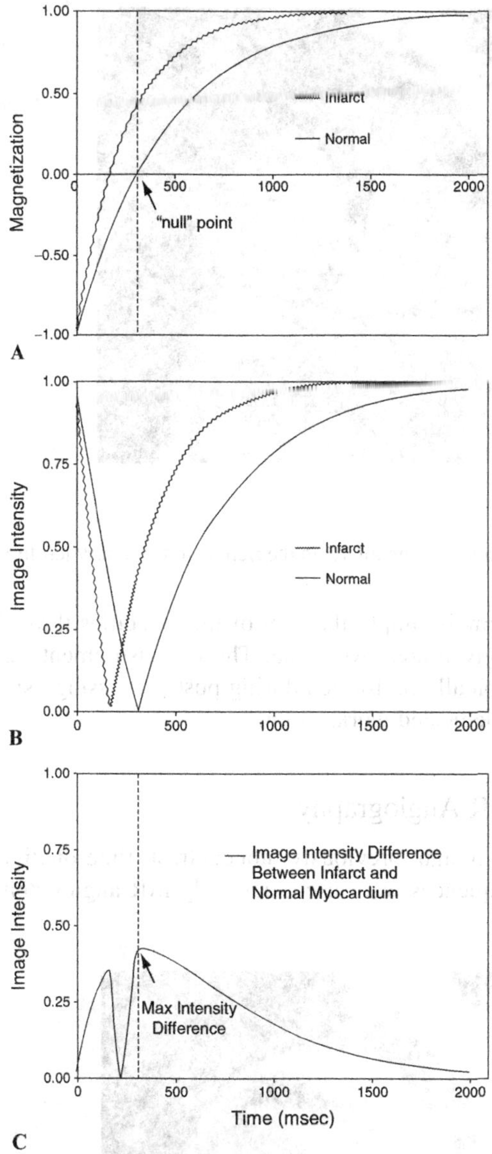

FIGURE 1.6. **(A)** Inversion recovery curves of normal and infarcted myocardium assuming T1 of normal myocardium is 450 msec and infarcted myocardium is 250 msec. The time at which the magnetization of normal myocardium reaches the zero crossing is defined as the inversion time to "null" normal myocardium. **(B)** Image intensities resulting from an inversion prepulse with various inversion delay times. Note that image intensities correspond to the magnitude of the magnetization vector and cannot be negative. **(C)** Difference in image intensities between infarcted and normal myocardium as a function of inversion time. The optimal inversion time is when the maximum intensity difference occurs. (From *J Cardiovasc Magn Reson* 2003;5:505–514, with permission)

Although predominately associated with the assessment of myocardial infarction and viability, the same delayed-enhancement sequences can also be helpful in a variety of other circumstances, such as the detection of viral myocarditis, identification of cardiac involvement by sarcoidosis, and the differentiation of ischemic from non-ischemic cardiomyopathy.[6, 33, 34]

Flow-Sensitive Imaging Using Velocity-Encoded Sequences

In this form of imaging, velocity-encoding phase shifts result from the sequential application of bipolar magnetic field gradients, which are composed of two lobes with opposite polarities. These opposed gradients will produce a phase shift with the first pulse that will be reversed by the second pulse. Therefore, stationary spins will acquire equal and opposite phases in the two gradients, and will have no net phase at the end of the sequence. However, flowing spins will acquire a net phase change, which will be dependent on their velocity in the direction of the flow-encoding gradients.[35–37] Gradients can be varied in amplitude or duration to sensitize the pulse sequence to fast or slow flow. The maximum velocity encoded by the sequence is termed the Venc and is selected by the operator.

Aliasing occurs when the maximum velocity sampled exceeds the upper limit imposed by the chosen Venc, resulting in apparent velocity reversal. To avoid aliasing the velocity threshold must be correctly selected (Case 20, series 43). Aliasing results in artifactual reduction of the measured flow, in direct proportion to the extent of aliasing, and therefore accurate flow measurements require its recognition. It is recognized in the velocity images where the voxels of assumed peak velocities have an inverted signal intensity compared with that of surrounding voxels.

The optimal Venc should just exceed the anticipated velocities to be measured. Setting the Venc too high will lead to increased noise or inaccuracy in the velocity or flow measurement. With sequences currently available, phase-contrast measurement can be performed in a breath hold using retrospective cardiac gating. Both the magnitude and phase images are often reviewed (Figure 1.9) (Case 20, series 46 and 47).

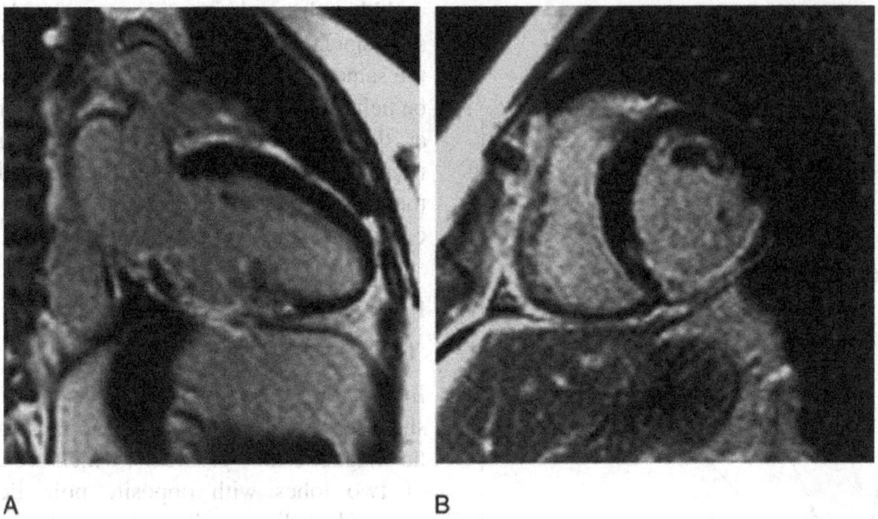

FIGURE 1.7. Inversion recovery delayed-enhancement images demonstrate an infarct in the right coronary artery territory

These sequences are typically used in two situations—quantification of gradients across stenotic valves, and for measurement of blood flow. The peak gradient across a stenotic valve can be calculated using the Bernouilli equation, $\Delta P = 4\ V^2$ where velocity V is in meters per second, and the gradient is given in mm Hg. On most scanners, the velocities are given in cm/sec, and must be converted to m/sec for the calculation. Flow is simply the sum of the velocities through a given area over time. These measurements are typically performed during post-processing using a dedicated workstation.

MR Angiography

Although previously noncontrast time-of-flight sequences were used, currently MR angiography

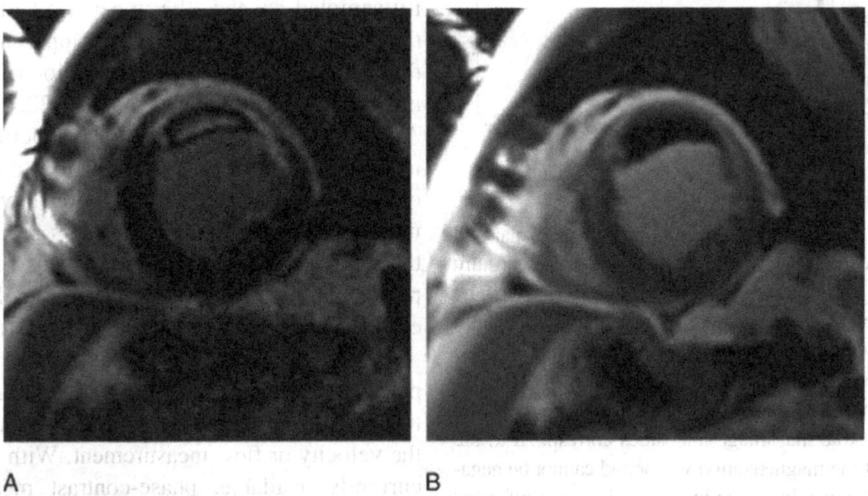

FIGURE 1.8. Short-axis single-shot inversion recovery delayed-enhancement images obtained with inversion times of 300 ms (**A**), and 600 ms (**B**). Note that the mural thrombus adherent to an anterior wall infarction appears high in signal intensity on the image where myocardium is nulled as it is well below the zero-crossing line. It is low in signal on the image with a long inversion time

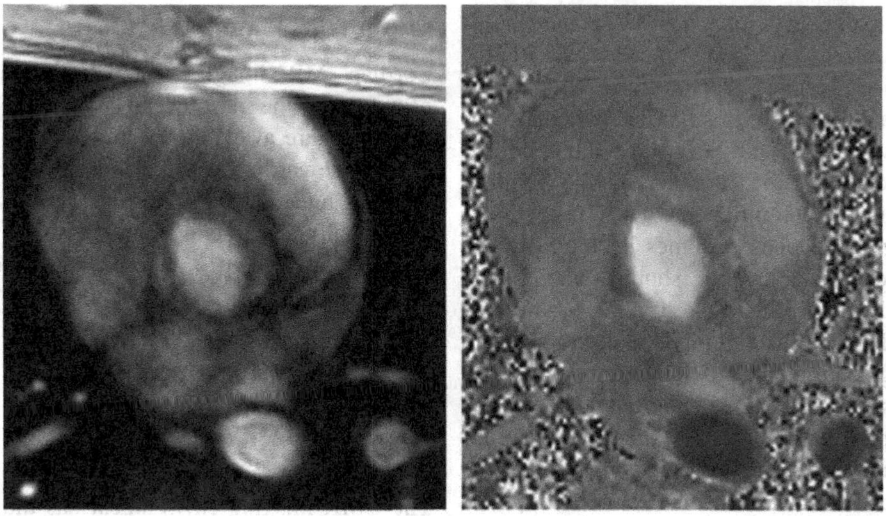

A B

FIGURE 1.9. Magnitude (A) and phase (B) images from a velocity-encoded study of a bicuspid aortic valve

is most often performed using thin section T1-weighted spoiled gradient-echo image acquisitions during the arterial passage of intravenously administered contrast.[38–43] Synchronization of image acquisition with the arterial passage of contrast is most often performed by using fluoroscopic monitoring of the contrast passage, with scan initiation triggered after visualization in the appropriate region (Case 15, series 40). Alternatively, a timing bolus technique may be used.[44] In this technique, a small (2 cc) bolus of contrast is administered and sequential images are obtained at a predetermined location at a rate of one per second. The arrival time of the contrast bolus is then used to calculate the appropriate time for scan triggering (Case 16, series 12).

Multiple thin slices are obtained in a 3-D volumetric technique, and are then assembled into maximum intensity projection images, as well as volume rendered images. Multi-planar review of the obtained images is also performed, in order to visualize the vessels in cross-section and to evaluate the vessel walls. This review is facilitated by the acquisition of the image data in isotropic voxels, which allow reformation into any desired plane without image degradation. The plane of imaging is freely selectable with MR angiography, but by convention, thoracic studies are usually performed in either the axial or sagittal plane. An oblique sagittal plane that provides a "candy cane" view of the thoracic aorta may be used to minimize breath hold time by reducing the thickness of the imaging slab. Abdominal, pelvic, and extremity studies are usually obtained in the coronal plane (Figure 1.10) (Case 16, series 13).

The in-plane image resolution, the slice thickness, and the volume of coverage are all freely

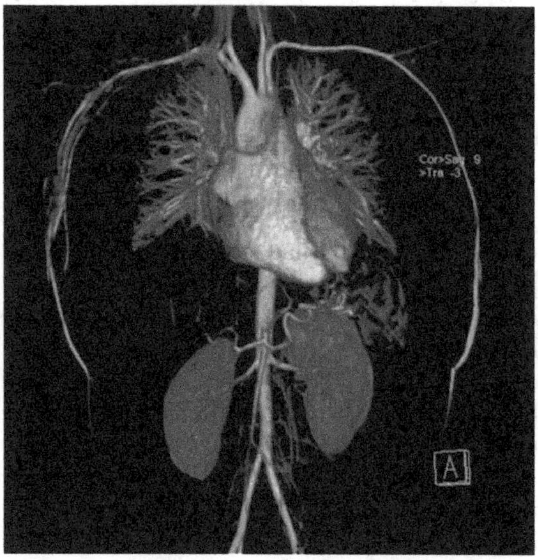

FIGURE 1.10. Volume-rendered image from a contrast-enhanced MR angiogram

selectable parameters. Increasing in-plane resolution will increase imaging time, as will diminishing slice thickness for a given volume of acquisition. Therefore, in situations where breath holding is required such as in chest and abdomen MR angiography, the duration of the acquisition becomes the limiting factor. A breath-hold exceeding 25 seconds becomes problematic for most patients, and imaging should generally be completed within this time frame. In circumstances where cardiac motion is likely to result in image degradation, such as imaging of the aortic root, the sequences can be acquired with electrocardiographic gating. In this situation, imaging can be timed to when cardiac motion is minimal (i.e. diastole), however, since data is acquired only during a portion of the cardiac cycle, voxel size is usually increased to maintain the same breath hold duration.

The use of MR angiography has been well validated in a variety of vascular regions, most notably for evaluation of renal artery stenosis where it compares favorably with digital subtraction angiography.[40,45] It is also been well accepted for abdominal, pelvic, and lower extremity runoff imaging for comprehensive multistation evaluation of the peripheral vasculature in patients likely to require revascularization.[46–48] It has advantages over conventional catheter and CT angiography in that no radiation or potentially nephrotoxic contrast is required. The examination can be performed in 30 minutes. No arterial puncture is required.

Parallel Imaging Acquisition Techniques

Although the different scanner manufacturers have their own proprietary implementations, all support parallel imaging techniques. These allow a reduction in image acquisition time, or improvement in spatial resolution with the same imaging time, but at a cost of mildly reduced signal-to-noise. This reduction is roughly proportional to the square root of the acceleration factor used, so that at the usual implementation of an acceleration factor of 2, the resultant signal-to-noise of the accelerated image is approximately 70% of the nonaccelerated image.[8,49] These techniques can be applied to all of the imaging sequences previously described, and are most helpful in cardiac imaging.

Summary

Cardiac MR imaging has made tremendous progress in the past decade. Multiple different sequences are available and provide the ability to interrogate cardiac structure, function, and viability with unparalleled precision. These sequences individually and in combination provide a diverse palette from which to choose. Recommendations for specific choices that will comprise a "Standard Cardiac Exam" follow in the next chapter.

CMR Safety

The CMR imaging environment has the potential to pose serious risks to patients and facility staff in several ways. Injuries can result from the static magnetic field (projectile impact injuries), very rapid gradient-field switching (induction of electric currents leading to peripheral nerve stimulation), RF-energy deposition (heating of the imaged portion of the body), and acoustic noise. The institution of policies that strictly limit access to the magnet room minimizes the risks of projectile injuries from the static magnetic field. For instance, patients are extensively screened prior to imaging, and all facility personnel undergo dedicated training in MR safety. The use of *MR-safe* or compatible equipment (stethoscopes, wheelchairs, gurneys, oxygen tanks, infusion pumps, monitors, etc.) with clear labeling of such in the scanner area reduces this risk further. The Food and Drug Administration (FDA) has placed limits on the rate of change of gradient magnetic fields (e.g. the slew rate) and the amount of RF energy (e.g., specific absorption rate [SAR]) that can be transmitted to patients. All scanners monitor the slew rate and calculate the SAR to help prevent nerve stimulation and heating. Acoustic noise of 100dB or more are generated from the vibration or motion of the gradient coils during image acquisition. The use of protective hearing devices, such as headphones or earplugs, reduces noise to levels that do not result in hearing impairment or patient discomfort. In practice, continuous communication with the patient throughout the examination is important for patent comfort and safety.

Patients with medical devices or implants can face additional potential hazards, including device heating, movement, or malfunction. For example, ferromagnetic aneurysm clips or electronic medical devices (e.g., neural stimulators, insulin pumps) are strict contraindications to MRI. However, there is a specific subset of patients with a metallic implants or devices that can safely undergo MRI. A comprehensive list of devices and implants that are compatible with undergoing MRI scanning can be found elsewhere.[50,51] Regarding cardiac devices, it is important to note that prosthetic valves and coronary artery stents are now considered safe for MRI scanning.[50–52] Indeed, recently, the FDA approved the use of MRI immediately after the implantation of paclitaxel and sirolimus drug-eluting stents. At most institutions, MRI scans are not performed in patients with implanted pacemakers or defibrillators because of the potential risk of device malfunction, excessive device or lead heating, or induction of currents within the leads. Recently, however, a few preliminary reports have emerged, suggesting that MRI can be possible in patients with modern pacemakers and defibrillators in whom the benefits are deemed greater than the risks.[53–55] In patients in whom devices have been extracted, but with the leads remaining (permanent or temporary transvenous), MRI is contraindicated as the risk of heating or induction of currents can be higher.

Recently, in several small case series, it has been reported that a small subset of patients with end-stage renal disease, receiving gadolinium contrast, may be at risk for developing nephrogenic systemic fibrosis (NSF)[56]. NSF is characterized by an increased tissue deposition of collagen, often resulting in thickening and tightening of the skin and predominantly involving the distal extremities. Additionally, fibrosis may affect other organs, including skeletal muscles, lungs, pulmonary vasculature, heart, and diaphragm. Although a definitive causal link with gadolinium contrast agents has yet to be established, gadolinium contrasts agents should be utilized cautiously (and alternative tests considered) in patients with severe renal disease, particularly those undergoing peritoneal dialysis or hemodialysis, or with acute renal failure. A policy statement regarding the use of gadolinium contrast agents in the setting of renal disease has been published by the American College of Radiology.[56]

References

1. Fuster V, Kim RJ. Frontiers in cardiovascular magnetic resonance. Circulation. 2005;112(1):135–144.
2. Edelman RR. Contrast-enhanced MR imaging of the heart: overview of the literature. Radiology. 2004;232(3):653–668.
3. Lima JA, Desai MY. Cardiovascular magnetic resonance imaging: current and emerging applications. J Am Coll Cardiol. 2004;44(6):1164–1171.
4. Finn JP, Nael K, Deshpande V, Ratib O, Laub G. Cardiac MR imaging: state of the technology. Radiology. 2006;241(2):338–354.
5. Elliott MD, Kim RJ. Late gadolinium cardiovascular magnetic resonance in the assessment of myocardial viability. Coron Artery Dis. 2005;16(6):365–372.
6. Mahrholdt H, Wagner A, Judd RM, Sechtem U, Kim RJ. Delayed enhancement cardiovascular magnetic resonance assessment of non-ischaemic cardiomyopathies. Eur Heart J. 2005;26(15):1461–1474.
7. Isbell DC, Kramer CM. The evolving role of cardiovascular magnetic resonance imaging in nonischemic cardiomyopathy. Semin Ultrasound CT MR 2006; 27(1):20–31.
8. Glockner JF, Hu HH, Stanley DW, Angelos L, King K. Parallel MR imaging: a user's guide. Radiographics. 2005;25(5):1279–1297.
9. Niendorf T, Sodickson DK. Parallel imaging in cardiovascular MRI: methods and applications. NMR Biomed. 2006;19(3):325–341.
10. Bellenger NG, Burgess MI, Ray SG, et al. Comparison of left ventricular ejection fraction and volumes in heart failure by echocardiography, radionuclide ventriculography and cardiovascular magnetic resonance; are they interchangeable? Eur Heart J. 2000;21(16):1387–1396.
11. Bellenger NG, Grothues F, Smith GC, Pennell DJ. Quantification of right and left ventricular function by cardiovascular magnetic resonance. Herz. 2000;25(4):392–399.
12. Wagner A, Mahrholdt H, Sechtem U, Kim RJ, Judd RM. MR imaging of myocardial perfusion and viability. Magn Reson Imaging Clin N Am. 2003;11(1):49–66.
13. Wagner A, Mahrholdt H, Holly TA, et al. Contrast-enhanced MRI and routine single photon emission computed tomography (SPECT) perfusion imaging for detection of subendocardial myocardial infarcts: an imaging study. Lancet. 2003;361(9355):374–379.
14. Francone M, Dymarkowski S, Kalantzi M, Bogaert J. Magnetic resonance imaging in the evaluation of the pericardium. A pictorial essay. Radiol Med (Torino). 2005;109(1–2):64–74; quiz 75–66.
15. Grizzard JD, Ang GB. Magnetic resonance imaging of pericardial disease and cardiac masses. Cardiol Clin. 2007;25(1):111–140.

16. Dembo LG, Shifrin RY, Wolff SD. MR imaging in ischemic heart disease. Radiol Clin North Am. 2004;42(3):651–673, vii.
17. Rajappan K, Bellenger NG, Anderson L, Pennell DJ. The role of cardiovascular magnetic resonance in heart failure. Eur J Heart Fail. 2000;2(3):241–252.
18. Reeder SB, Herzka DA, McVeigh ER. Signal-to-noise ratio behavior of steady-state free precession. Magn Reson Med. 2004;52(1):123–130.
19. Fuchs F, Laub G, Othomo K. TrueFISP–technical considerations and cardiovascular applications. Eur J Radiol. 2003;46(1):28–32.
20. Pereles FS, Kapoor V, Carr JC, et al. Usefulness of segmented trueFISP cardiac pulse sequence in evaluation of congenital and acquired adult cardiac abnormalities. AJR Am J Roentgenol. 2001;177(5):1155–1160.
21. Wu KC. Myocardial perfusion imaging by magnetic resonance imaging. Curr Cardiol Rep. 2003;5(1): 63–68.
22. Schwitter J. Myocardial perfusion imaging by cardiac magnetic resonance. J Nucl Cardiol. 2006;13(6): 841–854.
23. Slavin GS, Wolff SD, Gupta SN, Foo TK. First-pass myocardial perfusion MR imaging with interleaved notched saturation: feasibility study. Radiology. 2001;219(1):258–263.
24. Lee DC, Simonetti OP, Harris KR, et al. Magnetic resonance versus radionuclide pharmacological stress perfusion imaging for flow-limiting stenoses of varying severity. Circulation. 2004;110(1):58–65.
25. Klem I, Heitner JF, Shah DJ, et al. Improved detection of coronary artery disease by stress perfusion cardiovascular magnetic resonance with the use of delayed enhancement infarction imaging. J Am Coll Cardiol. 18 2006;47(8):1630–1638.
26. Cury RC, Cattani CA, Gabure LA, et al. Diagnostic performance of stress perfusion and delayed-enhancement MR imaging in patients with coronary artery disease. Radiology. 2006;240(1):39–45.
27. Kim RJ, Fieno DS, Parrish TB, et al. Relationship of MRI delayed contrast enhancement to irreversible injury, infarct age, and contractile function. Circulation. 1999;100(19):1992–2002.
28. Rehwald WG, Fieno DS, Chen EL, Kim RJ, Judd RM. Myocardial magnetic resonance imaging contrast agent concentrations after reversible and irreversible ischemic injury. Circulation. 2002;105(2):224–229.
29. Fieno DS, Kim RJ, Chen EL, Lomasney JW, Klocke FJ, Judd RM. Contrast-enhanced magnetic resonance imaging of myocardium at risk: distinction between reversible and irreversible injury throughout infarct healing. J Am Coll Cardiol. 2000;36(6): 1985–1991.
30. Simonetti OP, Kim RJ, Fieno DS, et al. An improved MR imaging technique for the visualization of myocardial infarction. Radiology. 2001;218(1):215–223.
31. Sievers B, Elliott MD, Hurwitz LM, et al. Rapid detection of myocardial infarction by subsecond, free-breathing delayed contrast-enhancement cardiovascular magnetic resonance. Circulation. 2007;115(2):236–244.
32. Huber A, Schoenberg SO, Spannagl B, et al. Single-shot inversion recovery TrueFISP for assessment of myocardial infarction. AJR Am J Roentgenol. 2006;186(3):627–633.
33. Mahrholdt H, Goedecke C, Wagner A, et al. Cardiovascular magnetic resonance assessment of human myocarditis: a comparison to histology and molecular pathology. Circulation. 2004;109(10):1250–1258.
34. Sechtem U, Mahrholdt H, Hager S, Vogelsberg H. New non-invasive approaches for the diagnosis of cardiomyopathy: magnetic resonance imaging. Ernst Schering Res Found Workshop. 2006(55):261–285.
35. Glockner JF, Johnston DL, McGee KP. Evaluation of cardiac valvular disease with MR imaging: qualitative and quantitative techniques. Radiographics. 2003;23(1):e9.
36. Lotz J, Meier C, Leppert A, Galanski M. Cardiovascular flow measurement with phase-contrast MR imaging: basic facts and implementation. Radiographics. May-Jun 2002;22(3):651–671.
37. Buonocore MH, Bogren H. Factors influencing the accuracy and precision of velocity-encoded phase imaging. Magn Reson Med. 1992;26(1):141–154.
38. Edelman RR. MR angiography: present and future. AJR Am J Roentgenol. Jul 1993;161(1):1–11.
39. Kramer U, Nael K, Laub G, et al. High-resolution magnetic resonance angiography of the renal arteries using parallel imaging acquisition techniques at 3.0 T: initial experience. Invest Radiol. 2006;41(2):125–132.
40. Zhang H, Prince MR. Renal MR angiography. Magn Reson Imaging Clin N Am. 2004;12(3):487–503, vi.
41. Krinsky GA, Rofsky NM, DeCorato DR, et al. Thoracic aorta: comparison of gadolinium-enhanced three-dimensional MR angiography with conventional MR imaging. Radiology. 1997;202(1):183–193.
42. Leung DA, McKinnon GC, Davis CP, Pfammatter T, Krestin GP, Debatin JF. Breath-hold, contrast-enhanced, three-dimensional MR angiography. Radiology. 1996;200(2):569–571.
43. Finn JP. MR angiography in the abdomen. Magn Reson Imaging Clin N Am. 1995;3(1):13–21.
44. Hany TF, McKinnon GC, Leung DA, Pfammatter T, Debatin JF. Optimization of contrast timing for breath-hold three-dimensional MR angiography. J Magn Reson Imaging.2007;3:551–556.

45. Leung DA, Hany TF, Debatin JF. Three-dimensional contrast-enhanced magnetic resonance angiography of the abdominal arterial system. Cardiovasc Intervent Radiol. 1998;21(1):1–10.
46. Hany TF, Carroll TJ, Omary RA, et al. Aorta and runoff vessels: single-injection MR angiography with automated table movement compared with multiinjection time-resolved MR angiography–initial results. Radiology. 2001;221(1):266–272.
47. Ruehm SG, Hany TF, Pfammatter T, Schneider E, Ladd M, Debatin JF. Pelvic and lower extremity arterial imaging: diagnostic performance of three-dimensional contrast-enhanced MR angiography. AJR Am J Roentgenol. Apr 2000;174(4):1127–1135.
48. Kreitner KF, Kalden P, Neufang A, et al. Diabetes and peripheral arterial occlusive disease: prospective comparison of contrast-enhanced three-dimensional MR angiography with conventional digital subtr-action angiography. AJR Am J Roentgenol. Jan 2000;174(1):171–179.
49. Wintersperger BJ, Nikolaou K, Dietrich O, et al. Single breath-hold real-time cine MR imaging: improved temporal resolution using generalized autocalibrating partially parallel acquisition (GRAPPA) algorithm. Eur Radiol. Aug 2003;13(8):1931–1936.
50. Shellock FG, Kanal E. Magnetic Resonance: Bioeffects, Safety, and Patient Management. New York: Raven Press; 1994.
51. Shellock FG. Reference Manual for Magnetic Resonance Safety, Implants, and Devices. 2006 ed. Los Angeles, CA: Biomedical Research Publishing Group; 2006.145.
52. Patel MR, Albert TS, Kandzari DE, et al. Acute myocardial infarction: safety of cardiac MR imaging after percutaneous revascularization with stents. Radiology. 2006;240:674–680.
53. Roguin A, Zviman MM, Meininger GR, et al. Modern pacemaker and implantable cardioverter/defibrillator systems can be magnetic resonance imaging safe: in vitro and in vivo assessment of safety and function at 1.5 T. Circulation. 2004,110. 475–482.
54. Roguin A, Donahue JK, Bomma CS, et al. Cardiac magnetic resonance imaging in a patient with implantable cardioverter-defibrillator. Pacing Clin Electrophysiol. 2005;28:336–338.
55. Nazarian S, Roguin A, Zviman MM, et al. Clinical utility and safety of a protocol for noncardiac and cardiac magnetic resonance imaging of patients with permanent pacemakers and implantable-cardioverter defibrillators at 1.5 tesla. Circulation. 2006;114: 1277–1284.
56. Kanal E, Barkovich AJ, Bell C, et al. ACR Guidance Document for Safe MR practices: 2007. Am J Radiology. 2007;188:1–27.

2
The Standard Cardiac Exam

Core Components and Common Modifications

Chapter 1 explained that an extensive array of MR sequences are available for cardiac imaging. Each of these sequences can provide complementary information, often of incremental value. The desire for the most comprehensive imaging possible, however, must be counterbalanced with the recognition of the limited time available for scanning based on patient tolerance and scanner availability. The judicious use of resources mandates that the essential information be acquired in the least amount of time possible.

At a minimum, a standard cardiac MR examination should provide a comprehensive evaluation of the structure and function of the heart. Additionally, in the vast majority of patients, myocardial tissue characterization—with an assessment of infarction, scarring, and viability—provides substantial clinical value at minimal time cost.

In light of the above, our standard cardiac examination includes the following:

1. **Localizer scout images.** (To localize the heart within the chest and determine the appropriate cardiac imaging planes).
2. **Cine images in the short-axis plane from above the mitral valve through the cardiac apex, as well as in the standard orthogonal long axis views–2-chamber, 4-chamber, and 3-chamber or left ventricular outflow tract views.** (For the analysis of global cardiac structure and function, regional wall motion, and the calculation of volumes and mass. NOTE: Also refer to "LV Structure and Function" module as described in the Protocols section of the Appendix) (Case 1).
3. **Delayed-enhancement images spatially matched to the cine images.** (For the evaluation of myocardial infarction and viability, and tissue characterization. This corresponds to the "Late Gadolinium Enhancement" module listed in the appendix) (Case 3).

At some centers, stress perfusion imaging using adenosine has become so commonplace as to become a part of the standard examination.[1–3] Thus, this will represent the first proposed modification. The standard examination would begin as usual and proceed through the acquisition of Cine images. At this point, the patient is moved partially out of the magnet to improve visibility during the administration

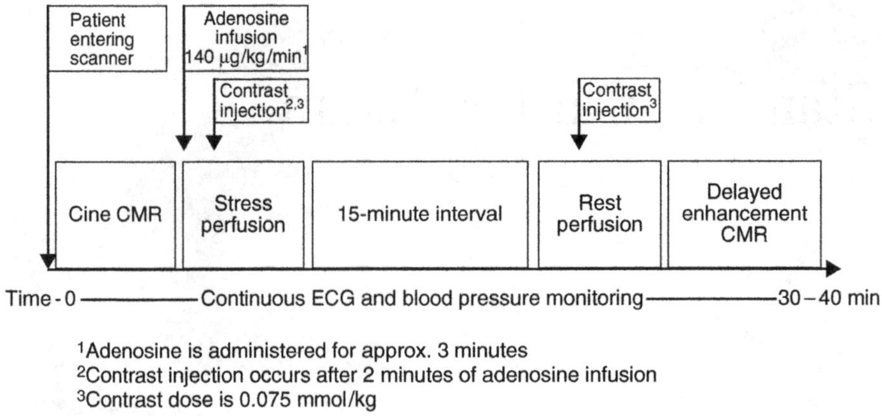

FIGURE 2.1. Timeline for adenosine stress perfusion MR

of adenosine. Adenosine is administered at a dose of 140ug/kg/min, for at least 2 minutes, at which time the patient is then returned to the scanner bore. Contrast is then administered (dose, 0.075–0.1 mmol/kg body weight) followed by a saline flush (~50 ml) at a rate of at least 3 ml/sec via an antecubital vein. On the console, the perfusion images are observed as they are acquired, with breath-holding starting from the appearance of contrast in the right ventricular cavity. If the scanner software does not provide real-time image display, breath-holding should be started no more than 5–6 seconds after beginning gadolinium injection. Breath-holding is performed to ensure the best possible image quality (i.e. no artifacts due to respiratory motion) during the initial wash-in of contrast into the LV myocardium. Once the contrast bolus has transited the LV myocardium, adenosine is stopped and imaging is completed 5–10 seconds later. Typically, the total imaging time is 40–50 seconds, and the total time of adenosine infusion is 3 to 3.5 minutes. During vasodilation, direct access to the patient is limited only during imaging of the first pass.

Prior to the rest perfusion scan, a waiting period of about 15 minutes is required for contrast to sufficiently clear from the blood pool. During this time, additional cine and or velocity/flow imaging for valvular or hemodynamic evaluation can be performed. Subsequently, the perfusion sequence with contrast is repeated without adenosine. Approximately 5 minutes after rest perfusion, delayed enhancement imaging can be performed. The total scan time for a comprehensive cardiac MR stress test, including cine imaging, stress and rest perfusion, and delayed enhancement is usually well under 45 minutes. The timeline is displayed in Figure 2.1 (Case 25).

Obviously, different clinical circumstances will result in appropriate modification of the basic cardiac MR examination, with additional modules added as needed. For example, in patients with angina referred for stress perfusion imaging from the emergency department, if this is their first evaluation, we typically add tomographic imaging of the entire chest. Single-shot dark-blood and/or bright-blood morphological imaging is performed to obtain an overview of the great vessels and juxtacardiac structures in recognition of the fact that chest pain is not always cardiac in origin. {Case 66, series 2 and 3}

Likewise, if a stenotic aortic valve is incidentally discovered during the core exam, velocity-encoded images through the aortic valve can be added. In the setting of congenital heart disease, MR angiographic images are frequently added to the standard morphologic images, and velocity-encoded flow studies are also usually necessary in this setting. Proposed standard protocols for a variety of cardiac disorders are included in the appendix.

Interpretation and Reporting

For general clinical reporting, we use the 17-segment model recommended by the American Heart Association.[4] This model divides the basal and mid-cavity levels into 6 segments each, an apical level into 4 segments and the true apex into 1 segment (Figure 2.2). For each segment, left

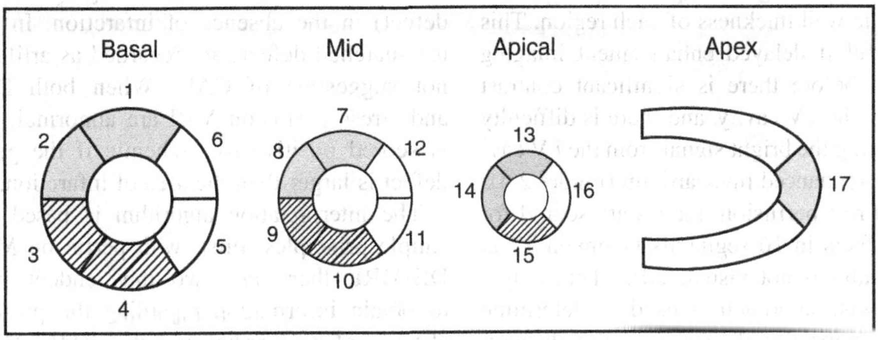

Cine Wall Motion:
0 = Normal / Hyperkinetic
1 = Mild / Moderate Hypokinesis
2 = Severe Hypokinesis
3 = Akinetic
4 = Dyskinetic

Delayed Hyperenhancement:
0 = None
1 = 1-25%
2 = 26-50%
3 = 51-75%
4 = 76-100%

FIGURE 2.2. Visual interpretation of cine and delayed enhancement images using the 17-segment model

ventricular systolic function is graded visually using a 5-point scale ranging from normal wall motion to dyskinesis. LV ejection fraction is also provided, and estimated from visual inspection of all the short- and long-axis views. Occasionally, LVEF is quantitatively measured by planimetry, such as in patients undergoing chemotherapy with potentially cardiotoxic agents.

The delayed enhancement images are also interpreted using a 5-point scale.[5] For each segment the area or transmural extent of hyperenhanced tissue is graded visually. Examples of myocardial segments with various transmural extents of hyperenhancement are shown in Figure 2.3. It is important that the delayed enhancement images are interpreted with the cine images immediately

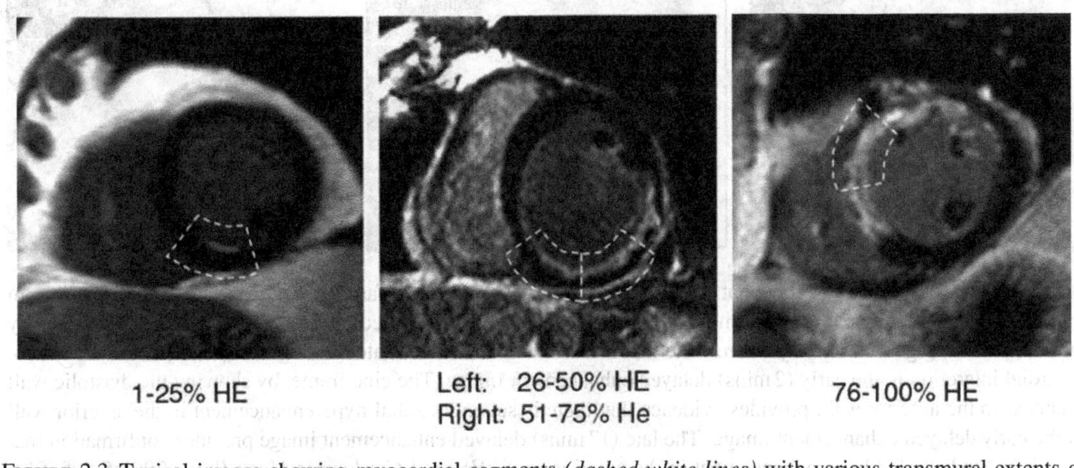

FIGURE 2.3. Typical images showing myocardial segments *(dashed white lines)* with various transmural extents of hyperenhancement. (From *J Cardiovasc Magn Reson* 2003;5:505–514, with permission)

adjacent. The cine images can provide a reference of the diastolic wall thickness of each region. This will be helpful if delayed enhancement imaging is performed before there is significant contrast washout from the LV cavity, and there is difficulty in differentiating the bright signal from the LV cavity from hyperenhanced myocardium (Figure 2.4).

Stress and rest perfusion images are scored for perfusion defects in 16 segments (segment 17 at the apex usually is not visualized). Then, a systematic stepwise approach is used to determine the presence or absence of coronary artery disease. Importantly, we use an interpretation algorithm that includes data from delayed enhancement imaging to improve the accuracy of detecting coronary artery disease over that of perfusion imaging alone (Figure 2.5).[3] Using this interpretation algorithm, a CMR stress test is deemed "positive for CAD" if myocardial infarction is present on DE-MRI ***OR*** if perfusion defects are present during stress imaging, but absent at rest ("reversible" defect) in the absence of infarction. Conversely, the test is deemed "negative for CAD" if no abnormalities are found (e.g. no MI and no stress/rest perfusion defects) ***OR*** if perfusion defects are seen at both stress and rest imaging ("matched" defect) in the absence of infarction. In the latter, matched defects are regarded as artifacts and not suggestive of CAD. When both DE-MRI and stress perfusion MRI are abnormal, the test is scored positive for ischemia if the perfusion defect is larger than the area of infarction.

The interpretation algorithm is based on two simple principles. First, with perfusion MRI and DE-MRI, there are two independent methods to obtain information regarding the presence or absence of myocardial infarction (MI). Thus, one method could be used to confirm the results of the other. Second, DE-MRI image quality (e.g. signal-to-noise ratio) is far better than perfusion MRI since it is less demanding in terms of scanner hardware (DE-MRI images can be built up over several seconds rather than in 0.1 seconds as is required for first-pass perfusion).[3] Thus, DE-MRI should be more accurate for the diagnosis of MI,[3] and the presence of infarction on DE-MRI favors the diagnosis of CAD, irrespective of the perfusion MRI results. Conceptually, it then follows that perfusion defects that have similar intensity and extent during both stress and rest ("matched"

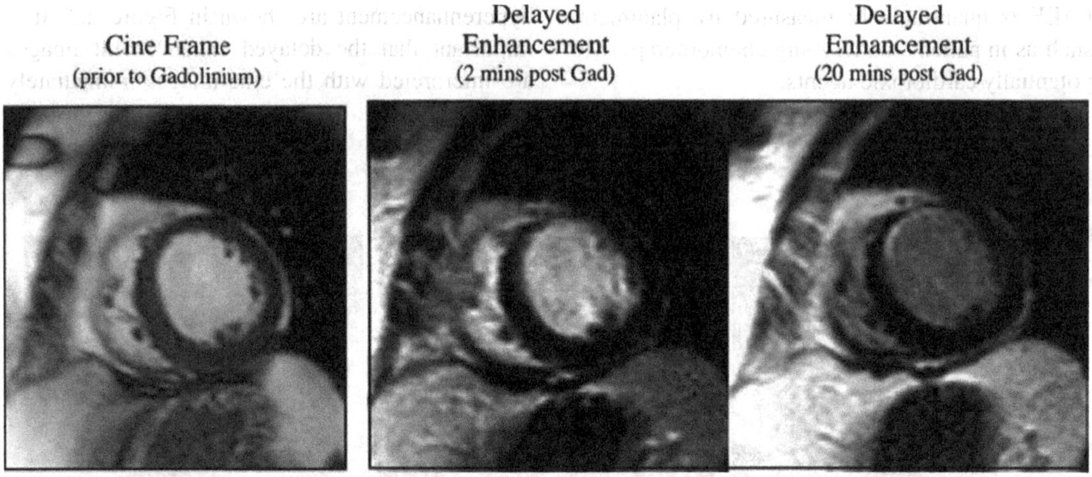

FIGURE 2.4. Short-axis view of a patient with an anterior wall myocardial infarction. Diastolic still-frame taken from the cine images before gadolinium administration is compared to the delayed enhancement image taken both early and late following gadolinium injection. Note that it is difficult to differentiate the bright LV cavity from the subendocardial infarction in the early (2 mins) delayed enhancement image. The cine frame, by showing the diastolic wall thickness in the anterior wall, provides evidence that there is subendocardial hyperenhancement in the anterior wall on the early delayed enhancement image. The late (17 mins) delayed enhancement image provides confirmation that there is subendocardial hyperenhancement in the anterior wall. (From, *J Cardiovasc Magn Reson* 2003;5:505–514, with permission)

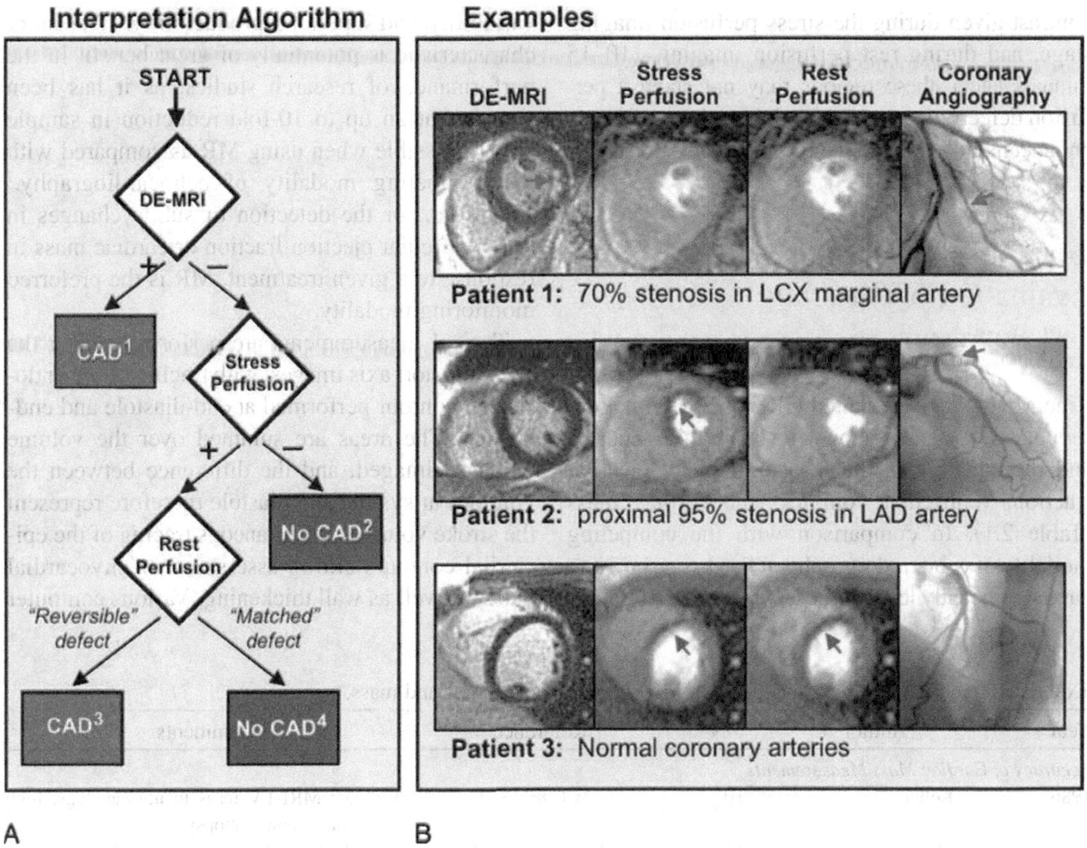

FIGURE 2.5. Interpretation algorithm for incorporating delayed enhancement imaging (DE-MRI) with stress and rest perfusion MRI for the detection of coronary disease. **(A)** Schema of the interpretation algorithm. **(1)** Positive DE-MRI Study: Hyperenhanced myocardium consistent with a prior myocardial infarction (MI) is detected. Does not include isolated midwall or epicardial hyperenhancement which can occur in nonischemic disorders. **(2)** Standard Negative Stress Study: No evidence of prior MI or inducible perfusion defects. **(3)** Standard Positive Stress Study: No evidence of prior MI but perfusion defects are present with adenosine that are absent or reduced at rest. **(4)** Artifactual Perfusion Defect: Matched stress and rest perfusion defects without evidence of prior MI on DE-MRI. **(B)** Patient Examples. **Top row:** Patient with a positive DE-MRI study demonstrating an infarct in the inferolateral wall (red arrow) although perfusion MRI is negative. The interpretation algorithm (step 1) classified this patient as positive for CAD. Coronary angiography verified disease in a circumflex marginal artery. Cine MRI demonstrated normal contractility. **Middle row:** Patient with a negative DE-MRI study but with a prominent reversible defect in the anteroseptal wall on perfusion MRI *(red arrow)*. The interpretation algorithm (step 3) classified this patient as positive for CAD. Coronary angiography demonstrated a proximal 95% LAD stenosis. **Bottom row:** Patient with a matched stress-rest perfusion defect *(blue arrows)* but without evidence of prior MI on DE-MRI. The interpretation algorithm (step 4) classified the perfusion defects as artifactual. Coronary angiography demonstrated normal coronary arteries. CAD=coronary artery disease. (Modified from Klem et al, *Circulation* 2006;47:1630–1638)

defect) but do not have infarction on DE-MRI are artifactual and should not be considered positive for CAD (with rare exceptions[2]). Concerning this latter point, it is important to recognize that the interpretation of stress/rest perfusion MRI is NOT analogous to stress/rest radionuclide imaging. For instance, "matched" defects on perfusion MRI are far more likely to represent artifact than prior myocardial infarction. Additionally, infarcted regions—particularly those that are large and transmural—often appear "reversible" on perfusion MRI. This is because infarcted regions will accumulate the contrast given during the stress perfusion imaging stage, and during rest perfusion imaging, (10–15 minutes later), these regions may not show a perfusion defect (hypointensity) since delayed "hyperenhancement" to some degree is already present.

General Applications – Quantitative Evaluation of Structure and Function

Cine MRI using segmented GRE or SSFP imaging sequences has been shown to be highly accurate and reproducible in the measurement of ejection fraction, ventricular volumes, and cardiac mass (Table 2.1). In comparison with the competing modality of echocardiography, it has been shown to have significantly less interobserver and intraobserver variability, and superior reproducibility.[6] This latter characteristic is potentially of great benefit in the performance of research studies, as it has been shown that an up to 10-fold reduction in sample size is possible when using MR as compared with the competing modality of echocardiography.[7] Therefore, for the detection of subtle changes in left ventricular ejection fraction or cardiac mass in response to a given treatment, MR is the preferred monitoring modality.

Typical measurements are performed using the stack of short axis images, with tracing of the endocardial contour performed at end-diastole and end-systole. The areas are summed over the volume of tissue imaged, and the difference between the volumes at systole and diastole therefore represent the stroke volume. Simultaneous tracing of the epicardial contours allows assessment of myocardial mass, as well as wall thickening. Various computer

TABLE 2.1. Accuracy and reproducibility of MRI for cardiac volumes and mass.

Year	Author	N	Reference	Comments
Accuracy of Cardiac Mass Measurements				
1986	Keller	10	JACC 8:113–7	Animals; MRI LV mass in normal dogs; high accuracy versus autopsy
1986	Florentine	11	JACC 8:107–12	Animals; MRI LV mass in normal dogs and cats; high accuracy versus autopsy and reproducible
1987	Caputo	13	AJR 148:33–8	Animals; MRI LV mass in normal (7) and hypertrophied LV (6) dogs; high accuracy versus autopsy and reproducible
1987	Maddahi	9	JACC 10:682–92	Animals; MRI LV mass in normal dogs, in-vivo and ex-vivo; high accuracy versus autopsy
1988	Katz	10/40	Radiology 169:495–8	Cadaver hearts / Pts; high accuracy of ex-vivo MRI measurements / high in-vivo reproducibility
1989	Shapiro	15	Circulation 79:706–11	Animals; MRI LV mass before and after MI in dogs; MRI mass accurate pre and post MI versus autopsy
1992	McDonald	10	JACC 19:1601–7	Animals; MRI LV and RV mass in dogs; high accuracy versus autopsy, high reproducibility for RV and LV mass
1993	McDonald	27	JACC 21:514–22	Animals; MRI LV mass in dogs post MI-model; postinfarct remodeling attenuation by nitrates detected by MRI
1995	Bottini	6/34	Am J Hypertens 8:221–8	Cadaver hearts / HTN, HCM pts; high accuracy of ex-vivo MRI / higher in-vivo reproducibility than echo
1999	Lorenz	10/75	JCMR 1:7–21	Animals / Pts; high accuracy of MRI LV mass in dogs; Pts scanned to obtain mean and variation in normals

(continued)

TABLE 2.1. (continued)

Year	Author	N	Reference	Comments
Accuracy of Cardiac Volume Measurements				
1985	Longmore	20/20	Lancet 1:1360–2	Normals / angina Pts; good correlation of MRI LV, RV stroke volumes, moderate correlation of MRI with x-ray VG
1985	Rehr	15	Radiology 156:717–9	Cadaver hearts; good correlation of MRI LV volumes with cadaver heart casts volumes
1987	Sechtem	10/5	Radiology 163:697–702	Normals; good correlation of MRI LV and RV stroke volumes, and with LV stroke volume by echo (n=5)
1995	Helbing	22/20	Am Heart J 130:828 37	Healthy and CHD children; good correlation of MRI LV and RV stroke volumes, and RV stroke volume with PA and tricuspid flow by phase contrast MRI
1987	Firmin	10	JCAT 11:751–6	Normals; good correlation of MRI LV stroke volume with aortic flow by phase contrast MRI
2000	Bellenger	52	EHJ 21:1387–96	HF Pts (CHRISTMAS substudy); modest agreement of MRI LV volumes and function with Echo, radionuclide VG
Reproducibility of Cardiac Mass and Volume Measurements				
1990	Semelka	19	Am Heart J 119:1367–73	DCM (11) and LVH (8) Pts; high reproducibility of MRI for LV mass, volumes, function
1990	Semelka	11	Radiology 174:763–8	Normals; high reproducibility of MRI for LV mass, volumes, function
1992	Germain	20	EHJ 13:1011–9	Angina (6), HTN (6), CMP (3), valvular lesion (3), SVT (2) Pts; higher reproducibility of MRI versus M-mode echo
1993	Yamaoka	20	Am Heart J 126:1372–9	Pts with various CV disorders; good correlation between MRI and CT for LV mass, high reproducibility of MRI
1993	Mogelvang	30	Clin Physiol 13:587–97	HTN (10), IHD (17), HCM (2), DCM (1) Pts; high reproducibility of MRI volumes and LV mass (11), moderate correlation between MRI LV mass and 2D-echo (13)
1995	Bogaert	12	MAGMA 3:5–12	Normals; higher reproducibility of MRI for LV volumes, mass, EF versus Echo
1996	Matheijssen	7	Int J Card Imag. 12:11–9	Pts with anterior MI; high reproducibility of MRI LV volumes, mass, EF
1998	Osterziel	50	Lancet 351:1233–7	DCM pts; MRI used as end-point for randomized trial of growth-hormone treatment
2000	Bellenger	20/20	JCMR 2:271–8	Normals / HF Pts; higher reproducibility of MRI for LV volumes, mass, EF versus Echo
2002	Grothues	20/40	Am J Cardiol 90:29–34	Normals / LVH, HF Pts; higher reproducibility of MRI for LV volumes, mass, EF versus Echo
2004	Bellenger	34	Heart 90:760–4	HF Pts (CHRISTMAS substudy); MRI used as end-point for randomized trial of carvedilol

CHD, congenital heart disease; CMP, cardiomyopathy; CT, computed tomography; CV, cardiovascular; DCM, dilated cardiomyopathy; Echo, echocardiography; EF, ejection fraction; HCM, hypertrophic cardiomyopathy; HF, heart failure; HTN, hypertension; IHD; ischemic heart disease; LV, left ventricle; LVH, left ventricular hypertrophy; MI, myocardial infarction; PA, pulmonary artery; Pts, patients; RV, right ventricle; SVT, supraventricular tachycardia, VG, ventriculography.

From, Kim et al, Magnetic Resonance Imaging of the Myocardium. In: Willerson et al, eds. *Cardiovascular Medicine (3rd ed.)*. New York, NY: Springer-Verlag; 2007.

workstations are available to facilitate the performance of these measurements.

References

1. Kim HW, Crowley AL, Kim RJ. A clinical cardiovascular magnetic resonance service: operational considerations and the basic examination. Cardiol Clin. 2007;25(1):1–13.
2. Kim HW, Klem I, Kim RJ. Detection of myocardial ischemia by stress perfusion cardiovascular magnetic resonance. Cardiol Clin. 2007;25(1):57–70.
3. Klem I, Heitner JF, Shah DJ, et al. Improved detection of coronary artery disease by stress perfusion cardiovascular magnetic resonance with the use of delayed enhancement infarction imaging. J Am Coll Cardiol. 2006;47(8):1630–1638.
4. Cerqueira MD, Weissman NJ, Dilsizian V, et al. Standardized myocardial segmentation and nomenclature for tomographic imaging of the heart: a statement for healthcare professionals from the Cardiac Imaging Committee of the Council on Clinical Cardiology of the American Heart Association. Circulation. 2002;105:539–542.
5. Kim RJ, Shah DJ, Judd RM. How we perform delayed enhancement imaging. J Cardiovasc Magn Reson. 2003;5:505–514.
6. Bellenger NG, Grothues F, Smith GC, Pennell DJ. Quantification of right and left ventricular function by cardiovascular magnetic resonance. Herz 2000;25(4):392–399.
7. Bellenger NG, Davies LC, Francis JM, Coats AJ, Pennell DJ. Reduction in sample size for studies of remodeling in heart failure by the use of cardiovascular magnetic resonance. J Cardiovasc Magn Reson. 2000;2(4):271–278.

3 Ischemic Heart Disease and Non-Ischemic Cardiomyopathies

Assessment of Myocardial Infarction and Viability

Myocardial infarction, scarring, and viability are simultaneously examined using the technique of delayed-enhancement MR. Multiple experimental studies have demonstrated an excellent spatial correlation between the extent of hyperenhancement on delayed-enhancement imaging, and areas of myocardial necrosis (acute MI) or scarring (chronic MI) at histopathology (Figure 3.1).[1] In patients, delayed-enhancement MR has been shown to be highly effective in identifying the presence, location, and extent of myocardial infarction in both the acute and chronic settings.[2,3] Additionally, it has been shown to be superior to SPECT for the detection of subendocardial myocardial infarction (Figure 3.2).[4]

Delayed-enhancement MR, in combination with cine imaging, allows identification of myocardial stunning following acute myocardial infarction,[5,6] or hibernating myocardium in the setting of chronic ischemic heart disease.[7,8] In the latter situation, it then follows that delayed-enhancement imaging can be performed before coronary revascularization procedures to predict the likelihood that there will be functional recovery after revascularization.[7,8] Specifically, there is an inverse relationship between the transmural extent of hyperenhancement, and the likelihood of wall motion recovery following revascularization. For instance, myocardial regions that demonstrate little or no evidence of hyperenhancement (i.e. infarction) have

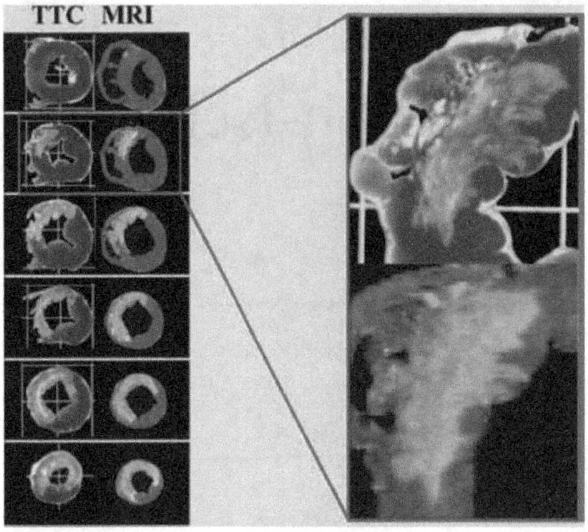

FIGURE 3.1. Comparison of ex-vivo, high resolution delayed enhancement MR images with acute myocardial necrosis defined histologically by triphenyltetrazolium chloride (TTC) staining. Note that the size and shape of the infarcted region *(yellowish-white region)* defined histologically by TTC staining is nearly exactly matched by the size and shape of the hyperenhanced *(bright)* region on the delayed enhancement image. (Modified from *Circulation* 1999;100:1992–2002, with permission)

high likelihood of recovery, whereas regions with transmural hyperenhancement have virtually no chance of recovery (Figure 3.3) Likewise, regions with intermediate levels of hyperenhancement (around 50%), have moderate chances of recovery. However, in this situation, it is important to remember that both myocardial viability and functional improvement are a continuum, and not simply a binary—yes or no—function.[9] Thus, since it most closely reflects reality, it is better to consider these regions as all having a high chance for an intermediate amount of improvement rather than 50% likely to have complete recovery and the other 50%, no improvement whatsoever.

In patients with acute myocardial infarction, delayed-enhancement imaging may also demonstrate "no reflow" zones. These regions are recognized as dark central areas surrounded by hyperenhanced necrotic myocardium (Figure 3.4) (Case 8). This finding indicates the presence of damaged microvasculature in the core of an area of infarction.[10] The presence of a "no reflow" zone appears to be associated with worse LV remodeling and outcome.[11–15]

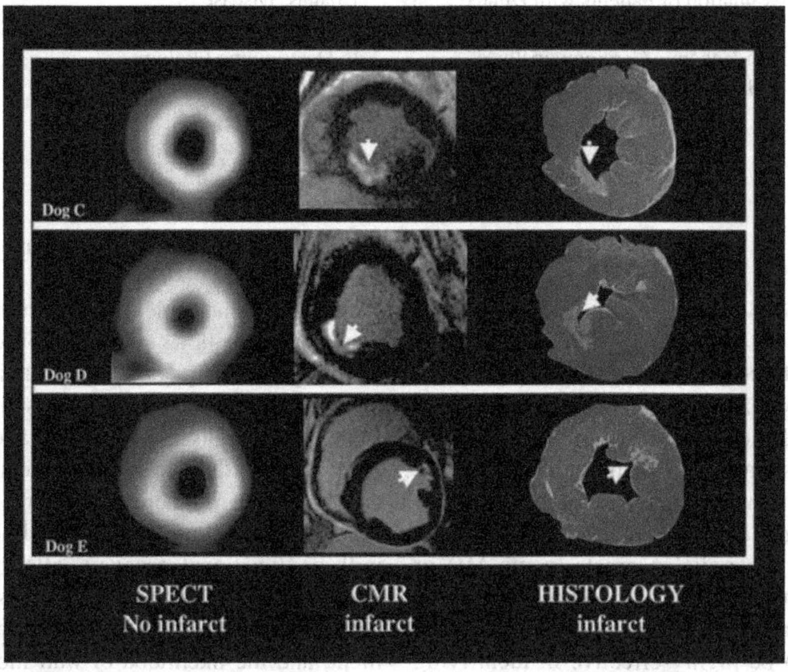

FIGURE 3.2. SPECT vs. delayed-enhancement CMR vs. histologic sections in a dog model of infarction demonstrate the superiority of DE-CMR relative to SPECT for the detection of subendocardial infarction. (From *Lancet* 2003;361:374–9, with permission)

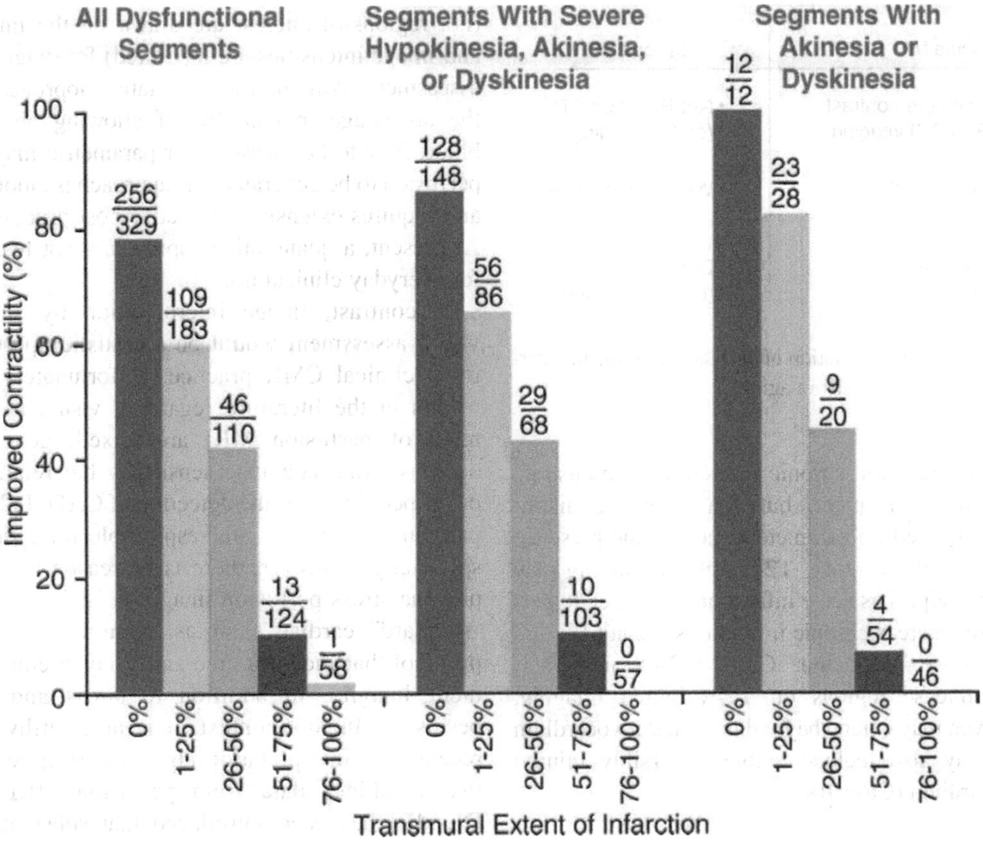

FIGURE 3.3. The likelihood of recovery of wall motion following revascularization is inversely related to the transmural extent of infarction (hyperenhancement) on delayed-enhancement imaging, even in severely hypokinetic, akinetic, or dyskinetic segments. (From *N Engl J Med* 2000;343:1445–53, with permission)

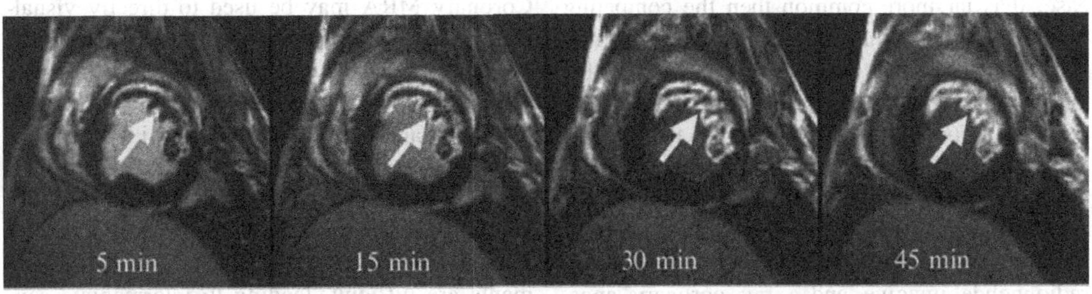

FIGURE 3.4. Sequential delayed-enhancement images demonstrate a "no-reflow" zone in an anterior infarction, manifested as a dark region surrounded by hyperenhancing myocardium. Labels refer to time after administration of gadolinium contrast. Note that the "no-reflow" zone fills in and becomes smaller over time. (From Kim RJ, et al. Assessment of myocardial viability by contrast enhancement. In: Higgins CB, de Roos A, (eds). *Cardiovascular MRI & MRA*. Philadelphia: Lippincott Williams & Wilkins, 2003;209–237, with permission)

Acute MI	Chronic MI
• Bright on pre-contrast STIR (or T2) imaging	• Not Bright on STIR (or T2) imaging
• Walls can be thicker than usual	• Walls can be thinned
• May have a "no-reflow" zone	• Does not have "no-reflow" zones

FIGURE 3.5. Differentiation of acute and chronic myocardial infarction on CMR imaging

Both acute and chronic infarctions demonstrate delayed-enhancement, but can often be distinguished based on parameters such as the presence of a "no reflow" zone. T2-weighted imaging may also be helpful as acute infarctions are often hyperintense whereas chronic infarctions are not (Figure 3.5) (Case 104-acute, Case 113-chronic).[16, 17] Hyperintense regions on T2-weighted imaging, however, may extend beyond infarcted myocardium and may also include viable, reversibly injured myocardium (Case 104).[18]

Detection of Coronary Artery Disease

Adenosine Stress Perfusion Imaging

Adenosine stress perfusion MR is increasingly used as a first line modality for the detection of hemodynamically significant coronary artery disease. It is far more common then the competing modality of dobutamine cine MR, and the patient is directly accessible (outside the scanner bore) for all but approximately 30 seconds of the adenosine infusion. (For a full discussion of the technical aspects of perfusion imaging, see Chapters 1 and 2). Its diagnostic performance has been evaluated in number of patient studies. Overall, these studies have shown good correlations with radionuclide imaging and x-ray coronary angiography, although there have been some variable results.[19] Table 3.1 summarizes the published literature on stress perfusion MRI in humans with coronary angiography comparison. Unfortunately, many of the studies used a quantitative approach (i.e. regions-of-interest are drawn on the images and image intensities are measured) for diagnostic assessment. Although a quantitative approach has the advantage, potentially, of allowing absolute blood flow to be measured or parametric maps of perfusion to be generated, the approach is laborious and requires extensive interactive post-processing. At present, a quantitative approach is not feasible for everyday clinical use.

In contrast, image interpretation by simple visual assessment would be a realistic approach for a clinical CMR practice. Unfortunately, the results in the literature regarding visual assessment of perfusion MRI are mixed, generally demonstrating adequate sensitivity but relatively poor specificity for the detection of CAD. In large part, image artifacts are responsible for reduced specificity. However, there is no reason to interpret the stress perfusion images in isolation. The "standard" cardiac exam is a multi-component protocol that includes cine and delayed-enhancement imaging in addition to stress and rest perfusion. In this context, it is noteworthy that recently an interpretation algorithm (Figure 2.5) that combines data from perfusion MRI and DE-MRI has been introduced that substantially improves the specificity and accuracy of rapid visual assessment for the detection of CAD.[20] It is this technique that is used throughout this teaching file (Case 73). The protocol and interpretation of stress perfusion imaging is reviewed in detail in Chapter 2.

Coronary MRA

Coronary MRA may be used to directly visualize coronary anatomy and morphology. However, coronary MRA is technically demanding for several reasons. The coronary arteries are small (3–5 mm) and tortuous compared with other vascular beds that are imaged by MRA, and there is nearly constant motion during both the respiratory and cardiac cycles. Thus, precise assessment of stenosis severity and visualization of distal segments are difficult, leading to intermediate sensitivity and specificity values for the detection of CAD in validation studies.[21, 22] Currently, the only clinical indication that is considered appropriate for coronary MRA is the evaluation of patients with suspected coronary anomalies.[23]

TABLE 3.1. Stress perfusion MRI studies in humans with coronary angiography comparison.

Year	Author	Reference	n	Pts with known CAD excluded	Protocol: MRI Perfusion Protocol[1]	Protocol: Gadolinium Dose (mmol/kg)	Protocol: Pulse-Sequence	X-Ray Angiography (CAD definition)	Analysis Method[2]	Sens	Spec
1993	Klein	AJR 161(2):257–63	5	no	Stress only	0.05	IR-GRE	>50	prospective	81*	100*
1994	Hartnell	AJR 163(5):1061–7	18	no	Rest/Stress	0.04	IR-GRE	≥70	prospective	83	100
1994	Eichenberger	JMRI 4(3):425–31	10	no	Rest/Stress	0.05	GRE	>75	retrospective	44*	80*
2000	Al-Saadi	Circ 101(12):1379–83	34	yes	Rest/Stress	0.025	IR-GRE	≥75	prospective[3]	90	83
2001	Bertschinger	JMRI 14(5):556–62	14	no	Stress only	0.1	SR-EPI	≥50	retrospective	85	81
2001	Schwitter	Circ 103(18):2230–5	48	yes	Stress only	0.1	SR-GRE-EPI	≥50	retrospective	87	85
2001	Panting	JMRI 13(2):192–200	22	no	Rest/Stress	0.05	IR Spin Echo-EPI	>50	retrospective	79	83
2002	Sensky	Int J CV Imaging 18(5):373–383	30	no	Rest/Stress	0.025	IR-GRE	>50	prospective	93*	60*
2002	Ibrahim	JACC 39(5):864–870	25	no	Rest/Stress	0.05	SR-GRE-EPI	>75	retrospective	69*	89*
2003	Chiu	Radiology 226(3):717–722	13	no[4]	Rest/Stress	0.05	IR-SSFP	>50	NS	92*	92*
2003	Ishida	Radiology 229(1):209–216	104	no	Stress/Rest	0.075	SR-GRE-EPI	≥70	prospective	90	85
2003	Nagel	Circ 108(4):432–437	84	no	Rest/Stress	0.025	SR-GRE-EPI	≥75	retrospective	88	90
2003	Doyle	JCMR 5(3):475–85	138	no	Rest/Stress	0.04	SR-GRE	≥70	prospective[3]	57	85
2004	Wolff	Circ 110(6):732–737	75	no	Stress/Rest	0.05–0.15	SR-GRE-EPI	≥70	prospective[5]	93	75
2004	Giang	EHJ 25(18):1657–65	80	no	Stress only	0.05–0.15	SR-GRE-EPI	≥50	retrospective[5]	93	75
2004	Paetsch	Circ 110(7):835–842	79	no	Stress/Rest	0.05	SR-GRE-EPI	>50	prospective	91	62
2004	Plein	JACC 44(11):2173–81	68	no[4]	Rest/Stress	0.05	SR-GRE[6]	≥70	prospective	88	83
2005	Plein	Radiology 235(2):423–430	92	no	Rest/Stress	0.05	SR-GRE[6]	>70	retrospective	88	82

(continued)

TABLE 3.1. (continued)

Year	Author	Reference	n	Pts with known CAD excluded	Protocol: MRI Perfusion Protocol[1]	Protocol: Gadolinium Dose (mmol/kg)	Protocol: Pulse-Sequence	X-Ray Angiography (CAD definition)	Analysis Method[2]	Sens	Spec
2006	Klem	JACC 47(8):1630–38	100	yes	Stress/Rest	0.063	SR-GRE[6]	≥70	prospective	84	58
2006	Cury	Radiology 240(1):39–45	47	no	Stress/Rest	0.1	SR-GRE-EPI	≥70	prospective	81[¤]	87[¤]
Total		20	1086								
Average										83	82

MRI, magnetic resonance imaging; CAD, coronary artery disease; n, number of patients; n, number of patients; IR, inversion recovery pre-pulse; SR, saturation recovery pre-pulse; GRE, gradient-recalled echo; EPI, echo-planar imaging; SSFP, steady-state free precession; DE-MRI, delayed enhancement MRI; Sens, sensitivity; Spec, specificity; NS, not stated.

[*] numbers based on a regional rather than per patient analysis.

[1] when both rest and stress imaging were performed the order is as listed.

[2] prospective studies were those in which the criteria for test abnormality were prespecified before data analysis.

[3] pilot study performed first to determine the best threshold for test abnormality.

[4] at enrollment all patients had the clinical diagnosis of non-ST elevation MI or acute coronary syndrome.

[5] reported sensitivity and specificity are from a fraction of the total cohort, a subgroup with the best results.

[6] with parallel imaging acceleration.

[†] sensitivity/specificity were higher after incorporating DE-MRI (89% and 87%, respectively).

[§] sensitivity/specificity were higher after incorporating DE-MRI (87% and 89%, respectively).

From Kim et al: Magnetic Resonance Imaging of the Heart. In Fuster V, O'Rourke, RA (eds). *Hurst's The Heart (12th ed.)*. New York: McGraw-Hill Medical, In Press.

More recently, SSFP sequences that offer superior signal-to-noise ratio in combination with whole-heart approaches[24, 25] analogous to multi-detector CT and parallel imaging to reduce scan times have improved the reliability of coronary MRA. These sequences typically can be run with submillimeter in-plane spatial resolution (0.8 × 1.0mm) and slice thickness just over 1 mm. In the authors' experience, the whole-heart approach is particularly powerful since it minimizes set-up time and operator interaction (Figure 3.6) (Case 37, Case 62). Additionally, with the use of modifications that compensate for respiratory drift,[26] imaging can usually be completed in under 10 minutes. Parallel imaging with undersampling in two rather than only one dimension will reduce scanning time further.

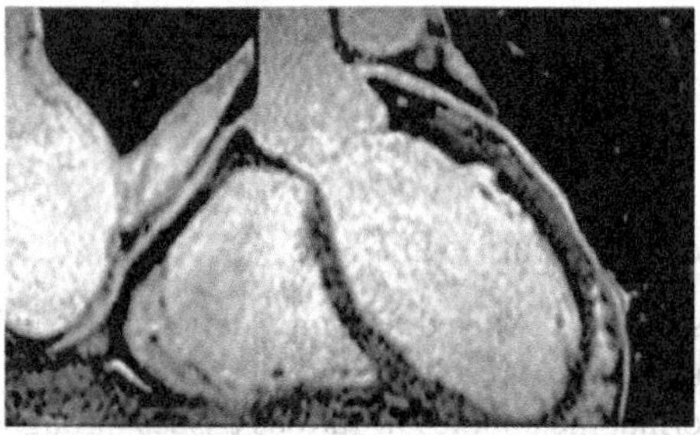

A

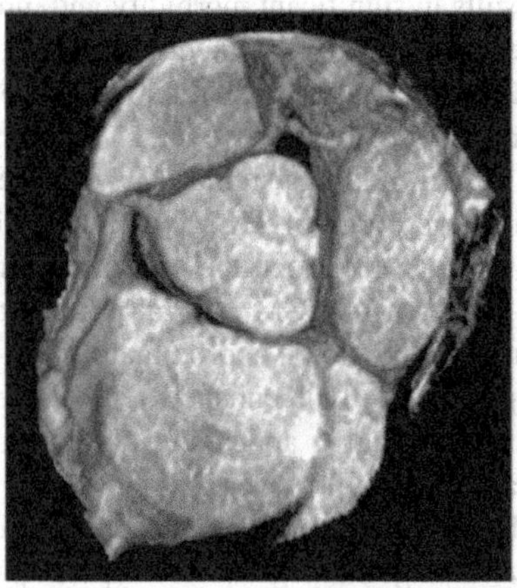

B

FIGURE 3.6. A curved MIP view from a whole-heart coronary MRA of a patient with normal coronaries (**A**). This acquisition took 8 minutes. A volume-rendered view from a whole-heart coronary MRA of a patient with an aneurysmal RCA (**B**)

Evaluation of Patients with Dilated Cardiomyopathy

As discussed, cine MR is arguably the "gold standard" technique for the evaluation of myocardial structure and function; and small changes in ejection fraction and cardiac mass are much more readily detected (and with greater precision) using MR than echocardiography.[27, 28] Therapeutic interventions for these patients, therefore, may be best assessed using MR.

Perhaps more importantly, in patients with dilated cardiomyopathy, delayed-enhancement imaging may be useful in distinguishing between ischemic and nonischemic etiology in the great majority of cases. Several studies have reported that virtually all patients with ischemic cardiomyopathy demonstrate delayed hyperenhancement in a typical "CAD" pattern, one in which the subendocardium is always involved. In contrast, patients with nonischemic dilated cardiomyopathy either demonstrate no hyperenhancement (60%), or a midwall stripe pattern in which the subendocardium is spared (25 to 30%) (Figure 3.7) (Case

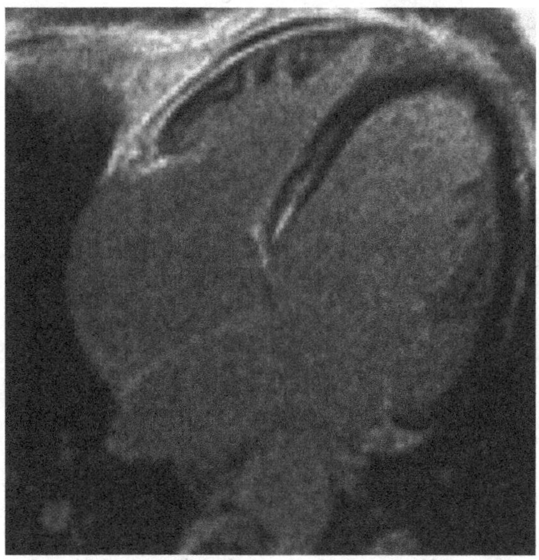

FIGURE 3.7. A 4-chamber delayed-enhancement image demonstrates the characteristic mid-wall "stripe" enhancement pattern of the septum in a patient with non-ischemic cardiomyopathy

121).[29, 30] Approximately 10 to 12% of patients with nonischemic dilated cardiomyopathy (with clean coronaries at cardiac catheterization) will paradoxically demonstrate subendocardial hyperenhancement. It has been speculated that these patients may have had prior episodes of coronary occlusion with recanalization.

Patients with dilated cardiomyopathy are subject to the development of ventricular thrombi (Case 136). Compared with transthoracic echocardiography, cardiac MR may have more than a two-fold increase in sensitivity for the detection of LV thrombus.[31, 32] Delayed-enhancement imaging using a long inversion time (550–600 msec) in our experience is the most sensitive technique for the detection of ventricular thrombi. In addition, delayed-enhancement imaging can be helpful in localizing regions where thrombi are prone to develop, as studies have demonstrated their frequent adherence to sites of prior infarction.[31, 32]

Non-Ischemic Cardiomyopathies

Hypertrophic Cardiomyopathy (HCM)

This is the most common genetic cardiac disease, with an estimated prevalence of 1 in 500. Given the advantages of a wide field of view, tomographic imaging with 3D coverage, and uniform image resolution, cine MR is capable of detecting regions of localized hypertrophy that are missed by echocardiography. Rickers et al. reported that in 6% of patients with suspected or known HCM, cine MR established the diagnosis of HCM, while no hypertrophy was seen on echocardiography.[33]

It has been shown by CMR that regions with the greatest hypertrophy are more likely to demonstrate significant impairment in contractile function.[34] In addition, a significant percentage of patients with HCM will demonstrate hyperenhancement (>80%).[34–38] In these patients, a characteristic pattern of enhancement is noted, often involving the regions of hypertrophy, and also frequently involving the junctions of the interventricular septum and the RV free wall (Figure 3.8) (Case 108).[34] Early reports suggest that the extent of hyperenhancement may correlate with the likelihood of the development of progressive disease.[38]

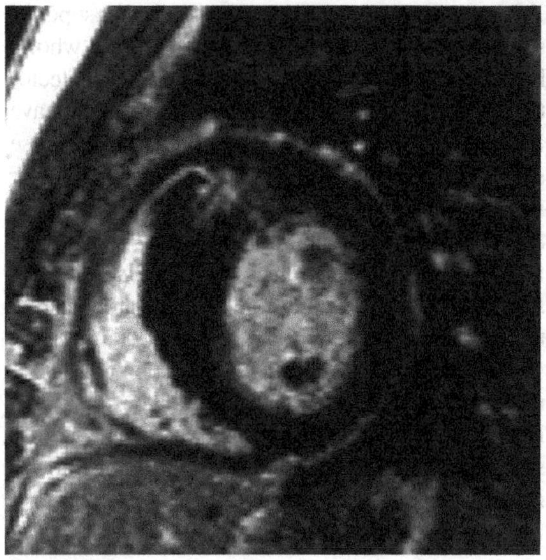

FIGURE 3.8. DE-CMR in a patient with hypertrophic cardiomyopathy. Note the characteristic hyperenhancement of the septum at the RV insertion site

Anderson-Fabry Disease

This is an X-linked enzyme deficiency (alpha-galactosidase) resulting in the accumulation of abnormal metabolites in various tissues throughout the body. Typically, involvement of the kidneys or heart results in significant morbidity and mortality. As expected from the X-linked inheritance, males are predominantly affected, but female carriers may sometimes be involved as well.[39] Cardiac involvement results in findings similar to those seen with the concentric form of HCM, and this disorder may mimic HCM. In fact, the prevalence of Fabry disease in a typical HCM referral population was found in one study to be approximately 5%.[40]

The pattern of hyperenhancement on delayed-enhancement imaging appears to be quite distinct from that of HCM, however. As opposed to HCM, which demonstrates patchy enhancement predominantly affecting the regions of hypertrophy and the RV-septal insertion sites, hyperenhancement in Fabry disease has a predilection for the inferolateral wall at the basal level (Figure 3.9) (Case 134). The reason for this finding is uncertain. Studies suggest that up to 50% of patients will demonstrate this finding on delayed-enhancement imaging.[41, 42] The presence of abnormal hyperenhancement as well as the degree of myocardial hypertrophy has

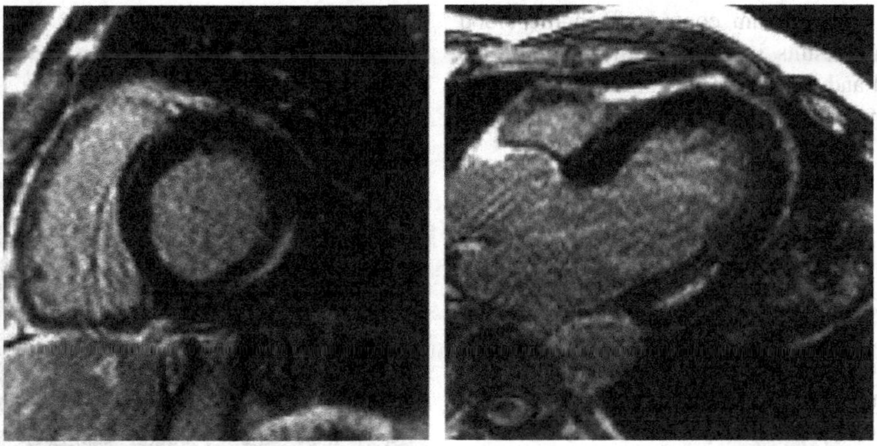

FIGURE 3.9. Delayed-enhancement images from a patient with Fabry's disease demonstrate the typical hyperenhancement pattern of the inferolateral wall at the base

been shown to correlate with the severity of cardiac involvement. In addition, given the availability of enzyme replacement,[43] follow-up studies to assess the effect of therapeutic intervention may be best performed with CMR.

Amyloidosis

Cardiac involvement is the most common cause of death in systemic amyloidosis, and cardiac amyloidosis is the most common identifiable cause of restrictive cardiomyopathy.[44–46] Cine imaging typically demonstrates global hypertrophy, often involving the right ventricle as well. Additionally, thickening of the interatrial septum and of the atrial walls are findings strongly suggestive of the diagnosis.[47, 48]

Delayed-enhancement imaging typically demonstrates diffuse LV hyperenhancement in these patients (Figure 3.10) (Case 41). Although often subendocardial, the pattern is clearly distinct from the usual CAD pattern in that the hyperenhancement does not follow a coronary artery distribution. From an imaging point-of-view, the presence of diffuse myocardial involvement may make setting the parameters for delayed-enhancement imaging problematic. Specifically, it may be difficult to determine the optimal inversion time that will null "normal" myocardium, as there may be few areas that are completely normal. Additionally, unlike the situation in normal patients, in whom the LV blood pool (post contrast administration) has far shorter T1 relaxation than myocardium, in patients with cardiac amyloidosis, the myocardium may have similar T1 to that of blood pool and image intensities may be similar on delayed-enhancement imaging. Reports indicate that this finding is likely due to profound expansion of the extracellular volume of the myocardium, as well as more rapid

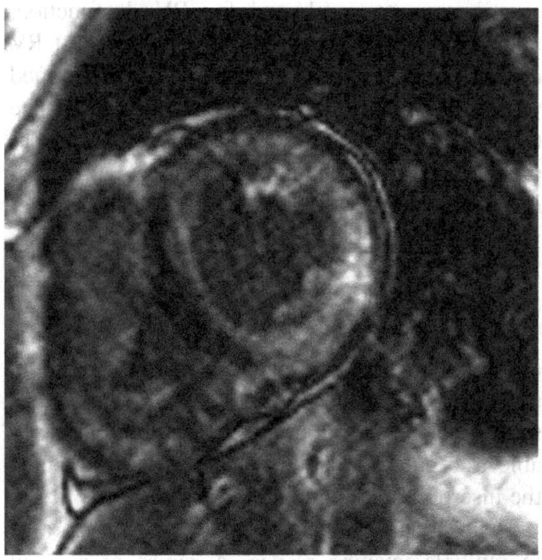

FIGURE 3.10. Diffuse subendocardial enhancement is noted on this delayed-enhancement short-axis image from a patient with amyloidosis

clearance of gadolinium contrast from the blood pool.[46] This results in near equilibration of the blood pool and myocardial gadolinium concentrations, and partially explains the difficulty in nulling.

ARVD

This is an inherited cardiomyopathy whose hallmark is fibrofatty replacement of the RV myocardium. The left ventricle is also involved in at least 15% of patients.[49] This disorder is thought to be due to pathologic mutations in the genes coding the formation of desmosomal proteins.[50]

The patients typically develop progressive RV failure, and have frequent arrhythmias. Historically, CMR examinations employed spin-echo pulse sequences in an attempt to visualize fatty infiltration of the RV myocardium as well as RV free-wall thinning. However, interpretation of these images was often difficult because of motion artifact, and volume averaging with adjacent epicardial and pericardial fat. As a result, relying on the presence or absence of fat on these images is a frequent cause of misdiagnosis,[51] and the presence or absence of fat and RV wall thinning by CMR are not included among the Task Force criteria for diagnosis.[52]

Currently, most centers evaluating patients with ARVD use a multi-modality approach in which cine images are evaluated for RV dysfunction, microaneurysm formation, and focal areas of RV dyskinesia.[53] Cine imaging should be performed with high spatial (<2mm in-plane, ≤6mm slice thickness) and temporal resolution (≤40msec per phase), and complete anatomical coverage including the RV outflow tract. A stack of four-chamber views is frequently helpful. Focal wall thinning, RV outflow tract dilatation, or trabecular disarray are all findings suggestive of the presence of ARVD. Although assessment of RV function is more reproducible and specific than fat infiltration, scans may still be overinterpreted since the RV has substantial normal variations including highly variable trabeculation and small outward bulges near the insertion of the moderator band.

Delayed-enhancement imaging is also performed in multiple imaging planes. A report of a small series of 12 patients indicated that 2/3 demonstrated abnormal hyperenhancement of the RV myocardium on delayed-enhancement imaging (Figure 3.11) (Case 53).[54] In addition, the presence of hyperenhancement correlated with the finding of inducible tachyarrhythmias. No normal patient demonstrated abnormal hyperenhancement of the right ventricle.

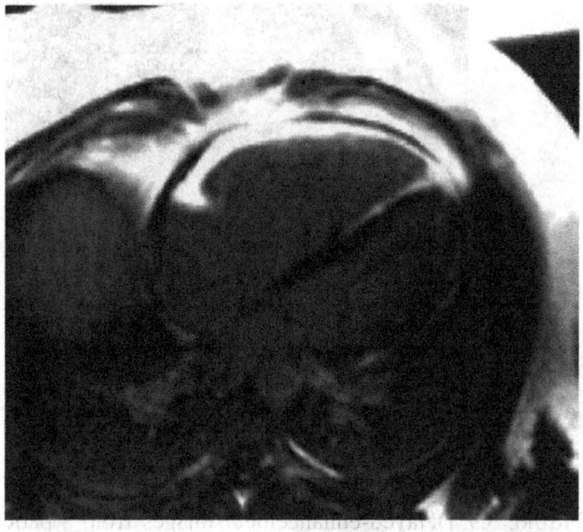

FIGURE 3.11. A 4-chamber delayed-enhancement image showing hyperenhancement of the RV free wall and the apical half of the interventricular septum in a patient with confirmed ARVD

Sarcoidosis

Although autopsy studies have frequently shown that cardiac involvement is found in approximately 25% of patients with sarcoidosis, cardiac involvement is recognized clinically in less than 10% of patients. This likely reflects the relative insensitivity of the most frequently used diagnostic tools.[55] Not detecting cardiac involvement may be important, as these patients are prone to sudden cardiac death. Recently, pilot studies have suggested the superiority of delayed-enhancement MR imaging compared with SPECT and PET imaging for the detection of cardiac sarcoidosis.[55, 56] In addition, significantly more patients were recognized using CMR than would have been diagnosed with the typical Japanese Ministry of Health criteria.

Typically, patchy hyperenhancement is typically found along the epicardium or mid-myocardium in a non-CAD pattern (Figure 3.12) (Case 85). Basal and septal involvement is frequent.[55–57] Approximately 10–30% of patients demonstrate a subendocardial or transmural hyperenhancement pattern that mimics CAD.

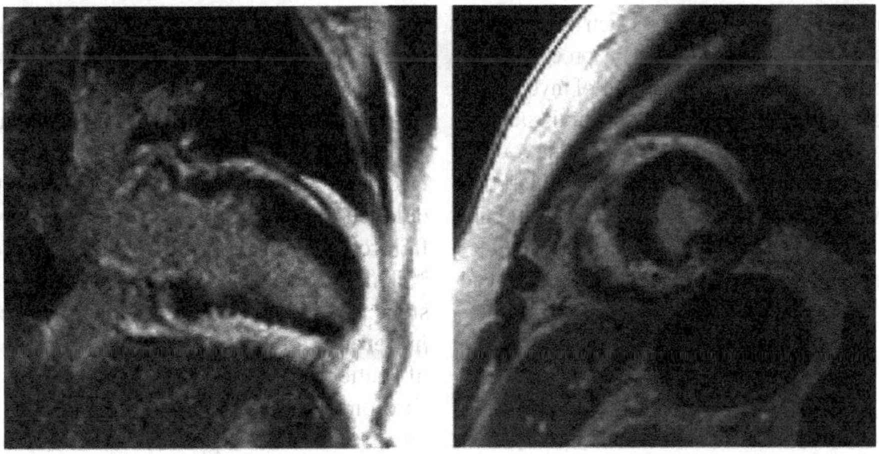

A B

FIGURE 3.12. A 2-chamber (**A**) and short-axis (**B**) delayed-enhancement images of a patient with sarcoid. Note the inferior wall epicardial enhancement in a non-CAD pattern

Myocarditis

Several different CMR pulse sequences have been used to evaluate patients with suspected acute myocarditis. Recent studies using delayed-enhancement inversion-recovery imaging demonstrated that hyperenhancement is a frequent finding in viral myocarditis, occurring in approximately 88% of patients.[58] Other researchers have suggested that T2-weighted sequences may demonstrate additional findings not apparent on delayed-enhancement imaging, and that the combination of sequences may be optimal (Figure 3.13) (Case 95).[59]

CMR studies evaluating the clinical course of myocarditis have demonstrated that hyperenhanced regions

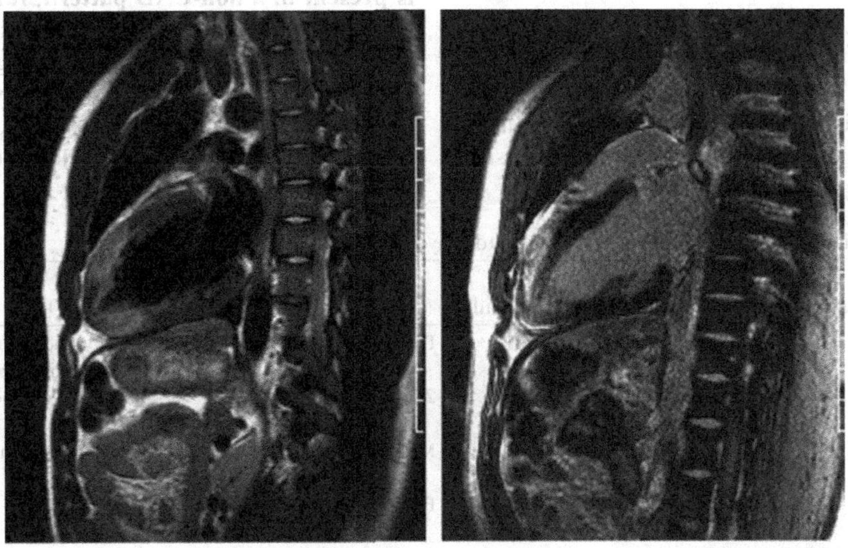

A B

FIGURE 3.13. T2-weighted (**A**) and delayed-enhancement (**B**) 2-chamber views images in a patient with myocarditis. Note the high signal in the anterior and inferior walls in the apical region in a non-CAD pattern on both images

observed during the acute setting often decrease in size significantly during follow up. This process likely represents myocardial healing as regions of myocardial necrosis are replaced with collagenous scar tissue.[60]

In the studies reported from Europe, parvovirus B19 was a frequent etiologic agent, particularly in cases involving the lateral free wall, and had generally favorable outcomes. Herpes simplex 6 had a predilection for septal involvement, and seemed to correlate with the development of progressive disease.[58, 60]

Chagas' Disease

This inflammatory disease is caused by the protozoa Trypanosoma Cruzi. Most patients survive the initial phase of illness, and remain asymptomatic for years. However, 20% of patients may develop chronic heart failure.[61] A recent report by Rochitte et al.[62] suggests that delayed-enhancement imaging is capable of detecting early involvement in Chagas' disease before the onset of symptoms. Additionally, delayed-enhancement imaging may provide unique information for clinical disease staging in Chagas' disease. Scarring occurred most commonly in the LV apex and inferolateral wall. Both non-CAD type (isolated epicardial or mid-wall involvement) and CAD type (indistinguishable from prior myocardial infarction) scar patterns were observed.

Summary: Systematic Approach to Determining Etiology of Cardiomyopathy

Table 3.2 lists the CMR findings of specific cardiomyopathies in a tabular format. The presence and pattern of scarring on delayed-enhancement imaging is often quite distinct, and a pattern recognition approach based on the visualization of abnormal enhancement will often provide useful diagnostic information as to the likely etiology. Recently, a systematic approach to interpreting delayed-enhanced images in patients with heart failure or cardiomyopathy has been proposed.[63, 64] This approach is based on the following three steps: **(Step 1) The presence or absence of hyperenhancement is determined.** In the subset of patients with longstanding severe ischemic cardiomyopathy, the data indicate that virtually all patients have prior MI.[65] The implication is that in patients with severe cardiomyopathy but without hyperenhancement, the diagnosis of idiopathic dilated cardiomyopathy should be strongly considered. **(Step 2) If hyperenhancement is present, the location and distribution of hyperenhancement should be classified as a CAD or non-CAD pattern.** For this determination, the concept that ischemic injury progresses as a "wavefront" from the subendocardium to the epicardium is crucial.[66] Correspondingly, hyperenhancement patterns that spare the subendocardium and are limited to the middle or epicardial portion of the LV wall are clearly in a non-CAD pattern. **(Step 3) If hyperenhancement is present in a non-CAD pattern, further classification should be considered.** As described above, there is emerging data that suggest certain nonischemic cardiomyopathies have predilection for specific scar patterns. For example, in the setting of LV hypertrophy, the presence of midwall

TABLE 3.2. Diagnostic CMR findings of specific cardiomyopathies.

Suspected diagnosis	Structure/ function module	Delayed enhancement module	Other
Amyloid	Thick ventricles, dilated atria	Diffuse subendocardial enhancement	Difficulty finding "null" point on inversion time scout sequence
ARVD	Large RV with poor function, microaneurysms	2/3rds show RV hyperenhancement	Look for RV enhancement, fat
Fabry	Concentric hypertrophy	Midwall HE inferolateral wall at the base	Predominantly men
HCM	Asymmetric, concentric or apical hypertrophy	Positive at RV insertion sites and in regions of thickening	
Myocarditis	Focal thickening, wall motion abnormality	Lateral epicardial or septal midwall HE common	T2-weighted imaging sometimes helpful
Sarcoidosis	Focal thickening, wall motion abnormality	Patchy uptake with slight basal/septal predominance	Mediastinal / hilar adenopathy often noted on morphologic images

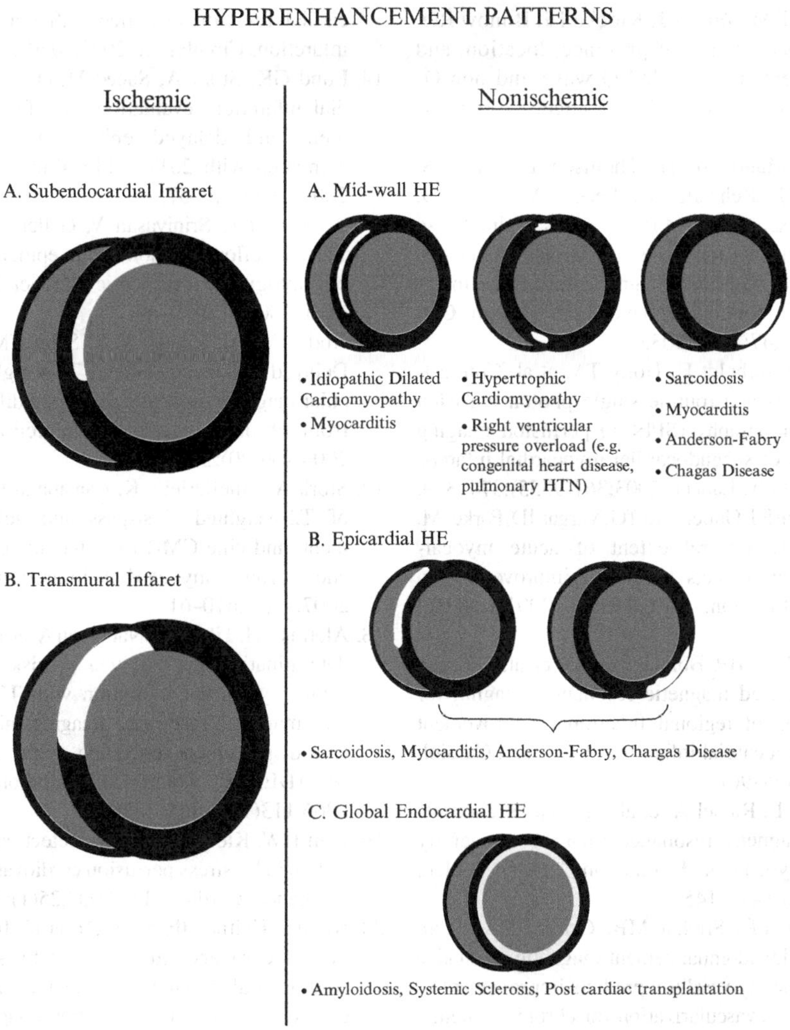

FIGURE 3.14. Hyperenhancement (HE) patterns that may be encountered in clinical practice. Since myocardial necrosis due to CAD progresses as a "wavefront" from the subendocardium to the epicardium, HE (if present) should always involve the subendocardium in patients with ischemic disease. Isolated mid-wall or epicardial HE strongly suggests a "non-ischemic" etiology. Additionally, endocardial HE that occurs globally (i.e. throughout the LV) is uncommon even with diffuse CAD and therefore a non-ischemic etiology should be considered. (From Shah et al. In: Edelman RR, et al., eds. *Clinical Magnetic Resonance Imaging*, *(3rd ed)*. New York: Elsevier Press; 2006, with permission)

hyperenhancement in one or both junctions of the interventricular septum and RV free wall is highly suggestive of hypertrophic cardiomyopathy, whereas midwall or epicardial hyperenhancement in the inferolateral wall is consistent with Anderson-Fabry Disease. Moreover, instead of there being an infinite variety of hyperenhancement patterns, it appears that a broad stratification is possible into a limited number of common delayed-enhancement phenotypes. Figure 3.14 illustrates potential hyperenhancement patterns that may be encountered in clinical practice along with a partial list of their differential diagnoses.

References

1. Kim RJ, Fieno DS, Parrish TB, et al. Relationship of MRI delayed contrast enhancement to irreversible injury, infarct age, and contractile function. Circulation. 1999;100(19):1992–2002.

2. Wu E, Judd RM, Vargas J, Klocke FJ, Bonow RO, Kim RJ. Visualization of presence, location, and transmural extent of healed Q-wave and non-Q-wave myocardial infarction. Lancet. 2001;357: 21–28.
3. Wagner A, Mahrholdt H, Thomson L, Hager S, Meinhardt G, Rehwald W, Parker M, Shah D, Sechtem U, Kim RJ, Judd RM. Effects of time, dose and inversion time for acute myocardial infarct size measurements based on magnetic resonance imaging—delayed contrast enhancement. J Am Coll Cardiol. 2006;47:2027–2033.
4. Wagner A, Mahrholdt H, Holly TA, et al. Contrast-enhanced MRI and routine single photon emission computed tomography (SPECT) perfusion imaging for detection of subendocardial myocardial infarcts: an imaging study. Lancet. 2003;361(9355):374–379.
5. Choi KM, Kim RJ, Gubernikoff G, Vargas JD, Parker M, Judd RM. Transmural extent of acute myocardial infarction predicts long-term improvement in contractile function. Circulation. 2001;104(10): 1101–1107.
6. Beek AM, Kuhl HP, Bondarenko O, et al. Delayed contrast-enhanced magnetic resonance imaging for the prediction of regional functional improvement after acute myocardial infarction. J Am Coll Cardiol. 2003;42(5):895–901.
7. Kim RJ, Wu E, Rafael A, et al. The use of contrast-enhanced magnetic resonance imaging to identify reversible myocardial dysfunction. N Engl J Med. 2000;343(20):1445–1453.
8. Schvartzman, PR, Srichai MB, Grimm RA, et al. Nonstress delayed-enhancement magnetic resonance imaging of the myocardium predicts improvement of function after revascularization for chronic ischemic heart disease with left ventricular dysfunction. Am Heart J. 2003;146:535–41.
9. Kim RJ, Manning WJ. Viability assessment by delayed enhancement CMR: will low-dose dobutamine dull the shine? Circulation. 2004;109:2476–2479.
10. Albert TS, Kim RJ, Judd RM. Assessment of no-reflow regions using cardiac MRI. Basic Res Cardiol. 2006;101(5):383–390.
11. Wu KC, Zerhouni EA, Judd RM, et al. Prognostic significance of microvascular obstruction by magnetic resonance imaging in patients with acute myocardial infarction. Circulation. 1998;97(8):765–772.
12. Gerber BL, Rochitte CE, Melin JA, et al. Microvascular obstruction and left ventricular remodeling early after acute myocardial infarction. Circulation. 2000;101(23):2734–2741.
13. Gerber BL, Garot J, Bluemke DA, Wu KC, Lima JA. Accuracy of contrast-enhanced magnetic resonance imaging in predicting improvement of regional myocardial function in patients after acute myocardial infarction. Circulation. 2002;106(9):1083–1089.
14. Lund GK, Stork A, Saeed M, et al. Acute myocardial infarction: evaluation with first-pass enhancement and delayed enhancement MR imaging compared with 201Tl SPECT imaging. Radiology. 2004;232(1):49–57.
15. Alfayoumi F, Srinivasan V, Geller M, Gradman A. The no-reflow phenomenon: epidemiology, pathophysiology, and therapeutic approach. Rev Cardiovasc Med. 2005;6(2):72–83.
16. Abdel-Aty H, Zagrosek A, Schulz-Menger J, et al. Delayed enhancement and T2-weighted cardiovascular magnetic resonance imaging differentiate acute from chronic myocardial infarction. Circulation. 2004;109(20):2411–2416.
17. Stork A, Muellerleile K, Bansmann PM, et al. Value of T2-weighted, first-pass and delayed enhancement, and cine CMR to differentiate between acute and chronic myocardial infarction. Eur Radiol. 2007;17(3):610–617.
18. Aletras AH, Tilak GS, Natanzon A, et al. Retrospective determination of the area at risk for reperfused acute myocardial infarction with T2-weighted cardiac magnetic resonance imaging: histopathological and displacement encoding with stimulated echoes (DENSE) functional validations. Circulation. 2006;113(15):1865–1870.
19. Kim HW, Klem I, Kim RJ. Detection of myocardial ischemia by stress perfusion cardiovascular magnetic resonance. Cardiol Clin. 2007;25(1):57–70.
20. Klem I, Heitner JF, Shah DJ, et al. Improved detection of coronary artery disease by stress perfusion cardiovascular magnetic resonance with the use of delayed enhancement infarction imaging. J Am Coll Cardiol. 2006;47(8):1630–1638.
21. Kim WY, Danias PG, Stuber M, et al. Coronary magnetic resonance angiography for the detection of coronary stenoses. N Engl J Med. 2001;345:1863–1869.
22. Manning WJ, Nezafat R, Appelbaum E, Danias PG, Hauser TH, Yeon SB. Cardiol Clin. 2007;25(1): 141–170.
23. Hendel RC, Patel MR, Kramer CM, et al. ACCF/ACR/SCCT/SCMR/ASNC/NASCI/SCAI/SIR 2006 appropriateness criteria for cardiac computed tomography and cardiac magnetic resonance imaging: a report of the American College of Cardiology Foundation Quality Strategic Directions Committee Appropriateness Criteria Working Group. J Am Coll Cardiol. 2006;48:1475–1497.
24. Weber OM, Martin AJ, Higgins CB. Whole-heart steady-state free precession coronary artery magnetic resonance angiography. Magn Reson Med. 2003;50(6):1223–1228.

25. Sakuma H, Ichikawa Y, Suzawa N, et al. Assessment of coronary arteries with total study time of less than 30 minutes using whole-heart coronary MR angiography. Radiology. 2005;237(1):316:321.
26. Hackenbroch M, Nehrke K, Gieseke J, Meyer C, Tiemann K, Litt H, Dewald O, Naehle CP, Schild H, Sommer T. 3D motion adapted gating (3D MAG): a new navigator technique for accelerated acquisition of free breathing navigator gated 3D coronary MR-angiography. Eur Radiol. 2005;15:1598–1606.
27. Bellenger NG, Burgess MI, Ray SG, et al. Comparison of left ventricular ejection fraction and volumes in heart failure by echocardiography, radionuclide ventriculography and cardiovascular magnetic resonance; are they interchangeable? Eur Heart J. 2000;21(16):1387–1396.
28. Bellenger NG, Davies LC, Francis JM, Coats AJ, Pennell DJ. Reduction in sample size for studies of remodeling in heart failure by the use of cardiovascular magnetic resonance. J Cardiovasc Magn Reson. 2000;2(4):271–278.
29. McCrohon JA, Moon JC, Prasad SK, et al. Differentiation of heart failure related to dilated cardiomyopathy and coronary artery disease using gadolinium-enhanced cardiovascular magnetic resonance. Circulation. 2003;108(1):54–59.
30. Soriano CJ, Ridocci F, Estornell J, Jimenez J, Martinez V, De Velasco JA. Noninvasive diagnosis of coronary artery disease in patients with heart failure and systolic dysfunction of uncertain etiology, using late gadolinium-enhanced cardiovascular magnetic resonance. J Am Coll Cardiol. 2005;45(5):743–748.
31. Srichai MB, Junor C, Rodriguez LL, et al. Clinical, imaging, and pathological characteristics of left ventricular thrombus: a comparison of contrast-enhanced magnetic resonance imaging, transthoracic echocardiography, and transesophageal echocardiography with surgical or pathological validation. Am Heart J. 2006;152(1):75–84.
32. Barkhausen J, Hunold P, Eggebrecht H, et al. Detection and characterization of intracardiac thrombi on MR imaging. AJR Am J Roentgenol. 2002;179(6):1539–1544.
33. Rickers C, Wilke NM, Jerosch-Herold M, et al. Utility of cardiac magnetic resonance imaging in the diagnosis of hypertrophic cardiomyopathy. Circulation. 2005;112:855–861.
34. Choudhury L, Mahrholdt H, Wagner A, et al. Myocardial scarring in asymptomatic or mildly symptomatic patients with hypertrophic cardiomyopathy. J Am Coll Cardiol. 2002;40(12):2156–2164.
35. Amano Y, Takayama M, Takahama K, Kumazaki T. Delayed hyper-enhancement of myocardium in hypertrophic cardiomyopathy with asymmetrical septal hypertrophy: comparison with global and regional cardiac MR imaging appearances. J Magn Reson Imaging. 2004;20(4):595–600.
36. Teraoka K, Hirano M, Ookubo H, et al. Delayed contrast enhancement of MRI in hypertrophic cardiomyopathy. Magn Reson Imaging. 2004;22(2):155–161.
37. Bogaert J, Goldstein M, Tannouri F, Golzarian J, Dymarkowski S. Original report. Late myocardial enhancement in hypertrophic cardiomyopathy with contrast-enhanced MR imaging. AJR Am J Roentgenol. 2003;180(4):981–985.
38. Moon JC, McKenna WJ, McCrohon JA, Elliott PM, Smith GC, Pennell DJ. Toward clinical risk assessment in hypertrophic cardiomyopathy with gadolinium cardiovascular magnetic resonance. J Am Coll Cardiol. 2003;41(9):1561–1567.
39. Whybra C, Kampmann C, Willers I, et al. Anderson-Fabry disease: clinical manifestations of disease in female heterozygotes. J Inherit Metab Dis. Dec 2001;24(7):715–724.
40. Sachdev B, Takenaka T, Teraguchi H, et al. Prevalence of Anderson-Fabry disease in male patients with late onset hypertrophic cardiomyopathy. Circulation. Mar 26 2002;105(12):1407–1411.
41. Moon JC, Sheppard M, Reed E, Lee P, Elliott PM, Pennell DJ. The histological basis of late gadolinium enhancement cardiovascular magnetic resonance in a patient with Anderson-Fabry disease. J Cardiovasc Magn Reson. 2006;8(3):479–482.
42. Moon JC, Sachdev B, Elkington AG, et al. Gadolinium enhanced cardiovascular magnetic resonance in Anderson-Fabry disease. Evidence for a disease specific abnormality of the myocardial interstitium. Eur Heart J. 2003;24(23):2151–2155.
43. Mignani R, Cagnoli L. Enzyme replacement therapy in Fabry's disease: recent advances and clinical applications. J Nephrol. 2004;17(3):354–363.
44. Kwong RY, Falk RH. Cardiovascular magnetic resonance in cardiac amyloidosis. Circulation. 2005;111(2):122–124.
45. vanden Driesen RI, Slaughter RE, Strugnell WE. MR findings in cardiac amyloidosis. AJR Am J Roentgenol. 2006;186(6):1682–1685.
46. Maceira AM, Joshi J, Prasad SK, et al. Cardiovascular magnetic resonance in cardiac amyloidosis. Circulation. 2005;111(2):186–193.
47. Celletti F, Fattori R, Napoli G, et al. Assessment of restrictive cardiomyopathy of amyloid or idiopathic etiology by magnetic resonance imaging. Am J Cardiol. 1999;83(5):798–801, A710.
48. Fattori R, Rocchi G, Celletti F, Bertaccini P, Rapezzi C, Gavelli G. Contribution of magnetic resonance imaging in the differential diagnosis of cardiac amyloidosis

and symmetric hypertrophic cardiomyopathy. Am Heart J. 1998;136(5):824–830.

49. Fletcher A, Ho SY, McCarthy KP, Sheppard MN. Spectrum of pathological changes in both ventricles of patients dying suddenly with arrhythmogenic right ventricular dysplasia. Relation of changes to age. Histopathology. 2006;48(4):445–452.
50. Sen-Chowdhry S, Syrris P, Ward D, Asimaki A, Sevdalis E, McKenna WJ. Clinical and genetic characterization of families with arrhythmogenic right ventricular dysplasia/cardiomyopathy provides novel insights into patterns of disease expression. Circulation. 2007;115(13):1710–1720.
51. Bomma C, Rutberg J, Tandri H, et al. Misdiagnosis of arrhythmogenic right ventricular dysplasia/cardiomyopathy. J Cardiovasc Electrophysiol. 2004;15(3):300–306.
52. Sen-Chowdhry S, Prasad SK, Syrris P, et al. Cardiovascular magnetic resonance in arrhythmogenic right ventricular cardiomyopathy revisited: comparison with task force criteria and genotype. J Am Coll Cardiol. 2006;48(10):2132–2140.
53. Tandri H, Castillo E, Ferrari VA, et al. Magnetic resonance imaging of arrhythmogenic right ventricular dysplasia: sensitivity, specificity, and observer variability of fat detection versus functional analysis of the right ventricle. J Am Coll Cardiol. 2006;48(11):2277–2284.
54. Tandri H, Saranathan M, Rodriguez ER, et al. Noninvasive detection of myocardial fibrosis in arrhythmogenic right ventricular cardiomyopathy using delayed-enhancement magnetic resonance imaging. J Am Coll Cardiol. 2005;45(1):98–103.
55. Smedema JP, Snoep G, van Kroonenburgh MP, et al. The additional value of gadolinium-enhanced MRI to standard assessment for cardiac involvement in patients with pulmonary sarcoidosis. Chest. 2005;128(3):1629–1637.
56. Tadamura E, Yamamuro M, Kubo S, et al. Effectiveness of delayed enhanced MRI for identification of cardiac sarcoidosis: comparison with radionuclide imaging. AJR Am J Roentgenol. 2005;185(1):110–115.
57. Vignaux O. Cardiac sarcoidosis: spectrum of MRI features. AJR Am J Roentgenol. 2005;184(1):249–254.
58. Mahrholdt H, Goedecke C, Wagner A, et al. Cardiovascular magnetic resonance assessment of human myocarditis: a comparison to histology and molecular pathology. Circulation. 2004;109(10):1250–1258.
59. Abdel-Aty H, Boye P, Zagrosek A, et al. Diagnostic performance of cardiovascular magnetic resonance in patients with suspected acute myocarditis: comparison of different approaches. J Am Coll Cardiol. 2005;45(11):1815–1822.
60. Mahrholdt H, Wagner A, Deluigi CC, et al. Presentation, patterns of myocardial damage, and clinical course of viral myocarditis. Circulation. 2006;114(15):1581–1590.
61. Punukollu G, Gowda RM, Khan IA, Navarro VS, Vasavada BC. Clinical aspects of the Chagas' heart disease. Int J Cardiol. 2006.
62. Rochitte CE, Oliveira PF, Andrade JM, et al. Myocardial delayed enhancement by magnetic resonance imaging in patients with Chagas' disease: a marker of disease severity. J Am Coll Cardiol. 2005;46(8):1553–1558.
63. Shah DJ, Kim RJ. Magnetic Resonance of Myocardial Viability. In: Edelman RR, ed. Clinical Magnetic Resonance Imaging. 3rd ed. New York: Elsevier; 2005.
64. Mahrholdt H, Wagner A, Judd RM, et al. Delayed enhancement cardiovascular magnetic resonance assessment of non-ischaemic cardiomyopathies. Eur Heart J. 2005;26:1461–74.
65. Schuster EH, Bulkley BH. Ischemic cardiomyopathy: a clinicopathologic study of fourteen patients. Am Heart J. 1980;100:506–512.
66. Reimer KA, Jennings RB. The "wavefront phenomenon" of myocardial ischemic cell death. II. Transmural progression of necrosis within the framework of ischemic bed size (myocardium at risk) and collateral flow. Laboratory Investigation. 1979;40:633–644.

4
Hemodynamic Assessment and Congenital Heart Disease

Introduction

Cardiac MR is the most accurate non-invasive means to characterize a variety of congenital cardiovascular malformations.[1–3] It also provides accurate hemodynamic measurements to detect and quantify a variety of valvular lesions as well as other lesions producing alterations of flow, such as coarctation of the aorta.[2] Assessment of altered hemodynamics is an integral part of the investigation of most forms of congenital heart disease and thus hemodynamic investigations and congenital heart disease will be considered together in this chapter.

Hemodynamics

Similar to other CMR protocols, hemodynamic assessment may comprise one or several pulse sequences, depending on the physiological parameters that should be appraised. For example, in valvular stenosis, morphologic characteristics (e.g. leaflet structure and mobility) and quantitative measurements, such as aortic valve area, can be directly assessed from the cine CMR images. Signal voids, which result from the dephasing of spins that occur with turbulent flow, can be used to qualitatively assess valvular regurgitation. First-pass perfusion imaging can be used to follow the transit of contrast media to determine the presence of intracardiac shunts in a manner analogous to a bubble study in echocardiography. Velocity-encoded imaging can be used to estimate pressure gradients and blood flow across an orifice.[4, 5]

This chapter first offers a brief comparison between velocity-encoded CMR and Doppler echocardiography will be provided. Then, it discusses a few select pathophysiological conditions as working examples.

Velocity-Encoded CMR versus Doppler Echocardiography

Although velocity-encoded CMR appears analogous to Doppler echocardiography, there are important differences. For instance, an advantage of velocity-encoded CMR is that blood flow through an orifice is directly measured on an en-face image of the orifice with "through-plane" velocity encoding. With echocardiography there are two limitations. First, the blood flow profile is not directly measured but assumed to be flat (i.e. velocity in the center of the orifice is the same as near the edges) so that, hopefully, one sampling velocity would indicate average velocity. Second, the cross-sectional area of the orifice is estimated from a diameter measurement of the orifice at a different time from when Doppler velocity was recorded using a different examination (M-mode or 2D imaging). On the other hand, velocity-encoded CMR has some disadvantages. Perhaps most importantly, velocity-encoded CMR is usually not performed in real time (because of current technical limitations) and requires breathholding to minimize artifacts due to respiratory motion. One consequence is that it is difficult to measure changes in flow that occur with respiration. A comparison of various imaging characteristics between velocity-encoded CMR and Doppler echocardiography is provided in Table 4.1.

TABLE 4.1. Comparsion of velocity-encoded CMR and doppler echocardiography.

Imaging characteristic	Velocity encoding CMR	Doppler echocardiography
Imaging during free breathing	Limited	Yes
Imaging during arrhythmias	Limited	Yes
Temporal resolution	~50 ms*	<10 ms
Peak velocity location	Yes	Location ambiguity (CW Doppler)
Angle dependence	Yes, 20 degrees	Yes, 20 degrees
Imaging planes	Any	Echocardiographic windows
Blood flow profile	Directly measured	Flat profile assumed
Flow quantification	En face	In-plane†

*Given temporal resolution is for breathhold imaging. Temporal resolution may be significantly improved for non-breathhold imaging, but artifacts due to respiratory motion artifact may be prominent.

†Conduit cross-sectional area is estimated from diameter measurement.

From Kim et al: Magnetic Resonance Imaging of the Heart. In Fuster V, O'Rourke, RA (eds). *Hurst's The Heart (12th ed.)*. New York: McGraw-Hill Medical, In Press.

Aortic Stenosis

Several validation studies have demonstrated good agreement of aortic valve area by planimetry on cine CMR images with measures derived using transesophageal and transthoracic echocardiography, and invasive hemodynamic measurements during cardiac catheterization.[6,7] Additionally, peak velocity measurements by velocity-encoded CMR appear to correlate well with Doppler echocardiography.[8,9] For both cine and velocity-encoded CMR, it is important to image in the correct short-axis plane across the leaflet tips. The correct plane is determined by first, obtaining at least 2 orthogonal long-axis views of the high velocity jet across the valve (by either cine or velocity-encoded CMR). Then, the short-axis plane is placed at the origin of the jet, and the plane is positioned to be orthogonal to the direction of the jet on all the long-axis views. Importantly, a stack of consecutive, parallel short-axis images (at least 3) is obtained in order to make sure that the plane with the highest peak velocity and the smallest peak systolic opening is not missed. Planimetry for valve area is performed on cine images with higher spatial and temporal resolution than usual for standard imaging. A small field-of-view image with high spatial resolution can be obtained with extensive oversampling in the phase encoding direction to prevent wraparound artifact (Figure 4.1) Planimetry on velocity-encoded images is not recommended as this usually leads to overestimation of valve area. Pulmonic and mitral valve stenosis is evaluated using a similar approach (Cases 20 and 43).

Regurgitant Valvular Lesions

Valvular regurgitation can be evaluated both qualitatively and quantitatively using cine CMR and velocity-encoded flow imaging. On cine CMR, regurgitant flow is visualized as a region of spin dephasing and resultant signal loss extending from the valve plane into the cavity into which the jet is directed (Case 13). An estimate of the size and extent of the signal loss can be performed by

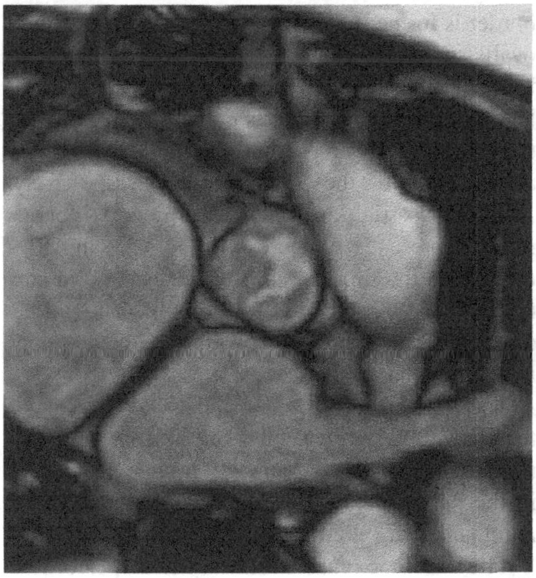

FIGURE 4.1. Still-frame during systole from an SSFP cine loop of an aortic valve demonstrating partial fusion of the cusps. A small field-of-view with extensive over-sampling in the phase encoding direction to prevent wraparound artifact was utilized to provide high spatial resolution. Note that planimetry of the valve can be readily performed

visual evaluation, and along with an evaluation of chamber sizes and other parameters such as cessation of antegrade flow in the pulmonary veins in the instance of mitral regurgitation, one can get an estimate of the severity of regurgitation.

For quantitative assessment of regurgitation, the regurgitation fraction may be calculated from data derived from velocity-encoded imaging, sometimes in combination with cine CMR.[5] For example, in the setting of pulmonic insufficiency, where flow is generally not turbulent, both stroke-volume and regurgitant volume can be directly measured from a single through-plane velocity-encoded acquisition of the valve in cross-section, and thus regurgitant fraction calculated (Figure 4.2).

However, with regurgitant lesions that result in more turbulent flow such as mitral or aortic regurgitation, the calculation of regurgitant volume and regurgitant fraction can be more complex.[10] This is related to the dephasing of spins that occurs in regions of turbulent flow, resulting in signal loss in the velocity-encoded images, which results in inaccurate data measurements. These errors typically result in an underestimation of the regurgitant

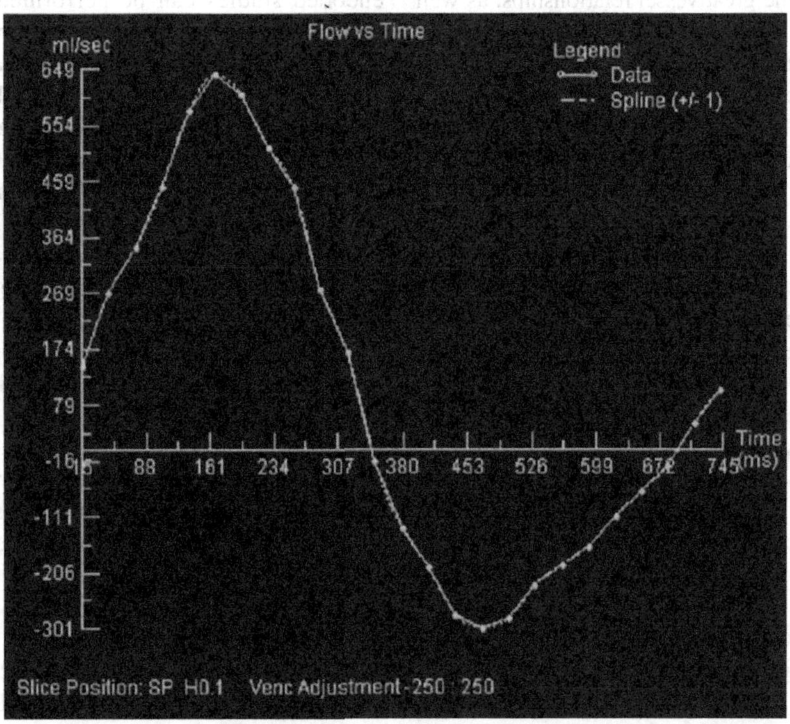

FIGURE 4.2. Velocity-encoded flow data obtained from a through-plane study of an incompetent pulmonic valve. The regurgitant fraction is calculated at 30%

volume. Therefore, to obtain the most accurate measurements, the regurgitant volume is measured indirectly for both mitral and aortic regurgitation. For example, with aortic regurgitation, the regurgitant volume may be calculated by subtracting the effective forward flow (antegrade – retrograde) through the pulmonic valve from the antegrade flow through the aortic valve using two separate through-plane velocity-encoded acquisitions. For mitral regurgitation, the regurgitant volume may be obtained by subtracting systolic flow through the aortic valve measured by velocity-encoded CMR from LV stroke volume measured by volumetric quantification of a stack of cine CMR images. For all velocity-encoded acquisitions, TE should be minimized to reduce dephasing and signal loss.

Congenital Heart Disease

Because of its capacity for multiplanar imaging, and the ability to comprehensively survey the heart and great vessels, MR imaging is quite helpful in the evaluation of known or suspected congenital heart disease. Standard morphologic imaging allows assessment of the great vessel relationships, as well as cardiac and abdominal situs. Cine imaging demonstrates global and regional cardiac structure and function. Velocity-encoded imaging allows quantitation of flow through the great vessels as well as through areas of possible stenosis.[11] Flow can also be calculated through surgically created shunts.

MR angiographic imaging is used to evaluate for the possibility of anomalous vessels, the structure and relationships of the great vessels, and the presence of collaterals. A brief discussion of specific defects follows. Suggested imaging protocols are described in the appendix.

Atrial Septal Defect

This refers to a group of disorders wherein there is abnormal communication between the atrial chambers. The most common form (~60%) is termed the secundum defect, which actually occur in the fossa ovalis formed by the primum septum. These may, however, extend beyond the fossa ovalis to involve a variable portion of the septum. The ostium primum ASD (~20%) is part of the atrioventricular septal defect complex. Its superior border is formed by the inferior border of the fossa ovalis and its inferior border is formed by the leaflets of the malformed atrioventricular valve. The less common sinus venosus defects (15%) involve the upper or lower portions of the atrial septum at the entry of the SVC and IVC respectively. Although partial anomalous pulmonary venous return is present with increased frequency in ASDs in general, the superior sinus venosus ASD in particular has a frequent association with anomalous drainage, particularly involving the right upper lobe pulmonary vein.

The left to right shunt occurring as a result of the atrial septal defect will result in right atrial and right ventricular enlargement. Increased volume in the pulmonary circuit may result in prominent main and hilar pulmonary arteries.

The CMR examination is often performed prior to anticipated closure of the defect, which currently is often performed using endovascular catheter techniques. A stack of four-chamber cine images as well as extension of the short-axis acquisitions through the interatrial septum will often allow depiction of secundum atrial septal defects, particularly if large. Velocity-encoded studies can be performed through the origins of the great vessels to allow calculation of the Qp/Qs ratio.[12] Through-plane velocity-encoded flow studies are particularly helpful. These can be performed to directly quantify transdefect flow and to visualize the morphology of the defect "en face" (Figure 4.3) (Case 139). The imaging plane is roughly parallel to the interatrial septum, but should be optimized to account for cardiac cycle interatrial septal motion and ASD flow direction. This en face view also provides excellent depiction of the anteroposterior and craniocaudal dimensions of the septal defect.[13]

MR angiographic data sets are obtained to evaluate for partial anomalous pulmonary venous return, which may be associated with atrial septal defects, particularly of the sinus venosus type.[14]

Ventricular Septal Defect

These lesions represent the most common form of left to right shunt, and are due to a deficiency of the septum between the ventricular chambers. They often arise as part of more complex congenital

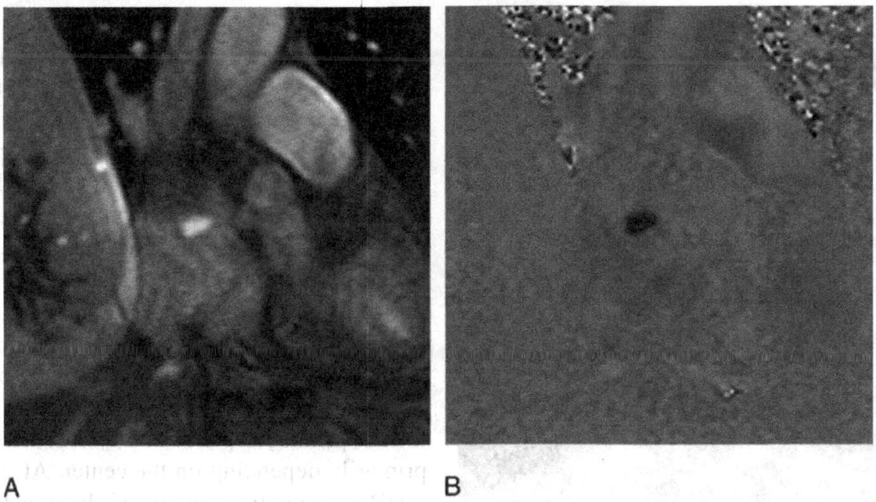

FIGURE 4.3. Morphology of a secundum atrial septal defect is visualized "en face" on a through-plane velocity-encoded acquisition resulting in magnitude (**A**) and phase (**B**) views of the defect

lesions. Small defects are known to undergo spontaneous closure, while large defects carry the risk of developing irreversible pulmonary hypertension. Morphologically, multiple forms exist and are classified by location (inlet, muscular, perimembranous, etc.) The defect itself can often be visualized on the cine images (Case 132). As in the case in an ASD, through-plane flow studies of the proximal great vessels can be obtained in order to calculate the Qp/Qs ratio. In cases where pulmonary hypertension has supervened, evaluation of the degree of abnormal interventricular septal curvature can often provide indirect evidence of pulmonary arterial hypertension.[15, 16]

Tetralogy of Fallot

This disorder is the most common cyanotic congenital defect, and is comprised of four findings: pulmonic stenosis (which may be valvular and/or subvalvular), ventricular septal defect (typically conoventricular in type), overriding of the aorta (that is, the aorta straddles the ventricular septum or extends across it), and right ventricular hypertrophy (which ensues from the outflow tract obstruction). All of these findings are related to the abnormal embryologic formation of the conal septum, which results in hypoplasia of the pulmonary infundibulum with over-riding of the aorta and a malalignment VSD. The surgical repair is directed to closure of the VSD and relief of the pulmonary outflow tract obstruction using an infundibular or transannular patch repair.

Most cases come to imaging after prior surgical repair in early childhood. Since these patients are at risk for postoperative pulmonic insufficiency or residual pulmonic stenosis, detailed evaluation of the right ventricular outflow tract and pulmonary valve is mandatory.[3] Right ventricular function is also of clinical importance and can be evaluated using cine imaging.[17] Recent studies have indicated that delayed-enhancement imaging of the right ventricular outflow tract can provide important prognostic information (Figure 4.4) (Case 30).[18] MR angiographic imaging can evaluate for coexisting pulmonary arterial abnormalities. Velocity-encoded imaging can be performed through the great vessels for calculation of any residual shunt. Additionally, given the frequent late presentation of aortic insufficiency, detailed evaluation of the aortic valve should also be performed.[19]

Coarctation of the Aorta

This disorder refers to a focal constriction of the proximal descending aorta just distal to the left subclavian artery, and opposite the site of the ductus arteriosus. In fact, aberrant ductal tissue

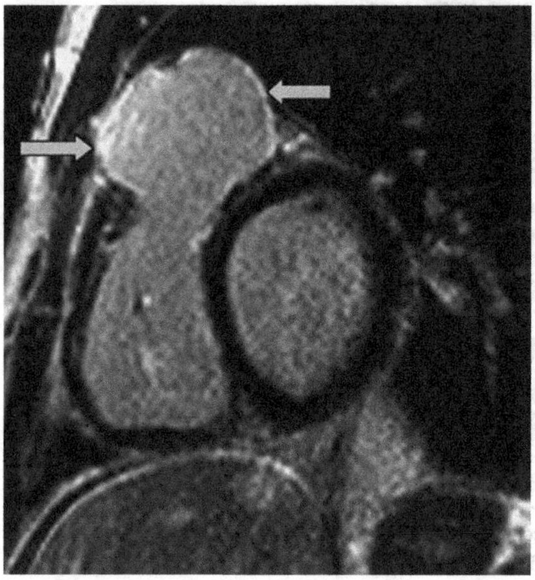

FIGURE 4.4. Delayed-enhancement short-axis view of the RV in a post-op Tetralogy patient demonstrating dilatation and hyperenhancement of the outflow tract (*arrows*)

present in the wall of the coarctation may have a role in its formation. It is often associated with varying degrees of hypoplasia of the transverse aortic arch, and also with bicuspid aortic valve (up to 85% of cases). Severe forms present in infancy while milder forms may not be discovered until adulthood. Upper extremity hypertension and diminished femoral pulses are frequently found in patients presenting in adulthood.

Repair in infancy is most commonly performed surgically, with primary end-to-end anastomosis when feasible. Endovascular repair is often used in cases of recoarctation or residual stenosis following primary repair, but is also sometimes used primarily depending on the center. At the time of CMR examination, many of these patients will have undergone prior surgical or endovascular repair. Late sequelae include the development of aneurysms at the site of the prior repair as well as recurrent coarctation. These findings are well evaluated using MR angiographic and cine imaging through the region of the proximal descending aorta (Figure 4.5) (Case 67).[2, 20, 21]

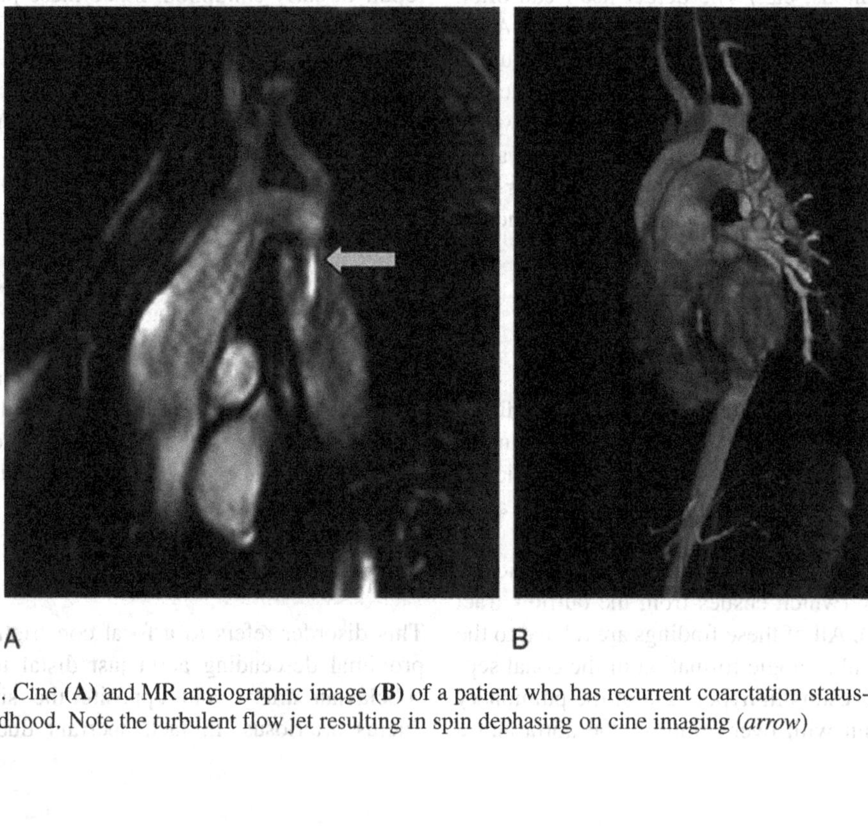

A B

FIGURE 4.5. Cine (**A**) and MR angiographic image (**B**) of a patient who has recurrent coarctation status-post correction in childhood. Note the turbulent flow jet resulting in spin dephasing on cine imaging (*arrow*)

Velocity-encoded imaging can be obtained just proximal to the region of coarctation, at the site of narrowing if present, and in the more distal descending thoracic aorta to evaluate for the presence of residual gradient, and for the detection of collateral flow.[22, 23] Small field-of-view cine imaging of the aortic valve as well as velocity-encoded data may be helpful in cases of associated bicuspid aortic valve.

Transposition of the Great Arteries

This entity is characterized by the presence of ventriculo-arterial discordance; that is, the aorta arises from the morphologic right ventricle and the pulmonary artery from the left ventricle. In the more common D-Loop arrangement, the ventricles are normally positioned and receive inflow in the usual way (RA>RV; LA>LV). As a result, the systemic and pulmonary circuits operate in parallel, instead of in series. Therefore, the patients are cyanotic and will not survive without a "mixing" lesion such as a VSD, ASD or PDA. Definitive repair is performed in infancy and most patients examined with CMR are status-post prior corrective surgery. The current surgical procedure of choice is the arterial switch (Jatene) procedure, but many older patients who were repaired using the atrial switch procedures (Mustard or Senning) are now adults and may present for imaging.[24] In these patients, MR imaging is tremendously helpful.[25] Standard morphologic and cine imaging provide a detailed assessment of the arterial and venous connections. Velocity-encoded information can be obtained through the origins of the great vessels to exclude any residual shunts.[26] MR angiographic imaging can be obtained to evaluate great vessel morphology and to exclude baffle stenosis. In these patients with a systemic right ventricle, cine imaging is helpful for the evaluation of right ventricular function (Case 36).

Other lesions, including complex defects and univentricular repairs using Fontan shunts can also be evaluated non-invasively with CMR (Case 148).

References

1. Valente AM, Powell AJ. Clinical Applications of Cardiovascular Magnetic Resonance in Congenital Heart Disease. Cardiol Clin. 2007;25(1):97–110.
2. Weber OM, Higgins CB. MR evaluation of cardiovascular physiology in congenital heart disease: flow and function. J Cardiovasc Magn Reson. 2006;8(4):607–617.
3. Dorfman AL, Geva T. Magnetic resonance imaging evaluation of congenital heart disease: conotruncal anomalies. J Cardiovasc Magn Reson. 2006;8(4):645–659.
4. Lotz J, Meier C, Leppert A, Galanski M. Cardiovascular flow measurement with phase-contrast MR imaging: basic facts and implementation. Radiographics. 2002;22(3):651–671.
5. Glockner JF, Johnston DL, McGee KP. Evaluation of cardiac valvular disease with MR imaging: qualitative and quantitative techniques. Radiographics. 2003;23(1):e9.
6. John AS, Dill T, Brandt RR, et al. Magnetic resonance to assess the aortic valve area in aortic stenosis: how does it compare to current diagnostic standards? J Am Coll Cardiol. 2003;42(3):519–526.
7. Kupfahl C, Honold M, Meinhardt G, et al. Evaluation of aortic stenosis by cardiovascular magnetic resonance imaging: comparison with established routine clinical techniques. Heart. 2004;90(8):893–901.
8. Kilner PJ, Manzara CC, Mohiaddin RH, et al. Magnetic resonance jet velocity mapping in mitral and aortic valve stenosis. Circulation.1993;87:1239–1248.
9. Caruthers SD, Lin SJ, Brown P, et al. Practical value of cardiac magnetic resonance imaging for clinical quantification of aortic valve stenosis: comparison with echocardiography. Circulation. 2003;108:2236–2243.
10. Nayak KS, Hu BS, Nishimura DG. Rapid quantitation of high-speed flow jets. Magn Reson Med. 2003;50(2):366–372.
11. Petersen SE, Voigtlander T, Kreitner KF, et al. Quantification of shunt volumes in congenital heart diseases using a breath-hold MR phase contrast technique–comparison with oximetry. Int J Cardiovasc Imaging. 2002;18(1):53–60.
12. Powell AJ, Tsai-Goodman B, Prakash A, Greil GF, Geva T. Comparison between phase-velocity cine magnetic resonance imaging and invasive oximetry for quantification of atrial shunts. Am J Cardiol. 2003;91(12):1523–1525, A1529.
13. Piaw CS, Kiam OT, Rapaee A, et al. Use of non-invasive phase contrast magnetic resonance imaging for estimation of atrial septal defect size and morphology: a comparison with transesophageal echo. Cardiovasc Intervent Radiol. 2006;29(2):230–234.
14. Valente AM, Sena L, Powell AJ, Del Nido PJ, Geva T. Cardiac magnetic resonance imaging evaluation of sinus venosus defects: comparison to surgical findings. Pediatr Cardiol. 2007;28(1):51–56.
15. Roeleveld RJ, Marcus JT, Faes TJ, et al. Interventricular septal configuration at mr imaging

and pulmonary arterial pressure in pulmonary hypertension. Radiology. 2005;234(3):710–717.
16. Dellegrottaglie S, Sanz J, Poon M, et al. Pulmonary hypertension: accuracy of detection with left ventricular septal-to-free wall curvature ratio measured at cardiac MR. Radiology. 2007;243(1):63–69.
17. Knauth AL, Gauvreau K, Powell AJ, et al. Ventricular Size and Function Assessed by Cardiac MRI Predict Major Adverse Clinical Outcomes Late After Tetralogy of Fallot Repair. Heart. Nov. 29 2006.
18. Oosterhof T, Mulder BJ, Vliegen HW, de Roos A. Corrected tetralogy of Fallot: delayed enhancement in right ventricular outflow tract. Radiology. 2005;237(3):868–871.
19. Niwa K. Aortic root dilatation in tetralogy of Fallot long-term after repair-histology of the aorta in tetralogy of Fallot: evidence of intrinsic aortopathy. Int J Cardiol. 2005;103(2):117–119.
20. Soler R, Rodriguez E, Requejo I, Fernandez R, Raposo I. Magnetic resonance imaging of congenital abnormalities of the thoracic aorta. Eur Radiol. 1998;8(4):540–546.
21. Wald RM, Powell AJ. Simple congenital heart lesions. J Cardiovasc Magn Reson. 2006;8(4):619–631.
22. Nielsen JC, Powell AJ, Gauvreau K, Marcus EN, Prakash A, Geva T. Magnetic resonance imaging predictors of coarctation severity. Circulation. 2005;111(5):622–628.
23. Araoz PA, Reddy GP, Tarnoff H, Roge CL, Higgins CB. MR findings of collateral circulation are more accurate measures of hemodynamic significance than arm-leg blood pressure gradient after repair of coarctation of the aorta. J Magn Reson Imaging. 2003;17(2): 177–183.
24. Warnes CA. Transposition of the great arteries. Circulation. 2006;114(24):2699–2709.
25. Laffon E, Latrabe V, Jimenez M, Ducassou D, Laurent F, Marthan R. Quantitative MRI comparison of pulmonary hemodynamics in mustard/senning-repaired patients suffering from transposition of the great arteries and healthy volunteers at rest. Eur Radiol. 2005:1–7.
26. Yoo SJ, Kim YM, Choe YH. Magnetic resonance imaging of complex congenital heart disease. Int J Card Imaging. 1999;15(2):151–160.

5 Pericardial Disease and Cardiac Masses

Introduction

For a variety of reasons, CMR is the reference standard for comprehensive imaging of pericardial disease and cardiac masses. CMR provides direct multiplanar imaging without the need for reconstructions, and in any freely selectable imaging plane. There are no limitations regarding acoustic windows. No radiation is required, and no nephrotoxic contrast media administered. Gadolinium is frequently administered, but is widely regarded as significantly safer than iodinated contrast material. Importantly, MR provides superior tissue characterization relative to both CT and echocardiography.[1,2] A variety of imaging sequences including standard and fast spin-echo T1-weighted, T2-weighted, cine and delayed-enhancement techniques provide a broad palette that the examiner can choose from to localize and characterize a variety of pericardial and cardiac disorders. Fat suppression can be added as needed in order to characterize suspected fatty tumors. Perfusion imaging can be performed for evaluation of tumor vascularity. Finally, CMR using real-time sequences can depict dynamic processes, thereby providing hemodynamic as well as structural information. Therefore, the multisequence, multiplanar capability of CMR makes it the ideal method for the evaluation of pericardial diseases, as well as the evaluation of pericardial and cardiac masses.[3,4] Although pericardial disease and cardiac masses are clearly separate and discrete entities, there are significant similarities in the utility of MR imaging for their diagnosis, as well as overlap in the MR techniques used. Thus, these disorders will be considered together in this chapter.

Technical Notes

A cardiac examination designed for evaluation of cardiac masses or pericardial disease should begin with the standard sequences used in essentially all cardiac MR imaging: initial static morphologic images as well as high resolution cine images of the heart. High-resolution morphologic imaging can be performed with both dark blood and bright blood sequences. Cine imaging through the entire myocardium in the short and long axis planes as routinely performed for cardiac evaluation is appropriate for the imaging of suspected pericardial disease and masses. In addition, newer scanners are able to perform real-time cine imaging, which allows acquisitions during free breathing. These acquisitions utilize single-shot steady state free precession sequences which can be ECG gated or non-gated. Real-time cine imaging is especially helpful for the evaluation of dynamic processes.[5]

Perfusion sequences are used to evaluate the vascularity of a lesion and can be obtained in multiple imaging planes with one injection. These are heavily T1-weighted sequences that can be helpful in identifying hypervascular tumors or in differentiating avascular thrombi from neoplasms.[6]

The delayed-enhancement sequences that are used for the detection of myocardial infarction are also used for the evaluation of neoplasms, which typically demonstrate hyperenhancement.[3, 7, 8] In addition, single-shot delayed-enhancement imaging using an inversion recovery SSFP sequence can provide similar information in a fraction of the time. It is often helpful to perform these sequences with a long inversion time (~600 ms) if thrombus is suspected, as will be described.

Pericardial Disease

Both loculated and circumferential pericardial effusions are readily identified by CMR. Simple (transudate) effusions typically appear bright and homogenous on T2-weighted images and dark on T1-weighted images. On SSFP cine imaging, which exhibits T2/T1 weighing, simple effusions appear bright with the same or even higher image intensity than epicardial fat (Figure 5.1) Complex effusions may appear heterogeneous and darker on T2 and SSFP imaging, and may indicate the presence of coexisting hemorrhage or inflammation. Additionally, unlike simple effusions, complex effusions may demonstrate increased image intensity on T1-weighted imaging after administration of gadolinium contrast. The ability of CMR to provide global three-dimensional imaging allows a comprehensive assessment of the volume of pericardial fluid present. {Case 109}

A common indication for CMR is the evaluation of possible constrictive pericarditis. In this disorder, circumferential or focal pericardial thickening is present, with resultant impairment of ventricular diastolic filling (Figure 5.2) (Case 59). Most of the literature regarding the evaluation of the pericardium has focused on morphological characterization using older spin echo (SE) sequences. Using these sequences, pericardial thicknesses of >4 mm were considered abnormal, while thicknesses <2 mm were normal.[9, 10] These thresholds were helpful in

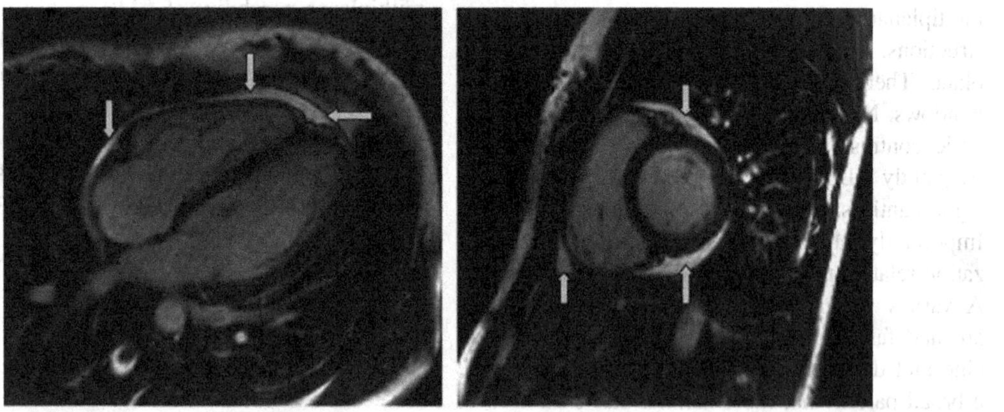

A B

FIGURE 5.1. Four-chamber (**A**) and short-axis (**B**) SSFP cine images demonstrate a small, simple pericardial effusion (*arrows*)

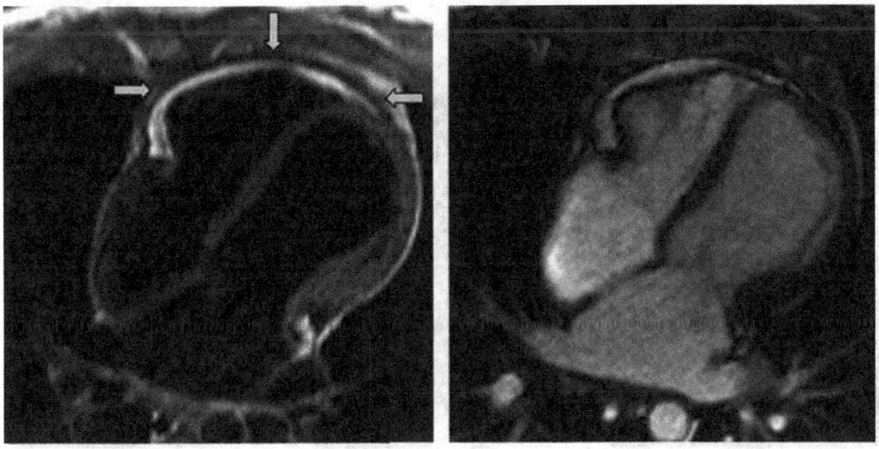

A B

FIGURE 5.2. Constrictive pericarditis. (**A**) T1-weighted gated fast spin-echo image shows extensive pericardial thickening (*arrows*). Cine image (**B**) obtained in early diastole demonstrates abnormal interventricular septal curvature

confirming a diagnosis of constrictive pericarditis, particularly when pericardial thickening was found to be extreme (>5 mm). However, it is important to note the limitations of spin-echo imaging and these threshold values. These older sequences were usually gated to the ECG, but because of long acquisition times (several minutes), imaging was performed during free-breathing. Thus, due to respiratory motion, effective in-plane pixel resolution may have been on the order of ≥4 mm. More recently, with the use of faster sequences with image acquisition during breathholding, in-plane resolution is routinely <2 mm and more subtle pericardial thickening can be appreciated. However, the published literature with regard to normal physiological values does not yet reflect these technical advancements.

Currently, pericardial constriction is best assessed using a combination of fast spin echo (FSE) morphology and SSFP cine imaging (Figure 5.2) The key advantage of FSE over conventional SE sequences is that acquisition time is substantially shorter, allowing an image to be acquired during a single breath. Importantly, however, to minimize motion artifacts and motion-related blurring, imaging should be gated to mid-diastole during relative cardiac standstill (<100 ms in length). SSFP cine imaging is also useful in evaluating the pericardium as it can provide both high spatial resolution and dynamic functional information. In addition to conventional cine imaging, tagged cine and real-time cine imaging may provide supplementary information. With cardiac tagging, discrete tissue points can be tracked throughout the cardiac cycle. This is accomplished using radiofrequency prepulses to label tissue (usually at end-diastole) with a dark grid pattern. Normally, gridlines at the interface between pericardium and epicardium (actually between parietal and visceral pericardium, as the latter is attached to the epicardium) should shear during systole since the two surfaces move independently and slide during contraction. Conversely, in the setting of pericardial adhesions, gridlines at the interface should remain intact, as motion of the two surfaces would be concordant.

Real time cine MRI can be used to demonstrate increased ventricular interdependence, a hemodynamic hallmark of pericardial constriction.[11] Specifically, abnormal ventricular septal motion towards the left ventricle in early diastole is seen during the onset of inspiration (Figure 5.3) (Case 117). Although the number of patients that have been studied is quite small, this finding appears helpful in distinguishing between constrictive pericarditis and restrictive cardiomyopathy.

Cardiac Masses

CMR is widely recognized as the imaging modality of choice in the evaluation of cardiac masses. Invasion into adjacent structures is easily recognized

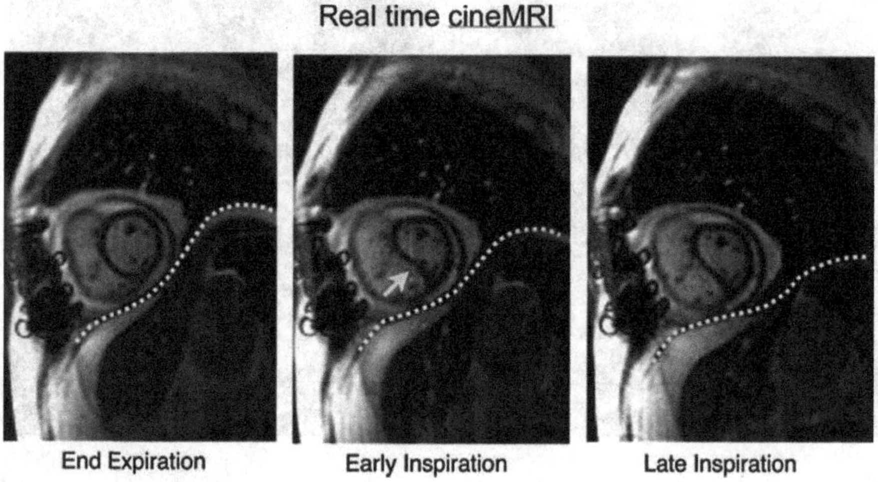

FIGURE 5.3. Real time cine imaging demonstrating septal displacement with inversion evident in response to augmentation of RV filling produced by a deep inspiration. Real time imaging thus demonstrates the abnormal interventricular dependence indicative of pericardial constriction

(Figure 5.4). Precise localization to a specific compartment (intracavitary, intramural, or epicardial) can easily be accomplished, significantly narrowing the differential diagnosis. In addition many normal variants can be mistaken for a cardiac mass, and CMR imaging can provide a definitive evaluation of these pseudomasses.

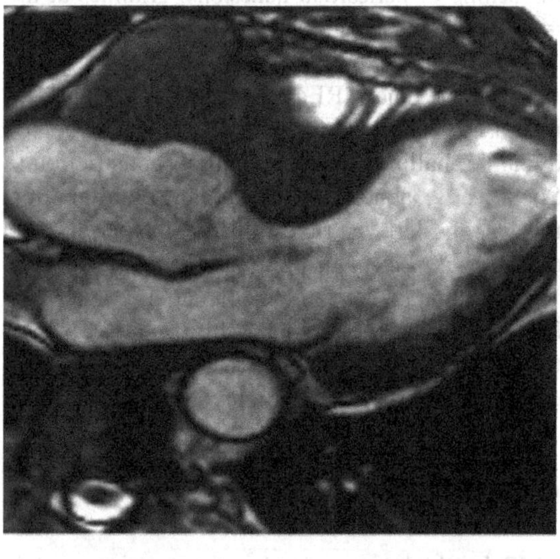

FIGURE 5.4. Still-frame image from a 3-chamber cine demonstrating infiltration of the RV outflow tract and the aortic root by invasive metastatic disease

Thrombus

Left ventricular thrombi represent an important subset of cardiac masses, and typically develop in the setting of myocardial dysfunction and impaired wall motion. Areas of prior infarction with adjacent stagnant cavity blood flow also provide a nidus for thrombus formation. As stated earlier, delayed-enhanced imaging may be one of the most definitive and sensitive means of detecting interventricular thrombi. Studies have demonstrated that delayed-enhancement imaging has at least twofold greater sensitivity for the detection of LV thrombi than echocardiography.[12, 13] Because of their lack of contrast uptake, thrombi demonstrate low signal intensity on inversion recovery delayed-enhancement images obtained with a long inversion time.[14] In our experience, these images are the most sensitive means of detecting ventricular thrombi (Case 11).

Benign Primary Neoplasms

True neoplasms of the heart, whether primary or secondary, are relatively uncommon in clinical practice. Metastatic tumors are 20–40 times more common than primary tumors. Of the primary cardiac tumors, 75% are benign, and at least 50% of these are atrial myxomas.[15–18]

Myxomas demonstrate a female predominance that is as high as 3 to 1 in some series, and closer to 1.5 to 1 in others. The average patient age at presentation is approximately 50, with the majority of cases occurring between the ages of 30 and 60. Myxomas are located in the left atrium in approximately 75% of cases, and are usually attached to the fossa ovalis. Approximately 15 to 20% arise in the right atrium, with a small percentage extending across the fossa ovalis to involve both atria. They are often mobile, and may prolapse through the mitral valve.[19] Myxomas are gelatinous tumors, and may be relatively high in signal on SSFP cine and static images (Figure 5.5) (Case 58). They typically demonstrate heterogeneous enhancement on delayed-enhancement imaging.[20]

Lipomas and lipomatous hypertrophy of the interatrial septum (LHIAS) are often grouped together in series describing cardiac masses, but are pathologically discrete entities. While both will demonstrate signal characteristics consistent with fat, they are histologically quite different. Lipomatous hypertrophy actually refers to a disorder characterized by unencapsulated hyperplasia of adipocytes in the interatrial septum while a lipoma is an encapsulated neoplasm composed of benign adipocytes. By definition, LHIAS involves the interatrial septum and is usually noted to spare the fossa ovalis, resulting in a characteristic "barbell" appearance (Figure 5.6) (Case 129). In contrast, lipomas are often epicardial or intramural.[17]

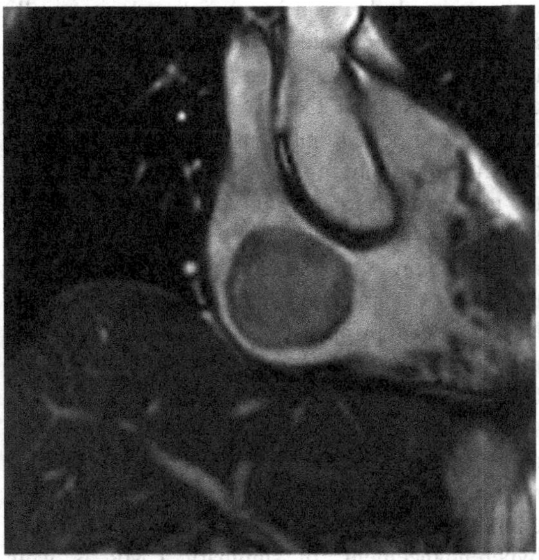

FIGURE 5.5. Right atrial myxoma. Note the relatively high signal intensity on SSFP cine imaging indicative of its gelatinous composition

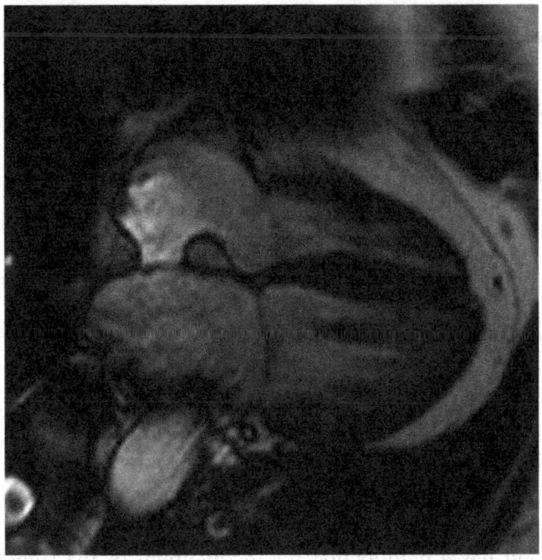

FIGURE 5.6. Lipomatous hypertrophy of the interatrial septum. The "barbell" appearance is due to infiltration of the septum by a hyperplasia of adipocytes with sparing of the fossa ovalis

The most common neoplasms in children include rhabdomyomas and fibromas, both of which are likely actually hamartomas rather than true neoplasms.[17] Both usually present as an intramural mass that distorts the myocardium. Rhabdomyomas are most often seen in infants and children with tuberous sclerosis, may be multiple, and often spontaneously regress. Rhabdomyomas most often involve the septum and are recognized as a focal mass of otherwise normal appearing muscle.

Fibromas are most often diagnosed in childhood, but may also be seen in adults. Approximately one-third of patients present with arrhythmias, one-third with heart failure or cyanosis, and one-third are incidentally detected. On standard dark blood imaging they are recognized as an intramural mass, often protruding into the ventricular cavity as well as distorting the epicardial surface of the heart. They are characterized by the presence of abundant collagen, and typically have low signal intensity on T1- and T2-weighted images.

Malignant Primary Neoplasms

Approximately 25% of primary cardiac neoplasms are malignant. The great majority represents some form of sarcoma, with lymphoma making up most of the remainder. The imaging characteristics of these malignant tumors are fairly similar, with the majority of the lesions demonstrating invasion of surrounding structures and normal myocardium, poor border definition, and frequent coexisting pericardial effusions. Most cannot be distinguished based on imaging characteristics as discrete entities, but findings favoring malignancy can usually be detected.

Angiosarcoma is the most common form of cardiac sarcoma, accounting for approximately 40% of cases, and most series demonstrate a slight male predominance. It is a tumor of endothelial origin, and has a predilection for involvement of the right atrium (Case 145). This location represents a differentiating feature in that most of the other sarcomas have a left atrial predilection (Figure 5.7).[16,17] These tumors infiltrate the myocardium and are usually accompanied by pericardial effusions. Sarcomas often demonstrate areas of internal hemorrhage and necrosis, resulting in complex signal characteristics. They usually demonstrate irregular enhancement on delayed-enhancement imaging.

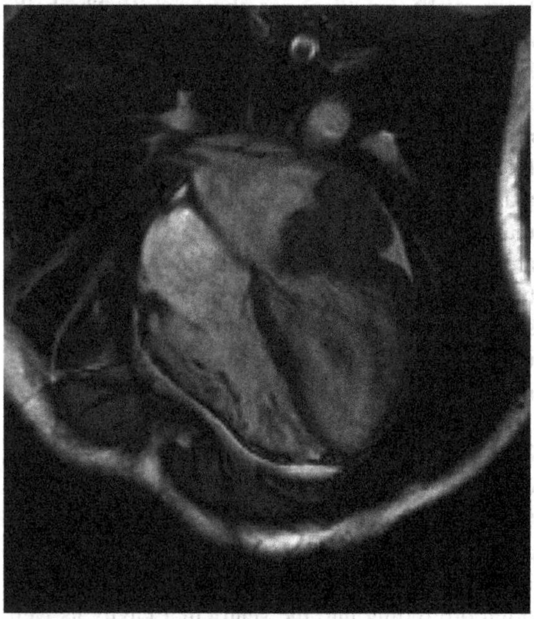

FIGURE 5.7. Osteosarcoma originating in the left atrium. Note the infiltration of the posterior wall of the left atrium and the mitral valve apparatus on this still frame from a cine acquisition

Metastatic Disease

Multiple series have demonstrated that approximately 10 to 12% of patients dying of cancer will demonstrate autopsy evidence of metastatic cardiac or pericardial disease. However, these lesions are rarely the presenting manifestation of the patient's malignancy, and are usually apparent only in the later phases of the patient's illness. Lung and breast carcinoma are common primary sites, but cardiac involvement by leukemia and lymphoma is also common.[21,22]

There are four pathways by which malignancy can reach the heart: direct extension from an adjacent primary tumor, retrograde extension via the lymphatics from adjacent mediastinal lymph node involvement, hematogenous spread, and transvenous extension. Many lesions demonstrate a combination of one or more of these pathways.

Given the variety of mechanisms of involvement, CMR findings of secondary cardiac malignancies span a broad range of possibilities. Pericardial effusion is probably the most common imaging manifestation of metastatic disease, although it may obviously be seen in other disorders as well. However, the presence of nodular implants upon the pericardium should be viewed with a high degree of suspicion. Complex pericardial effusions or loculated pericardial effusions are also suggestive findings. Intramural nodular deposits within the myocardium in an adult with a known primary malignancy would obviously be highly suspicious, and should prompt consideration of those disorders that tend to spread via hematogenous pathways. Metastases often produce extensive infiltration of normal structures, and cine imaging is very helpful for the depiction of altered myocardial and valvular function (Figure 5.8). These myocardial parenchymal lesions may demonstrate evidence of hypervascularity on perfusion imaging. Delayed enhanced imaging will also often demonstrate hyperenhancement. In summary, CMR is well suited to the evaluation and characterization of these secondary neoplasms, as well as determining their mode of spread (Cases 55 and 135).

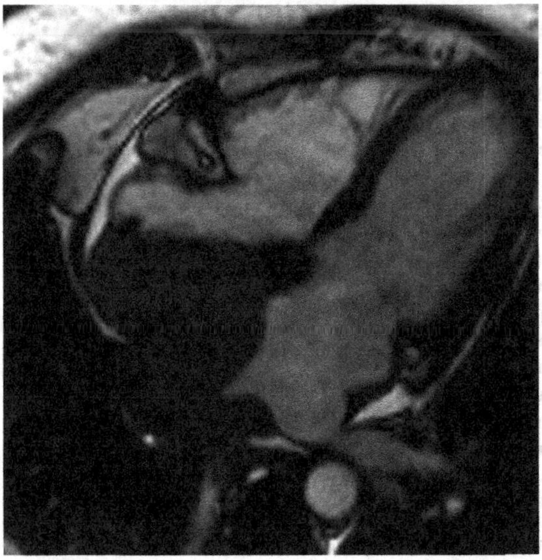

FIGURE 5.8. Still frame from a 4-chamber cine series demonstrating metastatic carcinoid tumor invading the interatrial septum, the posterior walls of both atria, and the pericardium

Differential Diagnosis

In the differential diagnosis of cardiac masses, location is everything. The diagnostic considerations can be significantly simplified if one has accurately localized the lesion. It should be noted that localizing the lesion also means assessing its boundaries, and whether it invades or simply displaces normal structures. Following localization, evaluation of the signal characteristics of the lesion is critically important, as many lesions have nearly pathognomonic features (e.g. tumors composed of fat or fibrous tissue). Finally, the contrast enhancement pattern can be quite helpful; for instance, myxomas and thrombi can have similar location (left atrium) and behavior (mobile), but myxomas demonstrate heterogenous enhancement while thrombi, by virtue of being avascular, have no enhancement. Although exceptions to these guidelines may occur, they represent a conceptual framework that will hopefully provide the reader with a starting point in forming an appropriate differential diagnosis (Table 5.1).

TABLE 5.1. Differential diagnosis of cardiac masses by location.

Location	Lesion	Typical MR imaging features	Specific diagnostic features
Intracavitary	Myxoma	Oval, mobile left atrial lesion, heterogenous enhancement	Attachment to fossa ovalis
	Thrombus	Left atrium/appendage or ventricles at sites of stasis/infarction	Low-signal (dark) on delayed enhancement images with a long inversion time
	Vegetations	Irregular nodules or masses arising along valvular surfaces and perivalvular tissues	Signal intensity similar to thrombus. May have associated septic pulmonary emboli
	Metastases	Transvenous extension of tumor	Lesions extend in continuity from primary lesion to heart
Intramural—Children	Rhabdomyomas	Multiple masses with signal intensity similar to muscle	Infants and children with tuberous sclerosis
	Fibromas	Solitary mass distorting normal anatomy	Low in signal intensity on T2 weighted images
Intramural—Adults	Metastases	Variable –pericardial effusions very common. Typically known late-stage malignancy. Lesions usually enhance	Melanoma metastases may show high signal on T1 weighted images.
	Lipomatous hypertrophy of interatrial septum	Thickening of septum to > 2cm; typically spares fossa ovalis. High signal on T1 weighted images	Signal drop-out on fat-saturation images
	Lipoma	Epicardial/ intramural lesion with high signal on T1 weighted images	Signal drop-out on fat-saturation images

(continued)

TABLE 5.1. (continued)

Location	Lesion	Typical MR imaging features	Specific diagnostic features
	Paraganglioma	Well-defined lesion arising in atrial walls or septum	"Light-bulb bright" on T2 weighted images
Epicardial/ Pericardial	Metastases	Variable, pericardial metastases more common than myocardial. Large pericardial effusions common	Direct tumor extension; extensive adjacent adenopathy very suggestive
	Pericardial cyst	Well-defined non-enhancing lesion contiguous with pericardium	Signal follows fluid on all sequences
	Hemangioma	Multicystic enhancing lesions, may involve epicardium and pericardium	High in signal on T1 and T2
	Lymphangioma	Rare multicystic lesions may be intramural, epicardial, or pericardial	Low in signal on T1 weighted images, high on T2

Source: Reprinted from Cardiology Clinics, Volume 25, Grizzard JD and Ang GB, Magnetic Resonance Imaging of Pericardial disease and Cardiac Masses, pages 111–140, Copyright (2007) with permission from Elsevier.

References

1. Gilkeson RC, Chiles C. MR evaluation of cardiac and pericardial malignancy. Magn Reson Imaging Clin N Am. 2003;11(1):173–186, viii.
2. Gulati G, Sharma S, Kothari SS, Juneja R, Saxena A, Talwar KK. Comparison of echo and MRI in the imaging evaluation of intracardiac masses. Cardiovasc Intervent Radiol. 2004;27(5):459–469.
3. Grizzard JD, Ang GB. Magnetic resonance imaging of pericardial disease and cardiac masses. Cardiol Clin. 2007;25(1):111–140.
4. Hoffmann U, Globits S, Schima W, et al. Usefulness of magnetic resonance imaging of cardiac and paracardiac masses. Am J Cardiol. 2003;92(7):890–895.
5. Kuhl HP, Spuentrup E, Wall A, et al. Assessment of myocardial function with interactive non-breath-hold real-time MR imaging: comparison with echocardiography and breath-hold Cine MR imaging. Radiology. 2004;231(1):198–207.
6. Fuster V, Kim RJ. Frontiers in cardiovascular magnetic resonance. Circulation. 2005;112(1):135–144.
7. Edelman RR. Contrast-enhanced MR imaging of the heart: overview of the literature. Radiology. 2004;232(3):653–668.
8. Luna A, Ribes R, Caro P, Vida J, Erasmus JJ. Evaluation of cardiac tumors with magnetic resonance imaging. Eur Radiol. 2005;15(7):1446–1455.
9. Sechtem U, Tscholakoff D, Higgins CB. MRI of the normal pericardium. AJR Am J Roentgenol. 1986;147(2):239–244.
10. Sechtem U, Tscholakoff D, Higgins CB. MRI of the abnormal pericardium. AJR Am J Roentgenol. 1986;147(2):245–252.
11. Francone M, Dymarkowski S, Kalantzi M, Bogaert J. Real-time cine MRI of ventricular septal motion: a novel approach to assess ventricular coupling. J Magn Reson Imaging. 2005;21(3):305–309.
12. Srichai MB, Junor C, Rodriguez LL, et al. Clinical, imaging, and pathological characteristics of left ventricular thrombus: a comparison of contrast-enhanced magnetic resonance imaging, transthoracic echocardiography, and transesophageal echocardiography with surgical or pathological validation. Am Heart J. 2006;152(1):75–84.
13. Barkhausen J, Hunold P, Eggebrecht H, et al. Detection and characterization of intracardiac thrombi on MR imaging. AJR Am J Roentgenol. 2002;179(6):1539–1544.
14. Shah DJ, Kim RJ. Magnetic Resonance of Myocardial Viability. In: Edelman RR, ed. Clinical Magnetic Resonance Imaging. 3rd ed. New York: Elsevier; 2005.
15. Araoz PA, Mulvagh SL, Tazelaar HD, Julsrud PR, Breen JF. CT and MR imaging of benign primary cardiac neoplasms with echocardiographic correlation. Radiographics. 2000;20(5):1303–1319.
16. Araoz PA, Eklund HE, Welch TJ, Breen JF. CT and MR imaging of primary cardiac malignancies. Radiographics. Dec 1999;19(6):1421–1434.
17. Grebenc ML, Rosado de Christenson ML, Burke AP, Green CE, Galvin JR. Primary cardiac and

pericardial neoplasms: radiologic-pathologic correlation. Radiographics. 2000;20(4):1073–1103; quiz 1110–1071, 1112.
18. Burke A VR. Tumors of the heart and great vessels Washington, DC: Armed Forces Institute of Pathology; 1996.
19. Grebenc ML, Rosado-de-Christenson ML, Green CE, Burke AP, Galvin JR. Cardiac myxoma: imaging features in 83 patients. Radiographics. 2002;22(3):673–689.
20. Fieno DS, Saouaf R, Thomson LE, Abidov A, Friedman JD, Berman DS. Cardiovascular magnetic resonance of primary tumors of the heart: A review. J Cardiovasc Magn Reson. 2006;8(6):839–853.
21. Klatt EC, Heitz DR. Cardiac metastases. Cancer. 1990;65(6):1456–1459.
22. Chiles C, Woodard PK, Gutierrez FR, Link KM. Metastatic involvement of the heart and pericardium: CT and MR imaging. Radiographics. 2001;21(2):439–449.

6
MR Angiography: General Principles

Introduction

Magnetic resonance angiography (MRA) has emerged over the last decade as the modality of choice for non-invasive vascular imaging. Although earlier time-of-flight techniques had significant limitations due to prolonged imaging times and image artifacts, currently available contrast-enhanced MRA is now a rapid and robust technique that consistently allows comprehensive imaging of virtually all vascular territories. Three-dimensional volumetric acquisitions are obtained at each station during the transit of gadolinium through the arterial system, and are subtracted from a preliminary, non-contrast mask image in order to maximize vessel conspicuity. Maximum intensity projection or MIP images are then prepared via post-processing, and are reviewed along with the source images. The acquisition of isotropic voxels (equal size in all 3 dimensions) allows 360 degrees rotation of the images into any obliquity, facilitating easy and accurate interpretation. Figure 6.1 is an example of the coverage and image quality now possible with MRA.

In considering the merits of MR angiography, it may be helpful to consider what might constitute an ideal vascular imaging technique. An ideal technique would be noninvasive, risk-free, fast and easy to acquire, and would not require an arterial puncture. Lack of ionizing radiation would be desirable. It should be painless and applicable to virtually all patients. Given the multifocal and progressive nature of atherosclerotic disease–the primary indication for such imaging–it should have the capability of providing extensive anatomic coverage. It should be easy to perform and interpret as well as cost effective. Three-dimensional rendering capabilities would be valuable. Finally, it should provide an accurate vascular roadmap for endovascular and surgical procedures.

Catheter angiography requires a painful arterial puncture, a four to six-hour convalescence, exposure to iodinated contrast and radiation, and results in a luminographic image. No imaging of the vessel wall is provided. Although accurate, the lack of three-dimensional imaging can be a potential source of error.

CT angiography provides extensive anatomic coverage, and does not require an arterial puncture, but does require ionizing radiation and the administration of iodinated contrast. Given that many patients with peripheral arterial disease also have preexisting renal compromise, this is obviously less than ideal. In addition, the frequent presence of calcification and the need to subtract the adjacent osseous structures often makes image interpretation complex, and may diminish accuracy.

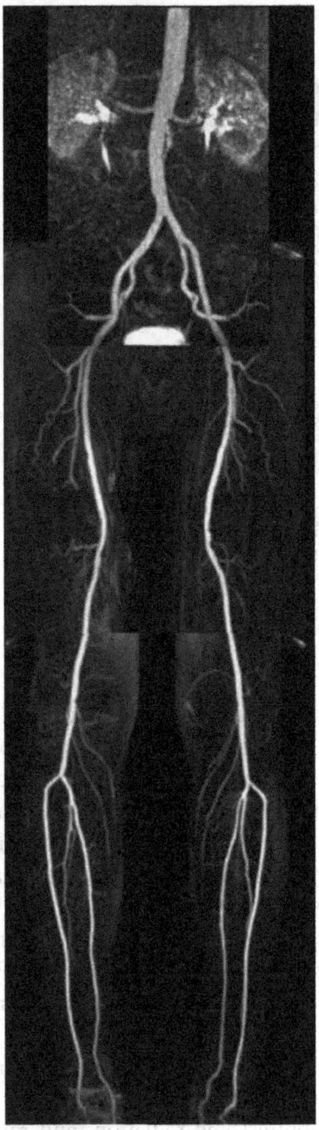

FIGURE 6.1. Normal three station MR runoff angiogram

MR angiography in many important respects fulfills the characteristics of an ideal imaging technique. It requires only venous administration of noniodinated contrast. It is quick and easy to perform, with exams typically requiring less than 30 minutes, and image interpretation is straightforward. Multiplanar displays are easily performed, and 3-D imaging is standard. There is no exposure to radiation or nephrotoxic contrast, but in patients with renal dysfunction, gadolinium use should be considered cautiously since they may be at risk for nephrogenic systemic fibrosis (see Chapter 1). Where available, it has assumed a premier role in performing noninvasive vascular imaging in a variety of vascular territories.[1–4]

Performing an MRA Study

Although the imaging protocols are tailored to the body region being examined, certain aspects of the exam remain constant.

First, localizer images are obtained, in order to determine the course and location of the vessels of interest. These are usually obtained with a series of low-resolution steady state free precession (SSFP) images obtained in the axial, sagittal, and coronal planes. These multiplanar images can be obtained in less than 30 seconds.

Second, dark blood and bright blood sequences are obtained in order to visualize the vessel walls, usually in the axial plane. These are obtained using standard double inversion-recovery dark blood techniques (HASTE), and bright blood SSFP imaging as previously described in Chapter 1. These sequences are typically performed with ECG gating in the thoracic region.

Third, the scan acquisition needs to be synchronized to the intra-arterial passage of an intravenously administered bolus of contrast. Synchronization can be performed with use of a timing bolus or with a bolus triggering technique.

A timing bolus acquisition consists of a series of rapid (typically one per second) T1-weighted image acquisitions obtained through a region of the vessel of interest. Generally, a one cm thick axial GRE acquisition is initiated simultaneously with the injection of 1 to 2 cc of contrast and 25 cc of flush, all administered at 2 cc/sec.[5, 6] The image with maximal opacification (not the first image with contrast) can be determined visually or by using a region of interest (ROI) placed in the vessel of interest. The appropriate time for the initiation of the scan is then calculated using the formula: Scan delay = Circulation time + (the injection duration / 2) – (the scan duration / 2).

For example, an MR angiogram of the abdominal aorta that takes 18 seconds to acquire might be performed using 20 cc of contrast administered at a rate of 2 cc/sec. The injection duration is 10 seconds, and the scan duration is 18 seconds. The circulation time obtained from visual evaluation of the images of a small test bolus is 19 seconds. Therefore, 19 + 5 − 9 equals 15 seconds. Thus, 15 seconds is the appropriate time for the scan delay. Thus, the 3-D MRA sequence is initiated 15 seconds after the start of the contrast injection. This results in alignment of the mid-point of the arterial phase of the contrast bolus with the mid-point (time when the center of k-space is acquired in a linear ordered sequence) of the image acquisition, with both occurring simultaneously at 24 seconds after the start of the contrast injection.

One advantage of the test bolus technique as outlined above is that there is no time lost switching from scan monitoring to image acquisition, and the arterial phase of contrast passage will perfectly coincide with the center of k-space acquisition. Therefore, in a multistation study, this scan will finish and the next position can be obtained more rapidly than when using a bolus triggering approach.

With the bolus triggering technique, contrast is administered as intended for the scan, and multiple one per second images of the vessel of interest are obtained in a predetermined imaging plane and displayed in real time on the scanner console. Scan triggering is then usually performed by the technologist based on the visualization of arterial contrast in the vessels of interest.[7] Automated triggering can also be performed, by monitoring signal intensity within a region of interest, with scan initiation occurring when the specified region of interest exceeds a predetermined signal intensity threshold.

When using the bolus triggering technique, since contrast is already present throughout the vasculature at the time of sequence initiation, centric ordering of k-space acquisition is advised. The main advantage of the bolus triggering technique is the ease of use; most technologists feel very comfortable with fluoroscopically monitored bolus triggered techniques. Also, variation from the patient's baseline for any number of reasons is accounted for by the real-time nature of the scan initiation. For these reasons, we typically use this method in the majority of our cases.

Fourth, following an initial noncontrast mask image, the angiographic data set is acquired using a heavily T1-weighted spoiled gradient echo sequence (SPGR or FLASH). It is T1-weighted in order to visualize the intra-arterial gadolinium based contrast, which produces shortening of the T1 of blood from 1200 ms to approximately 150 ms. Spoiling is used to destroy any residual transverse magnetization and to accentuate T1-weighting. The flip angle is variable, but is usually in the range of 15 to 35 degrees depending on TR (shorter the TR, the smaller the flip angle to maintain Ernst angle imaging). The administration of repetitive RF pulses to produce this flip angle every few milliseconds (typical TR 2.5–3.5 msec) results in nearly complete suppression of background tissue, while still producing high signal in the arterial structures that are filled with gadolinium contrast.[8] The sequence can be performed with fat saturation as needed, with only a slight increase in imaging time, and a slight decrease in signal to noise.

As in any MR sequence, the user must weigh the relative advantages and trade-offs between improved spatial resolution and prolongation of imaging time, but these issues take on special importance in vascular imaging.[9] In particular, when imaging the lower extremities the need to image small structures with adequate resolution must be balanced with the need to image these arterial structures before venous filling contaminates the image. Venous contamination can also present problems when imaging the renal arteries as the circulation time is quite rapid and the left renal vein is often superimposed over the left renal artery.

Parallel imaging techniques (IPAT/SENSE / ASSET) have improved the ability to perform high resolution imaging with fast acquisition time. This has resulted in fewer failed studies with improved robustness and overall image quality.[10] In its most common implementation, an acceleration factor of 2 is used, resulting in a decrease in imaging time (by nearly 50%) or an increase in spatial resolution (up to twofold). Most often, the improved efficiency is used to obtain some combination of both decreased time and improved resolution.[11] The cost of this improvement relative to the non-accelerated technique is a decrease in signal to noise by a factor of one divided by the square root of the acceleration factor (in this case 2). That is, for a two-fold increase in speed, the signal to noise drops to approximately 70% of the non-accelerated technique, not 50%. Since gadolinium-enhanced MR angiography is a signal-rich technique, this trade-off is quite advantageous. At facilities having this capability, MR angiography is almost always performed using parallel imaging technology.

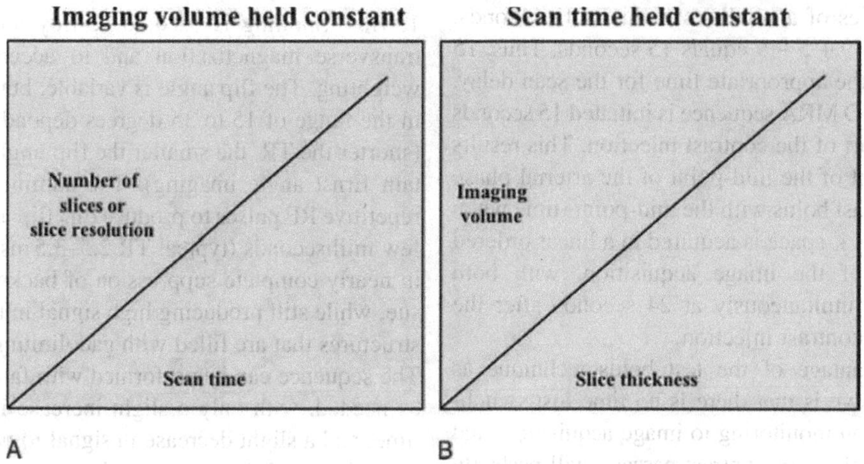

FIGURE 6.2. For a given imaging volume, as the number of slices or slice resolution increases, the scan duration increases (**A**). For a constant scan duration, as slice thickness increases (worse spatial resolution), the imaging volume increases (**B**)

The parameters used for the 3-D angiographic acquisition will depend on a variety of factors. The 3-D slab thickness must be sufficient to cover the vessels of interest, and the slice thickness, number of slices, and the desired resolution are selectable parameters that can be varied to achieve the desired blend of spatial resolution, signal-to-noise, and imaging speed. As can be seen in Figure 6.2, changes in imaging resolution, slice thickness, and number of slices all have an impact on scan duration. Imaging choices represent compromises between these competing priorities. Various other manipulations, including half-scanning techniques (useful if parallel imaging is not available, but not advisable in combination with parallel imaging), use of a rectangular field-of-view, and zero filling interpolation are available in most modern scanners. These will be considered in protocol selection (Case 130, series 17 and 18).

An additional parameter that should be considered is the ordering of k-space acquisition. Centrically ordered acquisitions are useful when the user wishes to acquire the central k-space lines of data (low spatial frequencies or general shapes and brightness) at the very beginning of the image acquisition. For example, when imaging the lower leg at the last station in a bolus chase acquisition, it is desirable to acquire the central k-space lines immediately at the start of image acquisition because there will be high arterial contrast concentration but minimal venous contrast concentration. If the central k-spaces lines were acquired in the middle of the image acquisition (as with a linearly ordered sequence), there is greater likelihood of an increased venous contrast concentration, resulting in venous contamination of the image.[12] As noted previously, when using a bolus-tracking or "fluoroscopic" synchronization technique where contrast media is already present throughout the vessels of interest, centric-ordering of k-space acquisition is advised.

Fifth, additional morphologic postcontrast images can be obtained to evaluate the vessel walls as well as adjacent organs of interest, often using a 3-D volumetric fat-suppressed T1 weighted technique.[13] Examples include the volumetric interpolated breath-hold exam or VIBE (Siemens) or the FAME sequence (General Electric) (Case 130, series 29). The addition of these sequences to the standard imaging protocol results in only a modest increase in total scan time, but can yield significant improvements in diagnostic ability. For example, these supplementary sequences are particularly useful in characterizing the extent of thrombus, atheroma, and vessel wall thickening in patients with aneurysms. They should be performed in regions where aneurysms are prevalent such as the abdomen, inguinal regions, and popliteal fossae, to screen for aneurysms that could be missed on luminographic images alone. Additionally, these supplementary sequences are very useful in the accurate detection of periaortic hemorrhage, inflammation, or fluid collections. In addition to allowing improved characterization of the vascular structures, these sequences can be helpful in evaluating associated abdominal and pelvic soft tissue pathology.

Post-Processing and Image Interpretation

In-line subtraction of the post contrast images from the pre contrast mask image can be programmed in advance to be automatically performed, along with creation of MIP images in various imaging planes. Typically, post processing will also include a series of coronal MIP images that are rotated through 360 degrees (Case 130, series 35.2).

The full volume MIP images provide a quick review of the arterial structures, but review of the source images is paramount, as the MIP algorithm can result in obscuration of important findings. Since a MIP image is created by performing a ray tracing through the volume of tissue, it can miss lesions that are enclosed by high signal structures along the ray path. For example, in Figure 6.3 the full-volume MIP image shows an irregularity of the proximal right common iliac artery that might easily be interpreted as atherosclerotic plaque. However, review of the thin section source images clearly demonstrates the presence of clot (Figure 6.3).

Therefore, complete assessment of the angiographic dataset entails simultaneous interrogation of the axial, sagittal, and coronal imaging planes using the source data reviewed in multi-planar reformation mode on a commercially available workstation. **Review of the unsubtracted dataset is recommended, as it allows visualization of the vessel wall, and not just the lumen, as may be the case on subtracted images.** In addition, other structures included in the study but poorly depicted by MIPs can also be better seen. Sliding thin submaximal MIP images also allow visualization of the arteries without overlap of overlying structures, and are often useful as well. Multiplanar curved reformations can be performed as needed.

Modern workstations can also create images using volume-rendering techniques, and allow endoscopic views. The volume rendered 3-D images can be impressive and are usually well received by clinicians (Figure 6.4). Although they can provide a unique global overview of the relevant anatomy, they are not well suited to primary

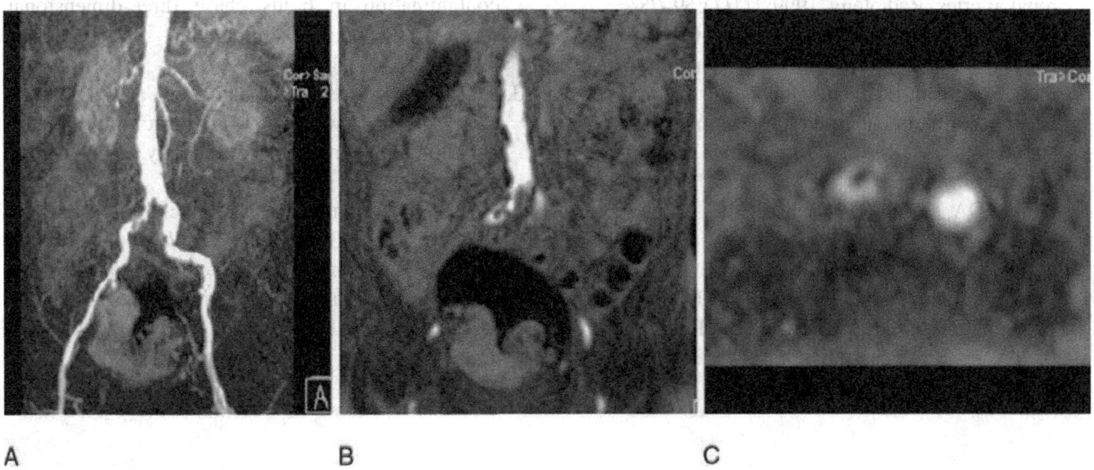

FIGURE 6.3. Full-thickness MIP image (**A**) shows irregularity of the right common iliac artery suggestive of atherosclerotic disease. Thin-section coronal (**B**) and axial (**C**) MPR images indicate that the finding is actually due to intraluminal thrombus

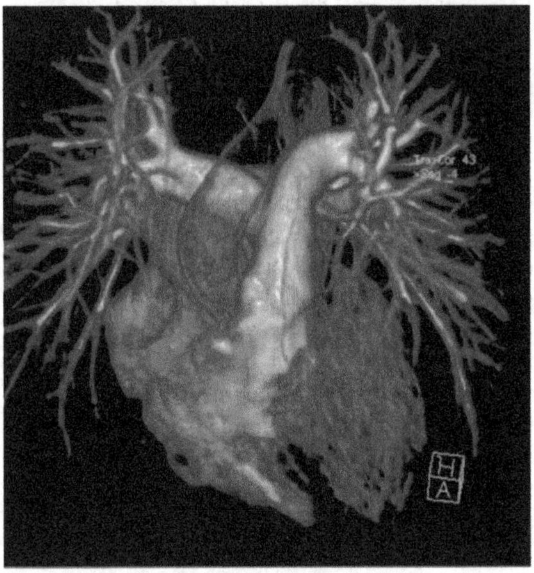

FIGURE 6.4. Color volume-rendered MR angiographic image of the main and branch pulmonary arteries

image analysis due to their tendency to either overestimate or underestimate lesions depending on the algorithm and thresholds used.[14]

References

1. Lee VS, Rofsky NM, Krinsky GA, Stemerman DH, Weinreb JC. Single-dose breath-hold gadolinium-enhanced three-dimensional MR angiography of the renal arteries. Radiology. 1999;211(1):69–78.
2. Krinsky GA, Reuss PM, Lee VS, Carbognin G, Rofsky NM. Thoracic aorta: comparison of single-dose breath-hold and double-dose non-breath-hold gadolinium-enhanced three-dimensional MR angiography. AJR Am J Roentgenol. 1999;173(1): 145–150.
3. Leung DA, Hany TF, Debatin JF. Three-dimensional contrast-enhanced magnetic resonance angiography of the abdominal arterial system. Cardiovasc Intervent Radiol. Feb 1998;21(1):1–10.
4. Hany TF, Schmidt M, Hilfiker PR, Steiner P, Bachmann U, Debatin JF. Optimization of contrast dosage for gadolinium-enhanced 3D MRA of the pulmonary and renal arteries. Magn Reson Imaging. 1998;16(8):901–906.
5. Hany TF, McKinnon GC, Leung DA, Pfammatter T, Debatin JF. Optimization of contrast timing for breath-hold three-dimensional MR angiography. J Magn Reson Imaging. 1997;7(3):551–556.
6. Earls JP, Rofsky NM, DeCorato DR, Krinsky GA, Weinreb JC. Breath-hold single-dose gadolinium-enhanced three-dimensional MR aortography: usefulness of a timing examination and MR power injector. Radiology. 1996;201(3):705–710.
7. Riederer SJ, Bernstein MA, Breen JF, et al. Three-dimensional contrast-enhanced MR angiography with real-time fluoroscopic triggering: design specifications and technical reliability in 330 patient studies. Radiology. 2000;215(2):584–593.
8. Maki JH, Chenevert TL, Prince MR. Three-dimensional contrast-enhanced MR angiography. Top Magn Reson Imaging. 1996;8(6):322–344.
9. Maki JH, Prince MR, Chenevert TC. Optimizing three-dimensional gadolinium-enhanced magnetic resonance angiography. Original investigation. Invest Radiol. 1998;33(9):528–537.
10. Glockner JF, Hu HH, Stanley DW, Angelos L, King K. Parallel MR imaging: a user's guide. Radiographics. 2005;25(5):1279–1297.
11. Chen Q, Quijano CV, Mai VM, et al. On improving temporal and spatial resolution of 3D contrast-enhanced body MR angiography with parallel imaging. Radiology. 2004;231(3):893–899.
12. Wang Y, Chen CZ, Chabra SG, et al. Bolus arterial-venous transit in the lower extremity and venous contamination in bolus chase three-dimensional magnetic resonance angiography. Invest Radiol. 2002;37(8):458–463.
13. Rofsky NM, Lee VS, Laub G, et al. Abdominal MR imaging with a volumetric interpolated breath-hold examination. Radiology. 1999;212(3): 876–884.
14. Persson A, Dahlstrom N, Engellau L, Larsson EM, Brismar TB, Smedby O. Volume rendering compared with maximum intensity projection for magnetic resonance angiography measurements of the abdominal aorta. Acta Radiol. 2004;45(4): 453–459.

7
Body MRA

Introduction

Advances in scanner hardware, coil technology, and software sequences have resulted in progressive improvement in the image quality provided by magnetic resonance angiography. The improvement in image quality has occurred concurrently with decreases in acquisition times, allowing comprehensive vascular imaging in a reasonable time frame. In the chest and abdomen, it has found a wide range of applications, which will be the subject of this chapter.[1–5] An initial discussion regarding the intrathoracic applications is followed by a similar discussion of the abdominal applications. Lastly, combined abdominal and thoracic imaging acquisitions will be discussed.

Thorax

Indications

MR angiographic imaging of the thorax is most often performed for the following indications:

- Acute aortic syndromes including aortic dissection, intramural hematoma, and penetrating atherosclerotic ulcer.[6]
- Thoracic atherosclerotic disease, including thoracic aortic aneurysm.
- Inflammatory disease of the thoracic aorta.
- Evaluation of congenital anomalies of the thoracic aorta (including heritable disorders of connective tissue such as Marfan and Ehlers-Danlos syndromes).
- Traumatic disruption of the thoracic aorta.
- Pulmonary vein studies.

Technical Notes

In virtually all indications for imaging of the thoracic aorta, visualization of the wall as well as lumen is important. In suspected dissections, visualization of the intimal flap is crucial to the diagnosis. Whether or not an intramural hemorrhage within the wall of the aorta communicates with the vessel lumen is what distinguishes an intramural hematoma from a localized dissection.[6,7] A penetrating atherosclerotic ulcer requires cross-sectional imaging through the area of abnormality for adequate diagnosis.[8]

Because of the need for high resolution imaging of the wall of the aorta, dark blood sequences such as single-shot HASTE are routinely obtained from the level of the thoracic inlet through the diaphragm in the axial plane.[9] These allow visualization of atherosclerotic plaque, as well as intimal flaps when present. Intramural hematoma is often better seen on dedicated fast spin-echo T1-weighted dark blood images, which can be obtained to supplement standard HASTE imaging in the evaluation of suspected acute aortic syndromes.

Cine images are routinely obtained through the base of the heart to visualize the wall motion in selected regions and to localize the aortic valve for dedicated high-resolution imaging. Small field-of-view imaging of the aortic valve in the cine mode is necessary to evaluate for incompetence as may be seen with a dissection, or the presence of a bicuspid valve which may accompany coarctation, and may predispose the patient to aneurysm formation and dissection.[10, 11] Cine images are also performed in the long axis of the aorta, in an oblique orientation that provides a "candy-cane" view (Case 106, series 24). The high temporal resolution of cine imaging makes this technique particularly valuable for delineating the location and presence of an intimal flap in cases of suspected dissection.

The 3-D MR angiographic data set is most often acquired in the sagittal or oblique sagittal plane, although occasionally coronal imaging is performed if visualization of the subclavian arteries is desired. In selected stable, cooperative patients cardiac gating may be elected in order to eliminate the image degradation that may be induced by cardiac motion. This is particularly true in the proximal ascending aorta.

As described earlier, an initial mask image is obtained without contrast, followed by either a timing bolus acquisition or bolus triggering acquisition. The contrast-enhanced data set is then obtained, and is subsequently subtracted from the precontrast data set for maximum vessel conspicuity. However, review of the unsubtracted data set is often helpful in evaluating for the presence of intramural abnormalities, and review of this data set is recommended. In cases of suspected dissection, repeat acquisitions are often helpful in visualizing the sequential opacification of the true and then false lumen.[12]

Additional postcontrast imaging with a fat-suppressed T1-weighted gradient echo volumetric data set (VIBE or FAME) is often helpful for further characterization of intramural hematoma, atherosclerotic plaque, and clot present within a thrombosed dissection (Case 106, series 31). Vessel wall enhancement may sometimes be appreciated in cases of inflammatory aortic disease.[13]

Velocity-encoded phase contrast imaging can be performed as needed to evaluate areas of suspected stenosis or flow alteration. These sequences are helpful in cases of aortic coarctation, and in cases of suspected subclavian steal, where reversal of flow can be demonstrated (Case 83, series 26).

Specific Disorders

Acute Aortic Syndromes

Acute aortic syndromes including aortic dissection, intramural hematoma, and penetrating atherosclerotic ulcer have a common propensity to present in an emergent fashion, with severe chest pain a frequent complaint. They are difficult to distinguish clinically, and sometimes at imaging as well.

Dissections are characterized by disruption of the intima with the development of a second, false channel for blood flow, usually through layers of the media. These remnants of media may sometimes be seen traversing the false lumen where they demonstrate a "web-like" appearance. When seen, they aid in recognition of the false lumen. Dissections may result in adverse consequences if they propagate to involve branch vessels, if they disrupt the aortic valve, or if they rupture into the pericardium.[14]

Comprehensive imaging should include the following:

1. The anatomic extent of involvement. Dissections that involve the ascending aorta are termed Type A dissections in the Stanford classification and are usually treated surgically. Those involving only the descending aorta are termed Type B (typically beginning just distal to the left subclavian artery) and are usually treated medically.
2. The presence of aortic valve pathology, as dissections may result in acute aortic insufficiency. In addition, bicuspid aortic valves are associated with an increased risk of dissection.[15]

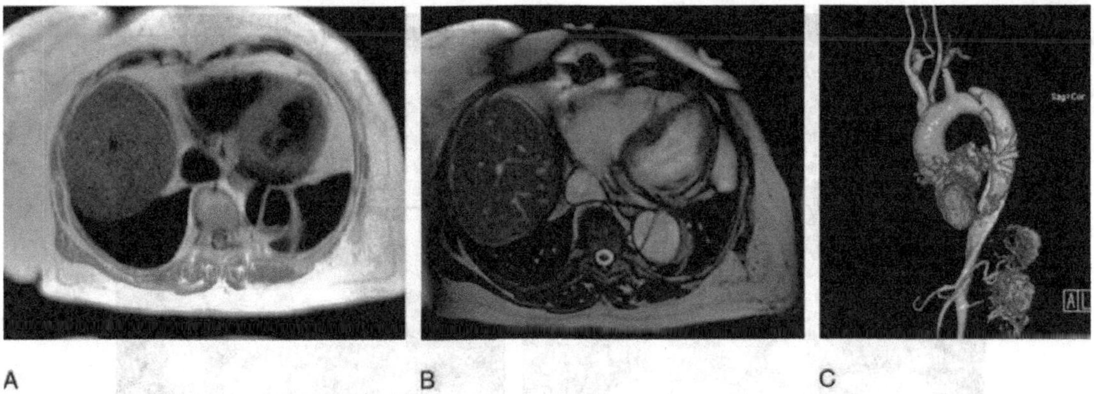

FIGURE 7.1. HASTE (A) and SSFP (B) static images show a dissection flap in the descending aorta. The MR angiographic image (C) displayed with volume-rendered technique demonstrates that this is a Type B dissection, beginning distal to the left subclavian artery.

3. Any evidence of an abnormal pericardial fluid collection, which may indicate intrapericardial rupture, a surgical emergency.
4. The presence of branch vessel involvement with resultant diminished end-organ perfusion.

The characteristic dissection flap separating the true and false lumens is usually evident on both dark blood and bright blood morphologic sequences (Figure 7.1) (Case 122). MR angiographic sequences often demonstrate the flap and are useful for assessing filling of branch vessels. Post-contrast VIBE images are helpful in assessing end-organ injury, and for demonstrating any associated thrombus in the wall of the aorta (Case 106, series 31).

Follow-up imaging after either surgical repair or after endovascular repair with stent-graft placement can also be performed with MRA (Case 143).[16]

Intramural hematoma is closely akin to dissection in that blood is also present in the wall of the aorta. However, it differs from dissection in that the intramural blood is not in communication with the lumen. Although it can present with severe chest pain, it does not always progress to more severe pathology. In some cases it progresses to classic dissection, in others to pseudoaneurysm formation, and in some it may regress completely.[17,18] Intramural hematoma involving the ascending aorta has been associated with a higher risk of progression to either dissection or pseudoaneurysm formation, and surgery is often recommended.[19] It is recognized as an area of focal or diffuse wall thickening on standard HASTE images, and precontrast fat-suppressed T1-weighted volumetric imaging (VIBE) is especially helpful in showing the abnormal intramural signal (Case 92).

Penetrating atherosclerotic ulcer (PAU) is characterized by the presence of an ulcerated plaque that disrupts the intima and extends for a variable distance into the media (Figure 7.2).[20,21] It can progress to rupture, and symptomatic ulcers or those that show deterioration may require intervention, particularly those involving the descending thoracic aorta.[22]

Penetrating atherosclerotic ulcers are recognized on imaging as focal ulcerations extending into the wall of the aorta, and most often involve the descending aorta. Morphologic imaging with dark and bright blood imaging is usually diagnostic, but angiographic images are also helpful. In particular, volume-rendered images will often demonstrate the outpouchings produced by the ulcerations with clarity (Case 147).

The more common atherosclerotic aneurysms of the thoracic aorta are readily depicted and characterized on MR imaging, with the multiplanar morphologic sequences of the standard exam facilitating accurate and reproducible measurements. Angiographic datasets provide visualization of the presence of associated thrombus and the filling of branch vessels.

Inflammatory Diseases

Inflammatory diseases of the aorta (Takayasu arteritis, giant-cell arteritis, and Ormond disease)

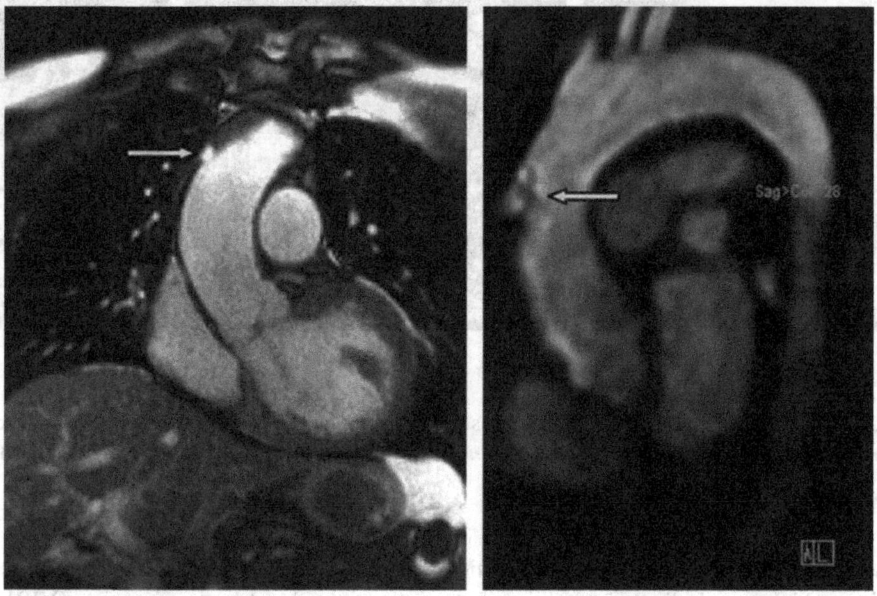

A B

FIGURE 7.2. Still-frame from cine loop (**A**) and source image (**B**) from an MR angiographic study of the ascending aorta demonstrating a focal penetrating ulcer of the anterolateral margin of the aorta (*arrows*)

typically result in wall thickening, which is readily detected on MR imaging.[23–25] Stenosis or occlusion of the arch vessels may occur, and is particularly common in Takayasu arteritis (Case 81).[26]

Congenital Aortic Disorders

Congenital aortic disorders such as coarctation or supravalvular aortic stenosis result in focal areas of narrowing of the aorta, often accompanied by significant gradients.[27,28] Although often repaired in childhood, recurrent or persistent narrowing may be observed in adulthood, and aneurysms may develop at the site of prior interventions. MRA provides accurate measurement of the aortic diameter and can depict any residual coarctation or postoperative aneurysm. Velocity-encoded imaging can be used to quantify any residual gradient (Case 67).

Certain hereditable disorders of connective tissue such as Marfan syndrome can predispose affected patients to the development of aortic aneurysms.[11,29] Marfan syndrome patients often demonstrate a characteristic "tulip-bulb" dilatation of the aortic root termed annulo-aortic ectasia (Figure 7.3) (Case 57). When the dilatation exceeds 5 cm, prophylactic surgical intervention is usually advised.[11] Certain subtypes

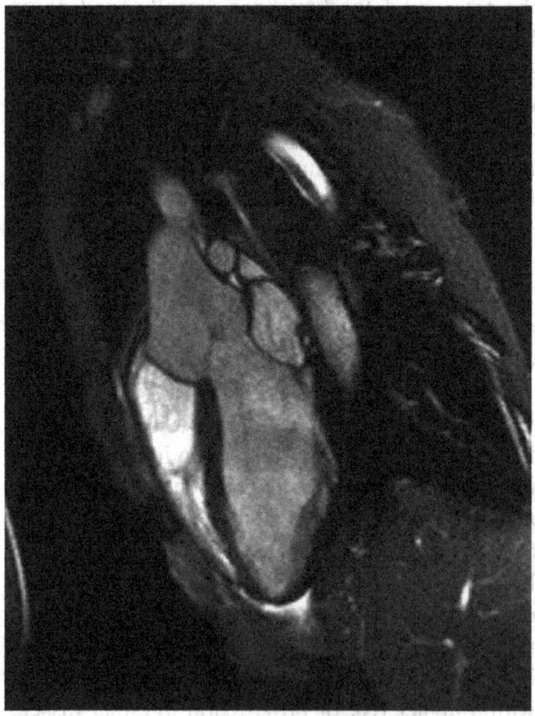

FIGURE 7.3. Still-frame from cine loop of a 17-year-old male with Marfan syndrome. Note the characteristic annulo-aortic ectasia

of Ehlers-Danlos syndrome (Type IV, the vascular variant) are also prone to the development of aneurysms and spontaneous dissections.[30–32] Surveillance imaging pre- and postoperatively in these patients can be performed with MRA (Case 48).

Traumatic Aortic Injuries

Traumatic aortic injuries most often affect the proximal descending aorta just distal to the left subclavian artery, and are life-threatening injuries that require urgent repair. In most facilities, they are usually diagnosed with CT, but occasionally they may present for CMR. Several small series of MR imaging findings have been reported.[33–35] In these reports as well as in our experience, MR demonstrates the characteristic intimal injury and associated pseudoaneurysm (Case 44).

Pulmonary Vein Studies

MR angiographic imaging of the pulmonary veins is often performed as part of pre-treatment planning prior to performance of pulmonary vein ablation for treatment of atrial fibrillation. Follow-up studies post-ablation may be obtained to exclude post-procedure stenosis. The studies are typically performed in the axial or modified coronal plane, and the 3D angiographic dataset obtained can be imported into software used in the electrophysiology lab to guide catheter placement (Figure 7.4) (Case 66). Reports should detail the size and number of pulmonary veins, as there is extensive normal variation.[36, 37] The location of the esophagus is also important to note, as it may be injured by the RF energy used to ablate the pulmonary veins if it passes in close proximity, with devastating consequences.[38]

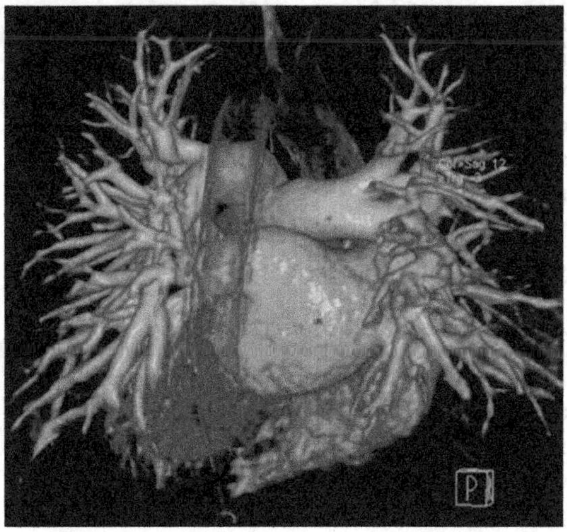

FIGURE 7.4. Posterior view of a 3D volume-rendered MR angiographic study of the pulmonary veins

Abdomen

Indications

MR angiography of the abdomen is most often performed for evaluation of the aorta and its major branch vessels. Given the excellent accuracy and favorable safety profile, it has assumed a primary role in the initial diagnostic evaluation of the abdominal aorta and the visceral arteries for a variety of indications.[2, 39]

Technical Notes

Initial localizer images are always followed by standard morphologic sequences. Dark blood imaging may be performed with single-shot techniques (HASTE) or with fast-spin echo techniques using breath-holding. Bright-blood imaging using SSFP sequences is also frequently helpful, and these may be performed without ECG-gating. Because of the multitude of organs and possible pathology, T1 fat-suppressed gradient-echo volumetric imaging (VIBE) is usually obtained both before and after administration of contrast material. Depending on the clinical circumstance, T1 in- and out-of-phase gradient echo imaging may also be obtained along with standard T2-weighted breath-hold sequences.

In general, MR angiographic imaging of the abdominal aorta and its branches is best performed in the coronal plane. Care must be taken to ensure that the imaging volume includes all the relevant vessels of interest. As in imaging of other regions, the desired spatial resolution, slice thickness, and acquisition time are interrelated variables that should be optimized for individual patients. In general, the study should be performed in less than 20–25 seconds to ensure patient cooperation for breath holding. The examination is repeated in multiple phases, to visualize succeeding vessels of interest. For example, imaging in the arterial phase is performed for evaluation of the hepatic arteries, with a 30 second delay before repeat imaging is obtained to visualize the portal vein. An even later acquisition can be performed for evaluation of the inferior vena cava.

Specific Disorders

Abdominal Aortic Aneurysm

Abdominal aortic aneurysms have usually been ascribed to atherosclerosis, and are especially common in current and former smokers. However, other etiologic factors probably also play a role in their genesis and enlargement. They usually begin below the level of the renal arteries, although perirenal and suprarenal aneurysms do occur, and present a formidable challenge to repair. Accurate measurements of the maximum transverse and sagittal diameters of the aorta are important, as the risk of rupture increases progressively as the diameter of the abdominal aorta exceeds 5 cm. Initial screening is often performed with ultrasound examination, but angiographic imaging is usually required for optimal characterization and for presurgical planning.[40, 41]

The relationship of the aneurysm to the origins of the renal arteries, and the presence of a definable "neck" often determine whether or not the patient may be a candidate for endovascular rather than surgical repair. Endovascular repair has been shown to have a favorable safety profile, although the patient remains at risk for the development of endoleak. Preoperative imaging is required to plan the therapeutic approach, and to assess the presence of associated atherosclerotic changes in the branch vessels.[41] Postoperative imaging is often required for follow-up surveillance, particularly if an endograft has been placed.[42]

It should be noted that follow-up MRA following endograft placement has been shown to be an accurate means for assessing the presence of endoleak and other complications. Current endografts are often composed of nitinol, which produces minimal MR artifact, and does not significantly impair subsequent lumen visualization.[42]

Dissection

Dissections of the abdominal aorta most often represent extension from the thoracic aorta (Figure 7.5).

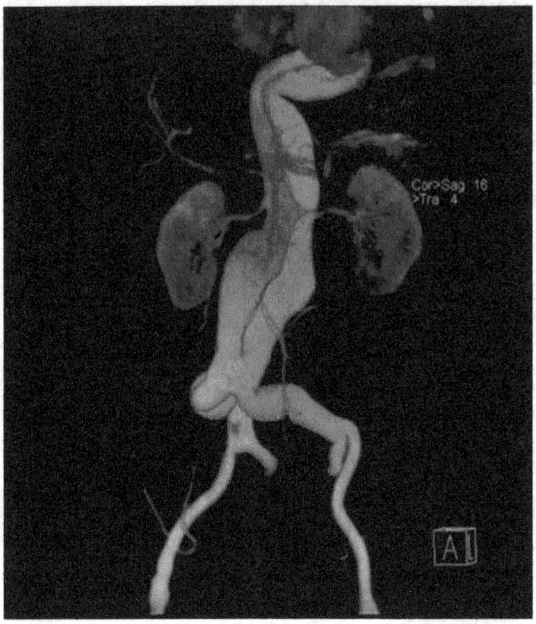

FIGURE 7.5. MR angiographic image of the intra-abdominal extension of a Type B thoracic aortic dissection

Primary abdominal dissections occasionally occur, but are uncommon (Case 48). The assessment of a dissection will focus on the presence of reentry sites, as well as whether branch vessels fill from the true or false lumen. Extension into the iliac and femoral vessels is also important to note.

Miscellaneous Aortic Disorders

Inflammatory aortitis may occasionally involve the abdominal aorta, although thoracic involvement is seen more commonly. Takayasu arteritis, as well as variant forms of retroperitoneal fibrosis may produce abdominal aortic involvement. Wall thickening is common in these entities, and enhancement may be noted on T1-weighted fat-suppressed gradient-echo imaging (VIBE).

Uncommon causes of aortic narrowing include abdominal coarctation, also known as mid-aortic syndrome.[43, 44] This syndrome may be associated with other systemic arterial abnormalities as may be seen with Williams syndrome, or may occasionally be seen in association with neurofibromatosis. In this disorder, an area of constriction is present in the midportion of the abdominal aorta, and is often associated with bilateral renal artery stenosis (Case 72).

Renal Arteries

Evaluation of the renal arteries is one of the most common indications for imaging of the abdominal aorta and its branches. Contrast-enhanced MRA has been shown to be quite accurate for the detection and quantification of renal artery stenosis,[45] which is most often due to atherosclerotic disease, and usually involves the proximal portions of the vessels. The 3-D nature of MRA frequently provides a diagnostic advantage over projectional imaging, such as digital subtraction angiography, as eccentric stenoses can be better visualized (Case 97).

Fibromuscular dysplasia is a less common cause of renal artery stenosis, predominantly affecting young women in their 30s. It should be suspected in more peripheral stenoses, or if the renal artery has a "beaded" appearance (Figure 7.6). It typically affects long segments of the midportion of the renal arteries and is frequently bilateral.

Potential kidney donors often undergo renal MRA, which has been shown to have comparable sensitivity for detecting accessory renal arteries as CTA.[46] Early branching of the renal arteries may occasionally complicate the performance of the surgical anastomosis required for transplantation, and should be noted in the report. Anomalies of the renal veins, particularly the left renal vein should also be noted as these may impact the surgical decision as to which kidney to harvest.[47]

MR angiography of the renal vessels is sometimes performed as part of the pretreatment planning for resection of a renal cell carcinoma, or in cases of suspected tumor invasion. Renal artery aneurysms are uncommon, but may occasionally be seen, and are typically located near the hilum of the kidney. In this pathology, morphologic in addition to luminagraphic imaging is suggested.

Splanchnic Arteries

Evaluation of the splanchnic vessels is most often performed for evaluation of suspected mesenteric ischemia. In this disorder, two of the three major vessels–celiac axis, superior mesenteric artery (SMA), and inferior mesenteric artery–must be narrowed in order to produce the anatomic substrate for bowel ischemia.[48] Patients with this disorder typically complain of postprandial pain, and frequently extensive weight loss is noted. MR angiography can clearly demonstrate the origins of the celiac axis, SMA, and inferior mesenteric artery, and provide accurate diagnosis (Figure 7.7) (Case 126).[49]

Living hepatic donors require preoperative angiography to assess the hepatic arterial vascular

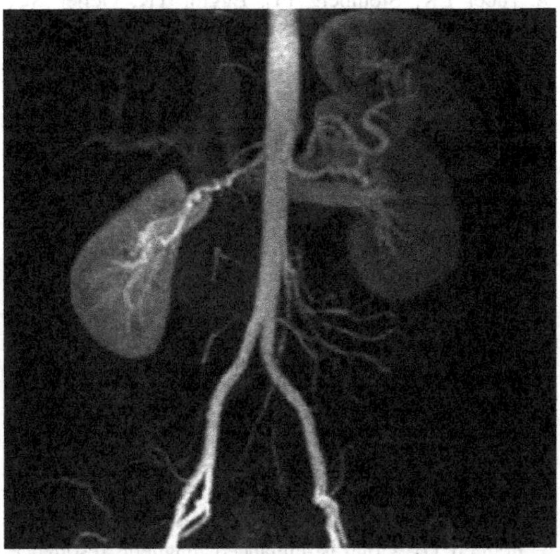

FIGURE 7.6. MR angiographic image demonstrating extensive irregularity of the renal arteries bilaterally consistent with fibromuscular dysplasia

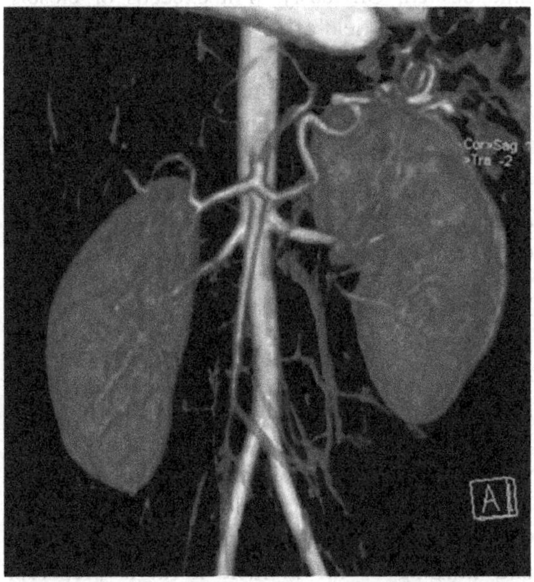

FIGURE 7.7. MRA showing patency of the celiac axis and the mesenteric vessels

supply of the liver and its various segments, as well as of the portal vein and its branching pattern.[50] It is often combined with MR cholangiographic imaging to visualize the biliary tree.[51] Extensive normal variation frequently complicates the evaluation, however, MR angiography is capable of providing high quality pretreatment planning.

Splenic and hepatic artery aneurysms are uncommon but potentially lethal manifestations of atherosclerosis. These are usually detected incidentally on another imaging study. MR angiography can provide accurate depiction of the relationship of the aneurysm to the parent vessel, and allow for pretreatment mapping. Splenic artery pseudoaneurysms are usually a complication of pancreatitis, and they have a high propensity to rupture. Therefore, their diagnosis and treatment is often a matter of some urgency once they are suspected.[52]

Combined Chest and Abdominal Angiographic Imaging

Not uncommonly, visualization of both the thoracic and abdominal aorta in a single patient visit is desired. In this instance, an assessment must first be made as to the extent of the imaging volume desired. Obviously, if it exceeds or closely approaches the field-of-view limits of the scanner, two separate acquisitions will be required. When in doubt, two separate acquisitions should be obtained. Although sequential imaging of the chest and the abdomen using a stepping table may be attempted, issues regarding contrast timing and optimum visualization can make this a cumbersome and complex endeavor. Often it is simpler and easier to perform two separate, sequential acquisitions.

In general, it is our preference to perform abdominal imaging first, followed by thoracic imaging. The reason for this choice is that prior administration of contrast will usually result in prolonged retention of contrast within the abdominal viscera, impairing visualization of the vessels of interest. However, if the abdomen imaging is performed first, by the time the patient is repositioned and imaging of the thoracic aorta is prepared, the intravascular contrast will usually have demonstrated significant washout from the intrathoracic vessels. Also, the thoracic MR angiographic acquisition will be obtained with a preinjection mask image, allowing subtraction of any minimal residual intravascular contrast present.

References

1. Prince MR, Narasimham DL, Jacoby WT, et al. Three-dimensional gadolinium-enhanced MR angiography of the thoracic aorta. AJR Am J Roentgenol. 1996;166(6):1387–1397.
2. Pereles FS, Baskaran V. Abdominal magnetic resonance angiography: principles and practical applications. Top Magn Reson Imaging. 2001;12(5):317–326.
3. Leung DA, Hany TF, Debatin JF. Three-dimensional contrast-enhanced magnetic resonance angiography of the abdominal arterial system. Cardiovasc Intervent Radiol. 1998;21(1):1–10.
4. Krinsky GA, Rofsky NM, DeCorato DR, et al. Thoracic aorta: comparison of gadolinium-enhanced three-dimensional MR angiography with conventional MR imaging. Radiology. 1997;202(1):183–193.
5. Krinsky G, Rofsky NM. MR angiography of the aortic arch vessels and upper extremities. Magn Reson Imaging Clin N Am. 1998;6(2):269–292.
6. Tsai TT, Nienaber CA, Eagle KA. Acute aortic syndromes. Circulation. 2005;112(24):3802–3813.
7. Macura KJ, Szarf G, Fishman EK, Bluemke DA. Role of computed tomography and magnetic resonance imaging in assessment of acute aortic syndromes. Semin Ultrasound CT MR. 2003;24(4):232–254.
8. Yucel EK, Steinberg FL, Egglin TK, Geller SC, Waltman AC, Athanasoulis CA. Penetrating aortic ulcers: diagnosis with MR imaging. Radiology. 1990;177(3):779–781.
9. Stemerman DH, Krinsky GA, Lee VS, Johnson G, Yang BM, Rofsky NM. Thoracic aorta: rapid black-blood MR imaging with half-Fourier rapid acquisition with relaxation enhancement with or without electrocardiographic triggering. Radiology. 1999;213(1):185–191.
10. Borger MA, David TE. Management of the valve and ascending aorta in adults with bicuspid aortic valve disease. Semin Thorac Cardiovasc Surg. 2005;17(2):143–147.
11. Boyer JK, Gutierrez F, Braverman AC. Approach to the dilated aortic root. Curr Opin Cardiol. 2004;19(6):563–569.
12. Mohiaddin RH, McCrohon J, Francis JM, Barbir M, Pennell DJ. Contrast-enhanced magnetic resonance angiogram of penetrating aortic ulcer. Circulation. 2001;103(4):E18–19.
13. Desai MY, Stone JH, Foo TK, Hellmann DB, Lima JA, Bluemke DA. Delayed contrast-enhanced MRI of the

aortic wall in Takayasu's arteritis: initial experience. AJR Am J Roentgenol. 2005;184(5):1427–1431.
14. Hagan PG, Nienaber CA, Isselbacher EM, et al. The International Registry of Acute Aortic Dissection (IRAD): new insights into an old disease. Jama. 2000;283(7):897–903.
15. Bonderman D, Gharehbaghi-Schnell E, Wollenek G, Maurer G, Baumgartner H, Lang IM. Mechanisms underlying aortic dilatation in congenital aortic valve malformation. Circulation. 1999;99(16):2138–2143.
16. Nienaber CA, Ince H, Petzsch M, et al. Endovascular treatment of thoracic aortic dissection and its variants. Acta Chir Belg. 2002;102(5):292–298.
17. Evangelista A, Mukherjee D, Mehta RH, et al. Acute intramural hematoma of the aorta: a mystery in evolution. Circulation. 2005;111(8):1063–1070.
18. Nienaber CA, Richartz BM, Rehders T, Ince H, Petzsch M. Aortic intramural haematoma: natural history and predictive factors for complications. Heart. 2004;90(4):372–374.
19. von Kodolitsch Y, Csosz SK, Koschyk DH, et al. Intramural hematoma of the aorta: predictors of progression to dissection and rupture. Circulation. 2003;107(8):1158–1163.
20. Hayashi H, Matsuoka Y, Sakamoto I, et al. Penetrating atherosclerotic ulcer of the aorta: imaging features and disease concept. Radiographics. 2000;20(4):995–1005.
21. Coady MA, Rizzo JA, Hammond GL, Pierce JG, Kopf GS, Elefteriades JA. Penetrating ulcer of the thoracic aorta: what is it? How do we recognize it? How do we manage it? J Vasc Surg. 1998;27(6):1006–1015; discussion 1015–1006.
22. Toda R, Moriyama Y, Iguro Y, Matsumoto H, Masuda H, Ueno T. Penetrating atherosclerotic ulcer. Surg Today. 2001;31(1):32–35.
23. Watanabe Y, Dohke M, Okumura A, et al. Dynamic subtraction contrast-enhanced MR angiography: technique, clinical applications, and pitfalls. Radiographics. 2000;20(1):135–152; discussion 152–133.
24. Hata A, Numano F. Magnetic resonance imaging of vascular changes in Takayasu arteritis. Int J Cardiol. 1995;52(1):45–52.
25. Bongartz T, Matteson EL. Large-vessel involvement in giant cell arteritis. Curr Opin Rheumatol. 2006;18(1):10–17.
26. Nastri MV, Baptista LP, Baroni RH, et al. Gadolinium-enhanced three-dimensional MR angiography of Takayasu arteritis. Radiographics. 2004;24(3):773–786.
27. Soler R, Rodriguez E, Requejo I, Fernandez R, Raposo I. Magnetic resonance imaging of congenital abnormalities of the thoracic aorta. Eur Radiol. 1998;8(4):540–546.
28. Nielsen JC, Powell AJ, Gauvreau K, Marcus EN, Prakash A, Geva T. Magnetic resonance imaging predictors of coarctation severity. Circulation. 2005;111(5):622–628.
29. Nollen GJ, Mulder BJ. What is new in the Marfan syndrome? Int J Cardiol. 2004;97(Suppl 1):103–108.
30. Germain DP, Herrera-Guzman Y. Vascular Ehlers-Danlos syndrome. Ann Genet. 2004;47(1):1–9.
31. Oderich GS, Panneton JM, Bower TC, et al. The spectrum, management and clinical outcome of Ehlers-Danlos syndrome type IV: a 30-year experience. J Vasc Surg. 2005;42(1):98–106.
32. Pinto YM, Pals G, Zijlstra JG, Tulleken JE. Ehlers-Danlos syndrome type IV. N Engl J Med. 2000;343(5):366–368.
33. Hughes JP, Ruttley MS, Musumeci F. Case report: traumatic aortic rupture: demonstration by magnetic resonance imaging. Br J Radiol. 1994;67(804):1264–1267.
34. Fattori R, Celletti F, Descovich B, et al. Evolution of post-traumatic aortic aneurysm in the subacute phase: magnetic resonance imaging follow-up as a support of the surgical timing. Eur J Cardiothorac Surg. 1998;13(5):582–586; discussion 586–587.
35. Fattori R, Celletti F, Bertaccini P, et al. Delayed surgery of traumatic aortic rupture. Role of magnetic resonance imaging. Circulation. 1996;94(11):2865–2870.
36. Takase B, Nagata M, Matsui T, et al. Pulmonary vein dimensions and variation of branching pattern in patients with paroxysmal atrial fibrillation using magnetic resonance angiography. Jpn Heart J. 2004;45(1):81–92.
37. Ghaye B, Szapiro D, Dacher JN, et al. Percutaneous ablation for atrial fibrillation: the role of cross-sectional imaging. Radiographics. 2003;23 Spec No: S19–33; discussion S48–50.
38. Cury RC, Abbara S, Schmidt S, et al. Relationship of the esophagus and aorta to the left atrium and pulmonary veins: implications for catheter ablation of atrial fibrillation. Heart Rhythm. 2005;2(12):1317–1323.
39. Glockner JF. Three-dimensional gadolinium-enhanced MR angiography: applications for abdominal imaging. Radiographics. 2001;21(2):357–370.
40. Prince MR, Narasimham DL, Stanley JC, et al. Gadolinium-enhanced magnetic resonance angiography of abdominal aortic aneurysms. J Vasc Surg. 1995;21(4):656–669.
41. Thurnher SA, Dorffner R, Thurnher MM, et al. Evaluation of abdominal aortic aneurysm for stent-graft placement: comparison of gadolinium-enhanced MR angiography versus helical CT angiography and digital subtraction angiography. Radiology. 1997;205(2):341–352.

42. Cejna M, Loewe C, Schoder M, et al. MR angiography vs CT angiography in the follow-up of nitinol stent grafts in endoluminally treated aortic aneurysms. Eur Radiol. 2002;12(10):2443–2450.
43. Lewis VD, 3rd, Meranze SG, McLean GK, O'Neill JA, Jr., Berkowitz HD, Burke DR. The midaortic syndrome: diagnosis and treatment. Radiology. 1988;167(1):111–113.
44. Messina LM, Reilly LM, Goldstone J, Ehrenfeld WK, Ferrell LD, Stoney RJ. Middle aortic syndrome. Effectiveness and durability of complex arterial revascularization techniques. Ann Surg. 1986;204(3):331–339.
45. Zhang H, Prince MR. Renal MR angiography. Magn Reson Imaging Clin N Am. 2004;12(3):487–503, vi.
46. Halpern EJ, Mitchell DG, Wechsler RJ, Outwater EK, Moritz MJ, Wilson GA. Preoperative evaluation of living renal donors: comparison of CT angiography and MR angiography. Radiology. 2000;216(2):434–439.
47. Israel GM, Lee VS, Edye M, et al. Comprehensive MR imaging in the preoperative evaluation of living donor candidates for laparoscopic nephrectomy: initial experience. Radiology. 2002;225(2):427–432.
48. Trompeter M, Brazda T, Remy CT, Vestring T, Reimer P. Non-occlusive mesenteric ischemia: etiology, diagnosis, and interventional therapy. Eur Radiol. 2002;12(5):1179–1187.
49. Laissy JP, Trillaud H, Douek P. MR angiography: noninvasive vascular imaging of the abdomen. Abdom Imaging. 2002;27(5):488–506.
50. Limanond P, Raman SS, Ghobrial RM, Busuttil RW, Saab S, Lu DS. Preoperative imaging in adult-to-adult living related liver transplant donors: what surgeons want to know. J Comput Assist Tomogr. 2004;28(2):149–157.
51. Freedman BJ, Lowe SC, Saouaf R. MR imaging in hepatic transplantation. Magn Reson Imaging Clin N Am. 2001;9(4):821–839, vii.
52. Agrawal GA, Johnson PT, Fishman EK. Splenic artery aneurysms and pseudoaneurysms: clinical distinctions and CT appearances. AJR Am J Roentgenol. 2007;188(4):992–999.

8 Peripheral MRA

Introduction

Peripheral arterial disease (PAD) is a vascular disorder that results in progressive narrowing of arteries of the lower extremities as a result of atherosclerosis. Although the initial evaluation for PAD consists of a basic physical examination including ankle-brachial indices and segmental pressures, many patients will require imaging to definitively establish the presence of PAD, and to provide an anatomic "roadmap" to aid in the performance of revascularization therapies.[1]

Indications

The clinical indications for peripheral vascular MR imaging can be categorized into two groups. Most studies will be performed in the setting of chronic stable disease, but occasionally the study will be requested for acute disease. Although special considerations may be needed in the evaluation of acute ischemic disease, peripheral vascular MR can be utilized in both settings since imaging can be performed quite rapidly.

Chronic Arterial Disease

Chronic forms of PAD include three general categories: atherosclerotic stenosis/occlusion, aneurysmal dilation, and congenital malformations.

1. Atherosclerotic stenosis/occlusion producing arterial insufficiency typically presents with classic claudication (pain induced by muscular activity such as walking that results in metabolic demands that exceed the delivery capacity of the supplying arterial circuit) but can occasionally present with claudication analogues such as leg cramping or fatigability. More severe forms of arterial insufficiency will present with rest pain, or nonhealing ulcers.
2. Aneurysmal dilation can occur in almost any arterial bed but most commonly will involve the aorta, iliac, common femoral and popliteal arteries.
3. Congenital malformations include persistent sciatic artery, popliteal entrapment syndrome, or Klippel-Trenaunay-Weber syndrome.

Acute Arterial Disease

Acute causes of vascular insufficiency may be imaged with MR angiography, provided that the patient is stable and capable of remaining motionless for this study. Pain control and coordination with the treating physician is important to allow optimal triage and treatment planning. Acute forms of PAD can be divided into 3 forms: "cold leg syndrome," dissection, or "blue toe syndrome."

1. "Cold leg" is the sudden, acute loss of perfusion to the lower extremity resulting in a pallor, coolness and pain of the leg. This is most often the result of embolism, usually from the heart or the upstream aorta. Expeditious performance of the exam is necessary to minimize tissue loss if MR angiography is performed prior to intervention.
2. Dissection. MR can be useful for visualizing the origin and extension of aortic dissection into the iliofemoral vessels. It can also help discriminate between true and false lumens.
3. "Blue-toe syndrome" is an acute, but not emergent disorder resulting in a bluish appearance to one or more toes. It usually results from peripheral embolization from a more proximal source, such as an abdominal aortic aneurysm with mural thrombus, or an ulcerated plaque. It can occasionally occur from embolism from the heart.

Technical Considerations

Scan Planning

The parameters used for the coronal 3-D acquisitions will depend on a variety of factors and specific recommendations will be given in the following sections. In general, the field-of-view should be maximized in order to obtain the greatest anatomic coverage possible for any given scanner, and to minimize the number of table movements required to encompass the desired anatomy.[2] Newer scanners with a 500 mm field-of-view allow scanning from the diaphragm to the pedal vessels in three stations in virtually all patients, but on scanners with a 400 mm field-of-view, four stations will often be needed in taller patients.

Automated table movement is now available on most scanners, along with dedicated peripheral phased array coils.[3] The table movement between stations should allow for overlap of the imaged anatomy, so that no gaps in coverage occur. For example, in a scanner with a 400 mm field-of-view, the table movement should be 300–350 mm between stations (therefore allowing 50 – 100 mm of overlap at each station). In cases where a short patient is imaged on a large field-of-view scanner, the degree of overlap can be increased.

Contrast Administration

Given the lengthy scan time for three or four stations in aggregate, and the desire to minimize venous opacification, most often a biphasic contrast administration is chosen with an initial rate of approximately 1.2 to 1.5 cc/sec for half the bolus administration followed by 0.4 to 0.5 cc/sec for the remainder of the injection. This latter rate approximates the tissue extraction rate, which would allow arterial opacification with minimal venous filling. This results in a prolonged arterial phase of injection, with slow and delayed filling of the venous structures.[4, 5] For combined imaging of the abdomen, pelvis, and lower extremities, typically 40 cc of contrast is administered. Synchronization of the image acquisition with the arterial phase of contrast passage can be performed with use of a timing bolus or with bolus triggering technique.

Minimizing Venous Contamination

Standard Techniques

The presence of venous contamination in run-off studies ranges in severity from the level of a nuisance that minimally complicates image interpretation to a complete disaster that renders interpretation impossible. In any case, the desire to minimize its presence drives much of the selection of imaging parameters and the bolus administration techniques that are used. Venous contamination can be minimized by:

1. Completing imaging within 60 seconds of study initiation.
2. Use of a biphasic administration of gadolinium, along with a slow prolonged infusion flush.
3. Use of venous compression devices at the level of the thighs (with pressures set to less than or equal to 50 mmHg) to delay venous filling.[6] NOTE: this technique should be used with caution in patients with bypass grafts, as the grafts are often superficial in location and vulnerable to compromise by the compression device.

Despite the optimization of imaging and contrast administration parameters, the frequent presence of venous contamination in the lower legs has stimulated the search for alternative techniques. Additionally, although most patients tolerate the venous compression techniques well, some find them objectionable, and as stated earlier, patients with prior bypass grafts should probably not undergo thigh compression. Therefore, alternative techniques have been sought that can minimize the problem of venous contamination in the lower leg station. Hybrid imaging techniques along with time resolved angiographic techniques have been utilized for this purpose.

Hybrid Imaging

A strategy that may solve the problem of venous contamination is the performance of a dedicated high-resolution acquisition at the lower leg level prior to imaging the abdomen and pelvis. In this technique, initial mask images of the lower legs are obtained, followed by a timing bolus acquisition centered on the popliteal arteries. Using this timing bolus, appropriate imaging delay is instituted, and 15 cc of contrast administered at a rate of 1 cc/sec with flush also administered at 1 cc/sec for 25 cc. Two sequential 3-D high-resolution coronal image acquisitions are then obtained. Subsequently, the abdomen-pelvis and upper legs are imaged in the standard fashion as previously described using approximately 25 cc of contrast. This technique was found to yield diagnostic images free of venous overlay in 95% of studies, and to demonstrate good agreement with selective DSA.[7] Other groups have reported similar findings, with a significant improvement in diagnostic accuracy at the calf level compared with standard bolus-chase methods.[8,9]

Time-Resolved Hybrid Imaging

Another strategy involves the use of a time-resolved imaging sequence in the lower leg station. In this situation, an initial scan with slightly lower resolution is repetitively performed in the lower legs, with a noncontrast image serving as the mask image. Each scan takes approximately 8 seconds, and is typically performed with a matrix size of 448 × 192. Sequential acquisitions (up to 15 or so depending on circulation time) are obtained during administration of 8 cc of contrast at 1 cc/sec followed by 30 cc of flush. Each scan is a complete 3-D angiographic data set. Starting from the second or third acquisition, each is subtracted from the mask, and the resulting MIP image in the coronal plane should be saved. The 15 MIP images that are generated can be subsequently viewed as a movie loop (Case 15, series 8). The study is then performed in the conventional fashion, with the lower leg high-resolution mask obtained followed by sequential table movement into the upper leg and abdomen-pelvis stations for the mask images. This strategy provides both moderate- and high-resolution images of the lower extremities, and with the combination can successfully image the arteries of the lower leg free of venous contamination. Additionally, since a series of images over time are acquired, these allow for visualization of discrepant flow if one leg is more severely diseased and has slower flow than the other (Figure 8.1).

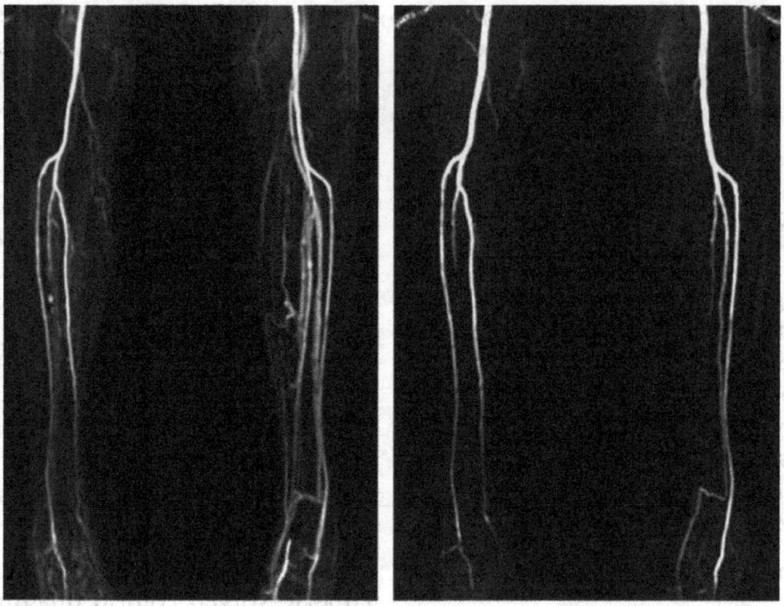

FIGURE 8.1. Standard image of the lower legs (**A**) is compromised by venous contamination on the left, but the time-resolved acquisition (**B**) clearly shows the left posterior tibial artery occlusion with reconstitution just above the ankle via collaterals from the peroneal artery

Findings in Specific Diseases

Atherosclerotic Peripheral Arterial Disease

Because of its systemic nature, atherosclerosis tends to be a multisegmental disease, affecting a variety of vascular territories. Nonetheless, recognized discrete syndromes are often found. Therefore, we will address the more common presentations of atherosclerotic peripheral arterial disease, recognizing that significant overlap occurs. In addition, given that such imaging is usually performed preparatory to either surgical or percutaneous intervention, emphasis will be placed on a discussion of findings relevant to planned interventions.

Aortoiliac Disease

High-grade occlusive disease of the terminal aorta or proximal iliac arteries often results in Leriche syndrome, a clinical entity characterized by the triad of diminished or absent femoral pulses, gluteal or thigh claudication, and impotence in males (Figure 8.2),

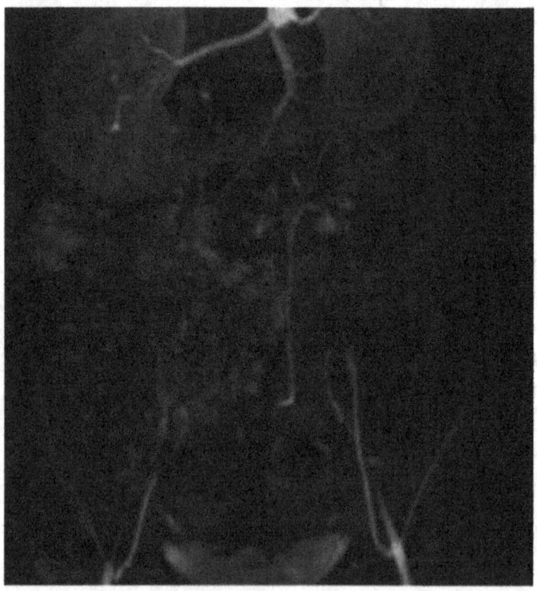

FIGURE 8.2. MR angiogram of aortic occlusion. Note the typical location just distal to the renal arteries. The femoral arteries are reconstituted via collaterals from the internal iliac arteries

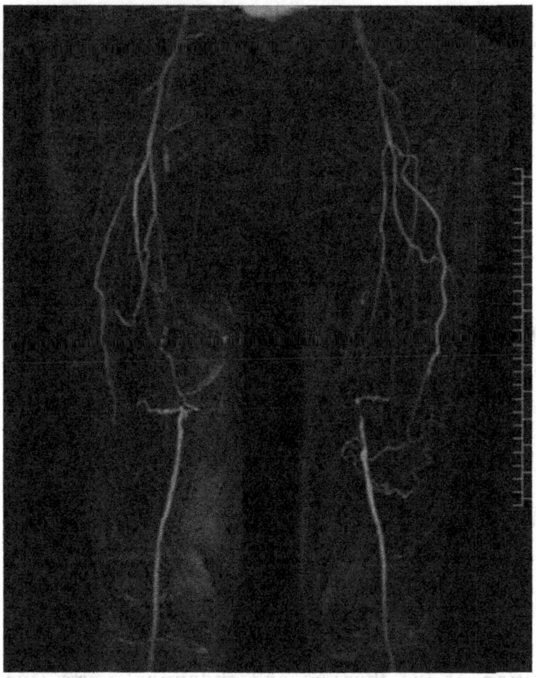

FIGURE 8.3. Bilateral superficial femoral artery occlusions. Note the surprising degree of symmetry of the findings

Pallor and wasting of the lower extremities may also be seen in extreme cases. More distal manifestations often coexist.

In analyzing MRA images in such patients, the severity of occlusive disease as well as the status of collateral vessels should be noted. The point at which the native circulation is reconstituted is quite important, as it will determine the feasibility of percutaneous or surgical approaches. In the treatment of long segment bilateral iliac occlusions, aortobifemoral open surgical repair is often preferred due to its superior patency.[10]

Superficial Femoral Artery Disease

Occlusive disease of the superficial femoral artery (SFA) is often surprisingly symmetric bilaterally (Figure 8.3). High-grade occlusions often result in claudication of the calf musculature on walking, and if accompanied by severe runoff disease, may progress to rest pain. The level of resumption of a normal caliber vessel is quite important as it serves as the likely site of distal anastomosis (Case 35). Also, if the anastomosis can be made proximal to the articular portion of the popliteal artery, synthetic graft material remains a viable choice, sparing the patient's native veins for future use if necessary.[11–13]

Runoff Disease

The usual patient with infra-articular runoff disease often presents with ischemic pain in the foot, progressing to rest pain and even gangrene. Diabetics in particular are at risk for this more peripheral, small vessel involvement (Figure 8.4) (Case 103).[14] Early venous filling and arteriovenous shunting is not uncommon in patients with severe runoff disease–often in those with cellulitis and coexisting soft tissue infection–which may complicate image interpretation. The status of the popliteal artery, the tibioperoneal trunk, and the vessels of the lower leg often determine whether or not the patient is a candidate for possible revascularization, or whether amputation is likely in the presence of rest pain.[13, 15]

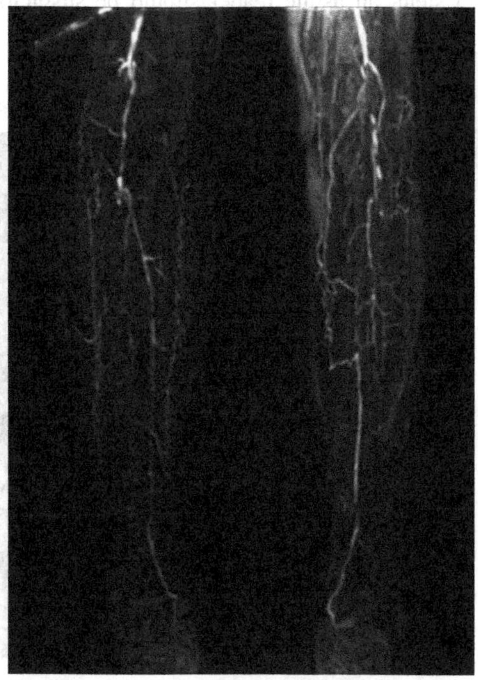

FIGURE 8.4. MRA of the lower legs in a diabetic patient with rest pain. Note the bilateral popliteal artery occlusions with no single vessel seen to extend continuously from the knee to the ankle

Post-Operative and Stent Imaging

Imaging of the post-operative patient is seldom performed simply as a surveillance procedure. More often there is suspected recurrence of occlusive disease, or progression of disease in the native vessels.[16]

Aorto-bifemoral grafts are widely used for the treatment of long segment iliac artery occlusions. Endovascular stent placement is frequently performed to increase the long-term patency of percutaneous interventions (Case 130). Visualization of luminal contrast in the presence of stents may be possible depending on the composition of the stent.[17–20] Nitinol containing stents usually produce minimal if any artifact. Stainless steel stents usually result in significant surrounding signal loss and as a result luminal visualization is not possible. If the presence of such a stent is unknown the reader may incorrectly assume that there is a short segmental occlusion (Figure 8.5). However, the true nature of the abnormality is easily clarified if radiographs are available. Even in the absence of radiographic or historical evidence of a stainless steel stent, an astute reader should be suspicious of this "pseudo-stenosis" based on the following: sharply marginated borders, the absence of collaterals, or the presence of stent artifact on thin section multiplanar images from the unsubtracted source images.

Embolic Disease

Peripheral arterial emboli affecting the lower extremity circulation typically originate either in the heart or the thoracic or abdominal aorta. Emboli will subsequently lodge in the more peripheral vessels, when their size precludes further migration, or at sites of preexisting stenosis. Depending on the abundance of collaterals, the degree of ischemia that results can be quite profound, and MR angiography is often performed in an urgent fashion (Case 42). When performing MR for evaluation of acute ischemic syndromes, meticulous attention should be paid to the evaluation of the thoracic and abdominal aorta (for potential sites of embolism), and a cardiac imaging study should be considered to exclude ventricular or atrial thrombi (Case 18).

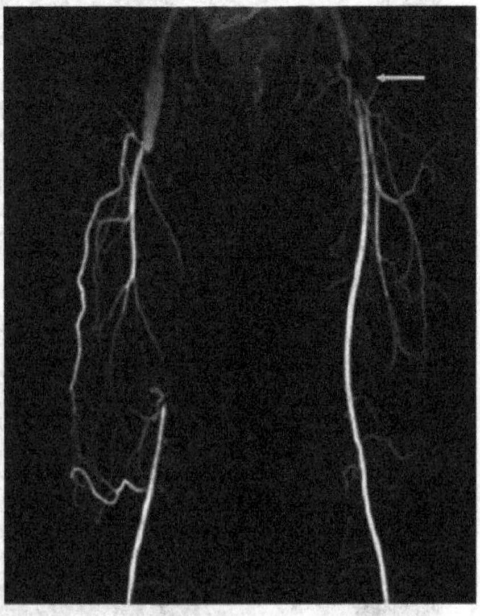

A

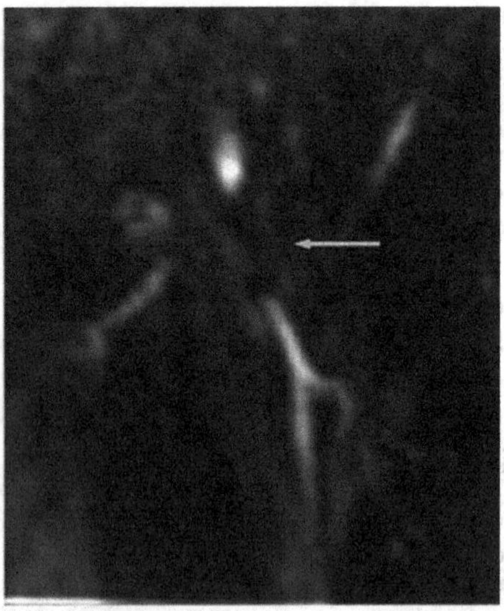

B

FIGURE 8.5. MIP image (**A**) shows an apparent occlusion of the left femoral artery (*arrow*). Thin-section multiplanar reformatted image (**B**) demonstrates the presence of a stent that has caused the signal loss. Patency of this segment is inferred from the excellent filling of the immediately distal segment and the absence of collaterals

Aneurysms and Dissection

An aneurysm is a localized area of dilation within any blood vessel to more than 150% of the native reference vessel diameter (i.e. a segment dilated to 1.5 cm or more in a vessel that has adjacent normal segment diameter of 1.0 cm would be considered an aneurysm). Aneurysms can be the result of trauma, infection, or connective tissue abnormality, but most frequently are a consequence of atherosclerosis. Atherosclerotic aneurysms predominately involve the infrarenal abdominal aorta, and are discussed in detail in the abdominal imaging section. Aneurysms can, however, be present in any of the vessels in the pelvis and lower extremity arterial circuit.

Dissections in the abdominal, iliac, or femoral vessels are usually the result of propagation of a dissection originating in the thoracic aorta (Case 122). Relative contributions of the true and false lumens to the supply of the abdominal and pelvic vasculature are important, and close attention should be paid to the relative perfusion patterns of the visceral organs. In particular, disparate perfusion of the kidneys is often evident in such patients and should be evaluated.

Isolated lower extremity dissections can be a result of mechanical trauma (e.g. a catheterization procedure), or can be spontaneous. Pseudoaneurysms are most often due to prior trauma, or may be a complication of surgical therapy.

Congenital and Miscellaneous Disorders

Uncommon causes of aortic narrowing include abdominal coarctation, also known as mid-aortic syndrome.[21, 22] This may be associated with other systemic arterial abnormalities as may be seen with Williams syndrome, or may occasionally be seen in association with neurofibromatosis. In this disorder, an area of constriction is present in the mid-portion of the abdominal aorta, and is often associated with bilateral renal artery stenosis.

Patients with Klippel-Trenaunay-Weber syndrome may occasionally present for angiographic imaging. In this disorder, abnormal arteriovenous connections may be present, and hemihypertrophy or hemiatrophy of the distal lower extremity is often seen. Abnormalities both of the arterial supply and of the draining veins may be present.[23] (Note: some authors separate Klippel-Trenaunay syndrome from Parke-Weber syndrome, while others lump the two together as Klippel-Trenaunay-Weber syndrome. The distinction is that classic KTS has only anomalous venous structures and is a low-flow disorder, while PWS patients have AV fistulae, high-flow lesions, and have a worse prognosis). Delayed imaging in the venous phase may be helpful in evaluation of such patients.

Popliteal entrapment syndrome is a disorder that results from abnormal medial placement of the medial head of the gastrocnemius muscle, resulting in compression of the popliteal artery in the popliteal fossa during exercise. This disorder may go unrecognized if imaging is not performed with the patient attempting plantar flexion. In cases where this disorder is suspected, dedicated imaging at the level of the popliteal arteries is suggested, both at rest and with provocative maneuvers.[24]

Cystic adventitial disease is an uncommon disorder resulting in localized arterial narrowing that may progress to occlusion, often involving the popliteal arteries. It is characterized by the development of myxoid cystic changes of the adventitia, with resultant compression of the vessel lumen.[25] Review of the axial source images is important in its recognition.

Arteriovenous malformations (AVMs) are congenital malformations in which there are abnormal connections between the arterial and venous structures without an intervening capillary bed. Both arteriovenous fistulas (AVF) and arteriovenous malformations (AVMs) result in abnormal early opacification of venous structures during the arterial phase of imaging.[26–28] Time resolved imaging may occasionally be helpful in such instances, but a rapid frame rate is necessary for this purpose (Case 140).[26]

Arteriovenous fistulas are more commonly traumatic in origin, and may result from iatrogenic intervention (Case 60).

References

1. Rajagopalan S, Prince M. Magnetic resonance angiographic techniques for the diagnosis of arterial disease. Cardiol Clin. 2002;20(4):501–512, v.
2. Carroll TJ, Grist TM. Technical developments in MR angiography. Radiol Clin North Am. 2002;40(4):921–951.
3. Ersoy H, Zhang H, Prince MR. Peripheral MR angiography. J Cardiovasc Magn Reson. 2006;8(3):517–528.

4. Prince MR, Chabra SG, Watts R, et al. Contrast material travel times in patients undergoing peripheral MR angiography. Radiology. 2002;224(1):55–61.
5. Wang Y, Chen CZ, Chabra SG, et al. Bolus arterial-venous transit in the lower extremity and venous contamination in bolus chase three-dimensional magnetic resonance angiography. Invest Radiol. 2002;37(8):458–463.
6. Zhang HL, Ho BY, Chao M, et al. Decreased venous contamination on 3D gadolinium-enhanced bolus chase peripheral mr angiography using thigh compression. AJR Am J Roentgenol. 2004;183(4):1041–1047.
7. Pereles FS, Collins JD, Carr JC, et al. Accuracy of stepping-table lower extremity MR angiography with dual-level bolus timing and separate calf acquisition: hybrid peripheral MR angiography. Radiology. 2006;240(1):283–290.
8. Morasch MD, Collins J, Pereles FS, et al. Lower extremity stepping-table magnetic resonance angiography with multilevel contrast timing and segmented contrast infusion. J Vasc Surg. 2003;37(1):62–71.
9. Meissner OA, Rieger J, Weber C, et al. Critical limb ischemia: hybrid MR angiography compared with DSA. Radiology. 2005;235(1):308–318.
10. Brothers TE, Greenfield LJ. Long-term results of aortoiliac reconstruction. J Vasc Interv Radiol. 1990;1(1): 49–55.
11. Muhs BE, Gagne P, Sheehan P. Peripheral arterial disease: clinical assessment and indications for revascularization in the patient with diabetes. Curr Diab Rep. 2005;5(1):24–29.
12. Al-Omran M, Tu JV, Johnston KW, Mamdani MM, Kucey DS. Outcome of revascularization procedures for peripheral arterial occlusive disease in Ontario between 1991 and 1998: a population-based study. J Vasc Surg. 2003;38(2):279–288.
13. Raffetto JD, Chen MN, LaMorte WW, et al. Factors that predict site of outflow target artery anastomosis in infrainguinal revascularization. J Vasc Surg. 2002;35(6):1093–1099.
14. Lapeyre M, Kobeiter H, Desgranges P, Rahmouni A, Becquemin JP, Luciani A. Assessment of critical limb ischemia in patients with diabetes: comparison of MR angiography and digital subtraction angiography. AJR Am J Roentgenol. 2005;185(6):1641–1650.
15. Ramdev P, Rayan SS, Sheahan M, et al. A decade experience with infrainguinal revascularization in a dialysis-dependent patient population. J Vasc Surg. 2002;36(5):969–974.
16. Bertschinger K, Cassina PC, Debatin JF, Ruehm SG. Surveillance of peripheral arterial bypass grafts with three-dimensional MR angiography: comparison with digital subtraction angiography. AJR Am J Roentgenol. 2001;176(1):215–220.
17. Ayuso JR, de Caralt TM, Pages M, et al. MRA is useful as a follow-up technique after endovascular repair of aortic aneurysms with nitinol endoprostheses. J Magn Reson Imaging. 2004;20(5):803–810.
18. Ersoy H, Jacobs P, Kent CK, Prince MR. Blood pool MR angiography of aortic stent-graft endoleak. AJR Am J Roentgenol. 2004;182(5):1181–1186.
19. Insko EK, Kulzer LM, Fairman RM, Carpenter JP, Stavropoulos SW. MR imaging for the detection of endoleaks in recipients of abdominal aortic stent-grafts with low magnetic susceptibility. Acad Radiol. 2003;10(5):509–513.
20. Cejna M, Loewe C, Schoder M, et al. MR angiography vs CT angiography in the follow-up of nitinol stent grafts in endoluminally treated aortic aneurysms. Eur Radiol. 2002;12(10):2443–2450.
21. Berkmen YM, Lande A. The midaortic syndrome: diagnosis and treatment. Radiology. 1989;170(2):571–572.
22. Messina LM, Reilly LM, Goldstone J, Ehrenfeld WK, Ferrell LD, Stoney RJ. Middle aortic syndrome. Effectiveness and durability of complex arterial revascularization techniques. Ann Surg. 1986;204(3):331–339.
23. Fontana A, Olivetti L. Peripheral MR angiography of Klippel-Trenaunay syndrome. Cardiovasc Intervent Radiol. 2004;27(3):297–299.
24. Elias DA, White LM, Rubenstein JD, Christakis M, Merchant N. Clinical evaluation and MR imaging features of popliteal artery entrapment and cystic adventitial disease. AJR Am J Roentgenol. 2003;180(3):627–632.
25. Wright LB, Matchett WJ, Cruz CP, et al. Popliteal artery disease: diagnosis and treatment. Radiographics. 2004;24(2):467–479.
26. Herborn CU, Goyen M, Lauenstein TC, Debatin JF, Ruehm SG, Kroger K. Comprehensive time-resolved MRI of peripheral vascular malformations. AJR Am J Roentgenol. 2003;181(3):729–735.
27. Bagga H, Bis KG. Contrast-enhanced MR angiography in the assessment of arteriovenous fistula after renal transplant biopsy. AJR Am J Roentgenol. 1999;172(6):1509–1511.
28. Rinker B, Karp NS, Margiotta M, Blei F, Rosen R, Rofsky NM. The role of magnetic resonance imaging in the management of vascular malformations of the trunk and extremities. Plast Reconstr Surg. 2003;112(2):504–510.

Part II
Cases

In this section, the discussions that accompany each case have been aggregated together. The first twenty cases are designed to introduce the reader to the display format and to the techniques used in CMR, including the mechanics and nuances of image acquisition. The subsequent cases are presented in the same random order as cases on the DVD, which is designed to allow readers to test themselves in interpreting "unknowns." However, each case is assigned to a category (congenital heart disease, adenosine stress perfusion, viability studies, and so on) and can be reviewed in a more structured fashion if desired.

Teaching File Case 1

51-year-old female with recent chest pain, rule out myocardial infarction

Category: Technical

Findings

Short-axis cine images in the top row demonstrate that the left ventricular cavity size is normal. The wall motion is normal throughout. This is confirmed on the 3-chamber or LV outflow tract view (first image of the second row), the 4-chamber view (second image of the second row), and the 2-chamber view (third image of the second row). The right ventricle is normal in size and function.

Evaluation of the valves demonstrates no significant abnormality. The aortic annulus is normal in appearance.

The aortic outflow tract view (fourth image of the second row) demonstrates that no dilatation of the aortic root is apparent. A small field-of-view cine series of the aortic valve is also obtained (fifth image of the second row).

Single-shot delayed-enhancement images (third row) show no evidence of scar. Segmented high-resolution delayed-enhancement images (fourth row) also show no scar. Static T2 weighted short-axis views are seen as the last three images of the fifth row and show no myocardial high signal to suggest the presence of edema.

Diagnosis

Normal study.

In the majority of the cases in this teaching file, the first row of images consists of a series of short-axis views arranged from the base to the apex as one proceeds from left-to-right. Given that there are six images per row, there are usually two short-axis images at the base, two at the mid-ventricle, and two at the apical level. Evaluation of these cine images in concert with the orthogonal 2-chamber and 4-chamber views provides an excellent means of evaluating the regional and global LV function. The 3-chamber view is the first image of the second row, followed by 4 and 2-chamber views. These are standard views that are almost always obtained as part of a comprehensive cardiac MR examination. Note that on the 4-chamber view in this case there is an apparent defect in the lower atrial septum and the upper ventricular septum. This represents partial-volume averaging of the adjacent aortic valve.

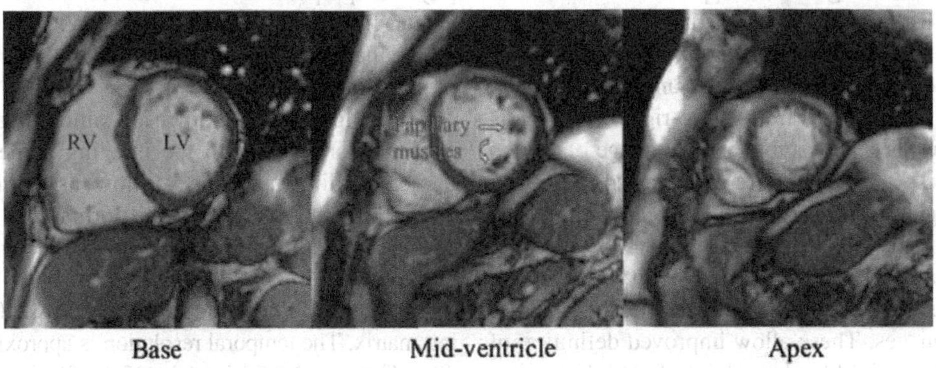

FIGURE 1.1. Still frame images from short-axis cine series at the base, mid-ventricle, and apical levels. Arrows point to the papillary muscles

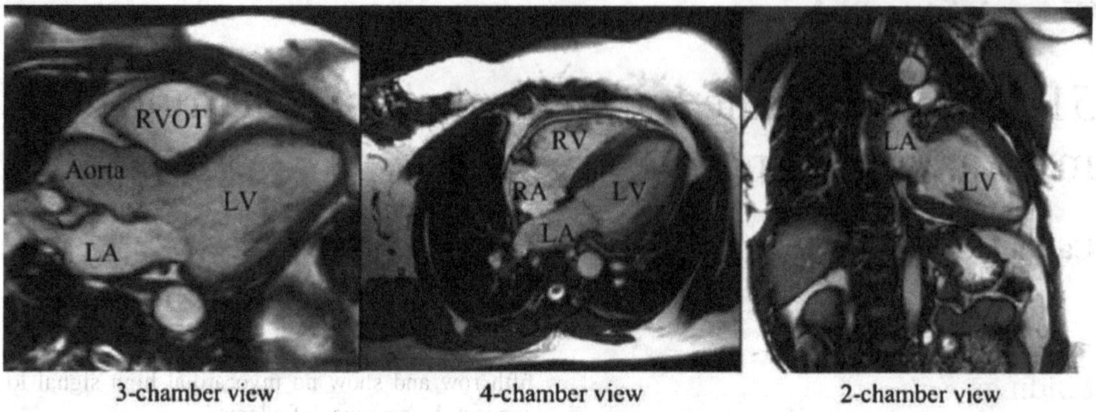

FIGURE 1.2. Still frame cine images in the 3-chamber, 4-chamber, and 2-chamber projections. The atria and ventricles are labeled

Teaching File Case 2

Normal volunteer

Category: Technical

Findings

The first five images of the upper row are short-axis images. The majority of image displays in this teaching file are arranged such that the short-axis views are displayed in the upper row, arranged from base to apex as one proceeds from left-to-right. In this case, the 4-chamber view is the far right image of the top row. These short-axis views are obtained by placing the imaging plane perpendicular to the septum and parallel to the mitral valve on a 4-chamber view.

Virtually all of the cine images in this teaching file are steady-state free precession (SSFP or True-FISP) images. These allow improved definition of the endocardial-blood pool interface when comparison is made with the older standard gradient echo images.

In SSFP images, the contrast between the blood pool and the myocardium is dependent on the physical properties of the tissues involved, and not on flow effects. Therefore, high signal will be maintained in the blood pool even in the presence of slow or turbulent flow.[1–3]

The imaging planes shown are similar in appearance and orientation to the imaging planes used in echocardiography. They allow assessment of cardiac structures in a standard format that can be easily cross referenced to other cardiac imaging modalities.

The standard cine sequence uses a 256 × 200 imaging matrix. The temporal resolution is approximately 40 ms/frames. Approximately 25 to 28 frames per cycle are displayed. The images are acquired using a segmented retrospectively gated technique.

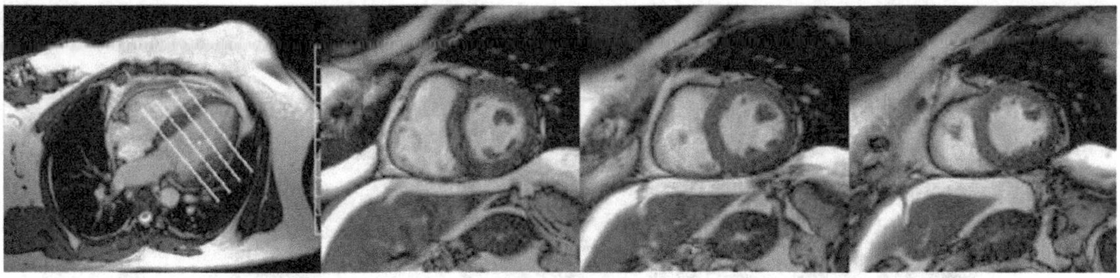

FIGURE 2.1. The 4-chamber scout view is used to prescribe the stack of short-axis cine images (not all images are shown)

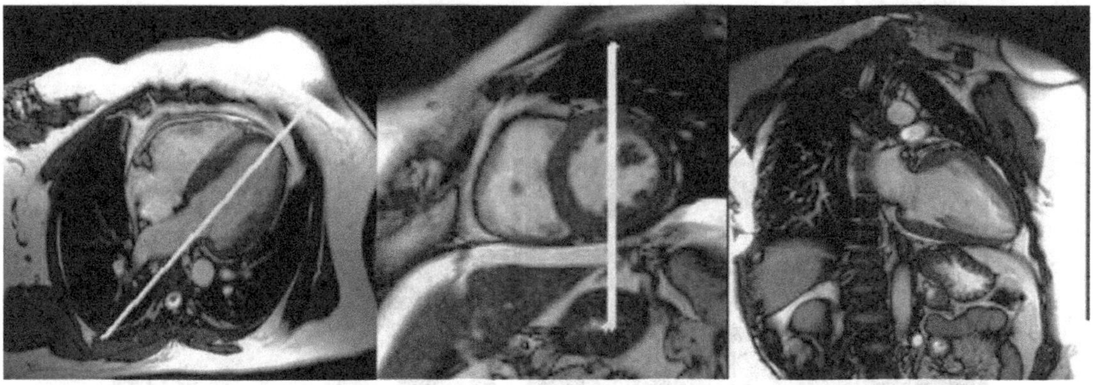

FIGURE 2.2. The 2-chamber view is obtained by placing a line through the left ventricle on an axial scout or a 4-chamber view parallel to the septum and bisecting the mitral valve and left ventricular apex. This view can also be planned by placing a line from the 12:00 position to the 6:00 position vertically through the left ventricle on the short-axis views

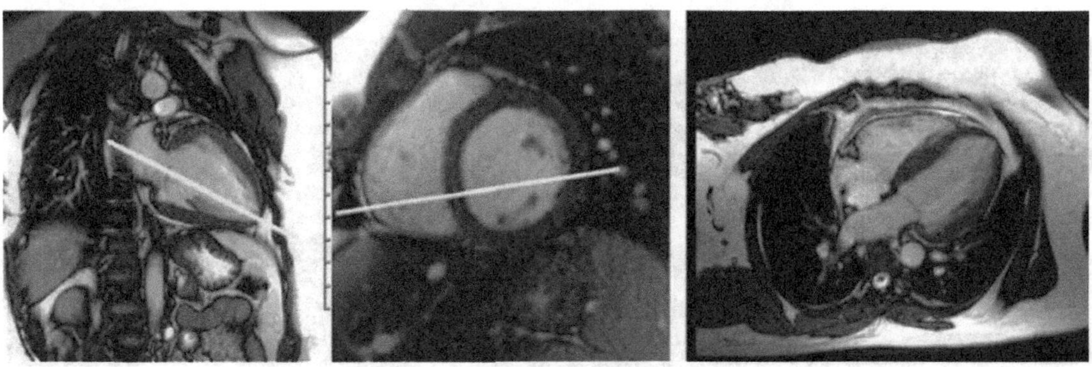

FIGURE 2.3. Using the 2-chamber view, the true 4-chamber view is obtained by placing a line through the apex and the atria as shown. Also, the true 4-chamber view can be prescribed from the short-axis view as shown

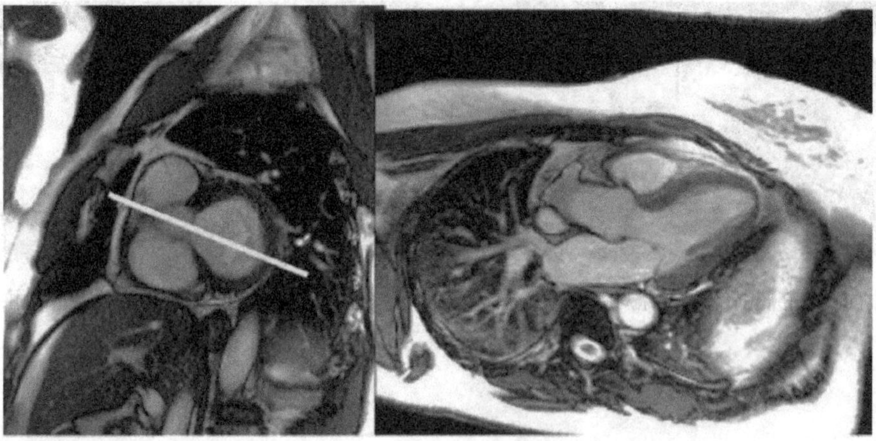

FIGURE 2.4. The 3-chamber view is obtained by placing a line through the aortic root and mitral valve, such that the line bisects the aortic and mitral valves

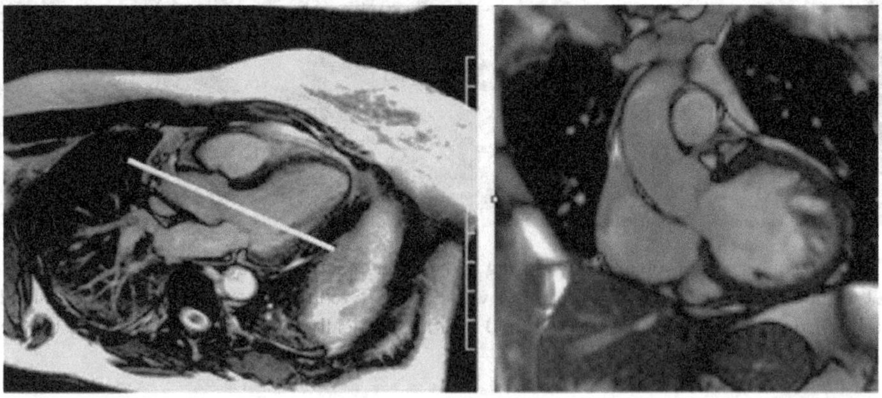

FIGURE 2.5. The aortic outflow tract view is obtained by placing a line in the center of the long axis of the aorta and bisecting the aortic valve. This results in a near coronal image including the aortic valve plane

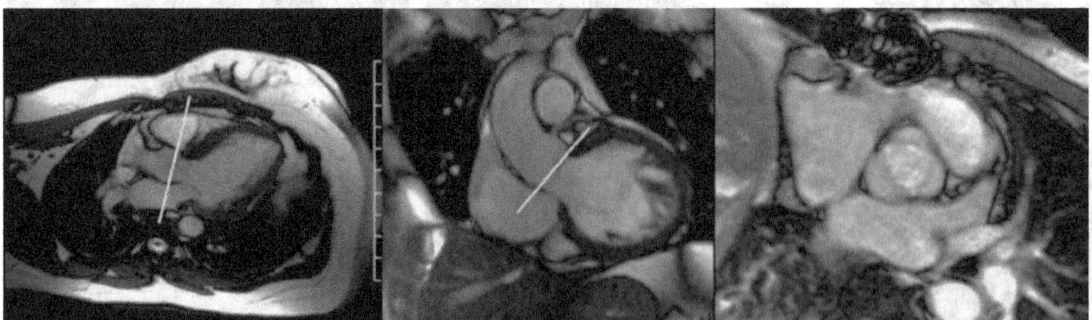

FIGURE 2.6. The small field-of-view image of the aortic valve is obtained by placing an imaging plane perpendicular to the aortic roat and parallal to the aortic valve in both the 3-chamber and the aortic outflow tract views

This technique works well in instances where the heart rate is regular. If there are frequent ectopic beats, or the cycle length varies excessively, prospectively triggered acquisitions may be used instead. In prospectively triggered acquisitions, the acquisition starts at the onset of the R wave, and terminates at a predetermined point after the R wave. The length of the acquisition is usually set to represent approximately 80 to 90% of the typical R–R interval, so as to exclude premature beats. Unfortunately, this technique will exclude the last portion of diastole, including atrial contraction in many cases.

Real-time acquisitions can also be performed in patients who have difficulty holding their breath or in whom there is excessive arrhythmia. In this technique, the entire cardiac cycle is acquired in real-time using a rapid true FISP technique.[4–6] These will be demonstrated in other exams.

References

1. Miller S, et al. MR Imaging of the heart with cine true fast imaging with steady-state precession: influence of spatial and temporal resolutions on left ventricular functional parameters. Radiology. 2002;223(1):263–269.
2. Pereles FS, et al. Usefulness of segmented trueFISP cardiac pulse sequence in evaluation of congenital and acquired adult cardiac abnormalities. AJR Am J Roentgenol. 2001;177(5):1155–1160.
3. Carr JC, et al. Cine MR angiography of the heart with segmented true fast imaging with steady-state precession. Radiology. 2001;219(3):828–834.
4. Lee VS, et al. Cardiac function: MR evaluation in one breath hold with real-time true fast imaging with steady-state precession. Radiology. 2002;222(3):835–842.
5. Kuhl HP, et al. Assessment of myocardial function with interactive non-breath-hold real-time MR imaging: comparison with echocardiography and breath-hold Cine MR imaging. Radiology. 2004;231(1):198–207.
6. Spuentrup E., et al. Quantitative assessment of left ventricular function with interactive real-time spiral and radial MR imaging. Radiology. 2003;227(3):870–876.

Teaching File Case 3

47-year-old male studied for evaluation of cardiac viability prior to possible bypass grafting

Category: Technical/Viability

History

The patient has a history of prior acute myocardial infarction with subsequent percutaneous coronary intervention (PCI) and stent placement.

Findings

The left ventricular cavity is mildly dilated to a diameter of 6 cm. The overall wall thickness is normal, but there is focal thinning of the anterior septum at the mid-ventricular level, extending to involve the apical level. Analysis of the regional and global wall motion indicates extensive hypokinesia of the anterior and antero-septal segments of the base, which become akinetic at the mid-ventricular level and dyskinetic at the apex. The remainder of the left ventricular myocardium demonstrates normal contractility.

The right ventricle is normal in size and function.

Mild dilatation of the left atrium is apparent.

Evaluation of the valvular structures demonstrates that there is no significant mitral or aortic regurgitation. The aortic valve is trileaflet and normal in appearance.

Rest perfusion imaging (first four images of the second row) demonstrates an area of diminished subendocardial enhancement (dark region) in the anteroseptal wall extending to involve the anterior wall at the basal level, as well as the anteroseptum in the mid-ventricular region.

The fourth row of images is comprised of delayed-enhancement images obtained in the short-axis plane. The viable myocardium is noted to be uniformly dark on these images, while infarcts are quite bright. These demonstrate extensive infarction (areas of bright signal) of greater than 75% transmural extent of the anterior septum at the basal and mid-ventricular levels, and approximately 50% transmural infarction of the anterior wall, and the inferior portion of the septum from the mid-ventricular level to the apex. The lateral wall is completely viable as is the inferior wall. Similar findings are noted in the single-shot delayed-enhancement images seen as the third, fourth and fifth image series of the third row. The sixth image series (far right) of this row is an inversion recovery single-shot image with a long inversion time (600ms) that shows no evidence of thrombus.

Diagnosis

A prior infarction of the anterior septum and the anterior wall is apparent, with nearly transmural involvement of the anterior septum at the basal and mid-ventricular levels, and approximately 50% transmural infarction of the anterior wall from the mid-ventricular level to the apex. Progressively greater involvement of the septum is noted as one proceeds from the mid-ventricular level to the apical region. The appearance is consistent with an infarction in the left anterior descending coronary artery (LAD) territory. The remainder of the myocardium is completely viable.

The delayed-enhancement sequence has become the gold standard for viability imaging. Its use is predicated on the underlying altered contrast dynamics present in areas of scarring relative to areas of viable myocardium. The MR pulse sequences used for infarct imaging were designed to maximize the imaging differences that result from the different contrast kinetics. For a detailed review of the use of the delayed-enhancement sequence for the evaluation of myocardial viability and scarring, please also refer to Chapter 1, Viability Imaging.

It is important to recall that both normal myocardium as well as infarcted and scarred myocardium will demonstrate contrast enhancement. However, contrast will wash out of normal myocardium at a much more rapid rate than it will infarcted or scarred myocardium.

In addition, areas of infarction, whether acute or chronic, will have a larger relative amount of extracellular space and therefore a greater volume of distribution for the gadolinium tracer than normal myocardium. Thus, areas of prior infarction will have higher concentrations of contrast on delayed images (after 5min). To see a schematic representation of this increased volume of distribution of gadolinium in areas of infarction, please refer to Chapter 1, Figure 1.5. The delayed-enhancement sequences used for infarct detection are designed to maximize the signal intensity differences between normal myocardium and infarcted myocardium. They do this by taking advantage of the different contrast kinetics present within areas of infarction and/or scar.

They are heavily T1-weighted gradient echo images, in which an inversion pulse has been applied. The inversion pulse serves to flip the magnetization 180 degrees. The recovery of magnetization back to baseline by areas that have a higher gadolinium concentration will be more rapid than those with a lower concentration of gadolinium, such as normal myocardium. Therefore, the increased concentration of gadolinium in an area of scar will be reflected by more rapid return above the zero-crossing line and back to baseline. In other words, it will recover magnetization quickly and become high in signal intensity. The time after the inversion pulse at which normal myocardium is at the zero-crossing line (and is therefore dark) is chosen in order to maximize the conspicuity of infarction. Infarctions by virtue of their increased contrast content will recover above the zero-crossing line more rapidly (contrast accelerates the recovery back to baseline longitudinal magnetization), and therefore will appear bright on these images where the signal from normal myocardium is "nulled."[1–3]

To see a diagrammatic representation of the process of using the inversion recovery sequence to null normal myocardial signal and maximize infarct conspicuity, please refer to Chapter 1, Figure 1.6.

Other entities besides infarction including infiltrative disorders as well as inflammatory processes can also result in hyperenhancement on delayed-enhancement images. Subsequent cases will demonstrate these findings.

It should be noted that areas of ischemic injury without infarction will not demonstrate contrast enhancement. The areas that appear bright on the delayed-enhancement images reflect areas of necrosis and not ischemia. This has been shown repeatedly in a variety of experimental models.[3] To see a figure demonstrating this excellent spatial correlation of DE-MR and tissue pathology, please refer to Chapter 3, Figure 3.1.

Both acute and chronic infarctions will hyperenhance, as they both have an increased volume of distribution of contrast. Therefore, the delayed-enhancement sequence does not distinguish between these entities. T2-weighted images are helpful in making this distinction.

The standard delayed-enhancement images are segmented acquisitions, meaning they are acquired over several heartbeats. Single-shot delayed-enhancement images are acquired in a single heartbeat, and thus are relatively impervious to breathing artifact, as well as arrhythmia. These are inversion-recovery SSFP images and are slightly lower in contrast to noise ratio than the segmented inversion-recovery gradient echo images, but are sufficiently accurate as to be useful in a variety of circumstances.[4, 5] For interest, compare the single-shot delayed-enhancement images in the third row with the high-resolution segmented images in the fourth row.

The delayed-enhancement single-shot inversion recovery images with a long inversion time are very helpful in demonstrating the presence of thrombi. Thrombi will appear dark on these images, whereas the normal myocardium and areas of infarction will be medium to high in signal intensity.

References

1. Kim RJ, Shah DH, Judd RM, How we perform delayed-enhancement imaging. J Cardiovasc Magn Reson. 2003;5(3):505–514.
2. Simonetti, O.P., et al. An improved MR imaging technique for the visualization of myocardial infarction. Radiology. 2001. 218(1):215–23.
3. Fieno, D.S., et al. Contrast-enhanced magnetic resonance imaging of myocardium at risk: distinction between reversible and irreversible injury throughout infarct healing. J Am Coll Cardiol. 2000; 36(6):1985–91.
4. Sievers, B., et al. Rapid detection of myocardial infarction by subsecond, free-breathing delayed contrast-enhancement cardiovascular magnetic resonance. Circulation. 2007;115(2):236–44.
5. Huber, A., et al. Single-shot inversion recovery TrueFISP for assessment of myocardial infarction. AJR Am J Roentgenol. 2006;186(3):627–33.

Teaching File Case 4

55-year-old female with a history of chest pain and abnormal enzymes

Category: Technical/Viability

History

She had a cardiac catheterization that was read as negative. Her ECG was also negative. The study is performed for further evaluation.

Findings

The left ventricular cavity size and wall thickness are within normal limits. The wall motion at the basal level appears normal. There appears to be slight hypokinesia of the inferolateral wall at the mid-ventricular level. The apical region appears unremarkable.

The right ventricle is normal in size and appearance.

Evaluation of the valvular structures demonstrates no significant abnormalities.

Delayed-enhancement images demonstrate a focal area of subendocardial infarction in the inferolateral wall at the mid-ventricular level. This is best appreciated on the fourth short-axis image as well as on the 3-chamber view.

Note the signal present within the myocardium on the second and third delayed-enhancement short-axis images. These were obtained with an incorrect inversion time of 250 ms. The fourth image that best demonstrates the infarction was obtained with an inversion time of 300 ms.

Diagnosis

Inferolateral infarction is noted at the mid-ventricular level, consistent with a circumflex artery territory lesion. An incorrect inversion time is evident on several of the delayed-enhancement images.

Review of the patient's cardiac catheterization demonstrated that although the study had been read as negative, an occluded branch of the obtuse marginal from the left circumflex was noted (See Figure 4.1).

In the appropriate patient with a non-ST-segment elevation MI, MR imaging prior to cardiac catheterization may be quite helpful in determining the likely culprit artery. Given the fact that many patients have several subtotal occlusive lesions that could potentially be responsible for the non-ST-segment elevation infarction, this determination may be quite helpful in guiding appropriate intervention.

MR imaging has been shown to demonstrate excellent sensitivity for the detection of subendocardial infarctions. Many of these may be missed at SPECT imaging. In one study, SPECT failed to detect 41% of the subendocardial infarctions detected by MR.[1] This is not surprising given the roughly 40-fold improvement in spatial resolution with MR relative to nuclear imaging. For a an image demonstrating these findings, please refer to Chapter 3, Figure 3.2. These infarctions, though small, are not insignificant as they indicate that the patient is at high-risk for future events. In one CMR study of patients not known to have had a prior MI, the presence of any focus of delayed-enhancement indicative of prior infarction conveyed a >7-fold increased risk for major adverse cardiac events relative to those not demonstrating delayed-enhancement.[2]

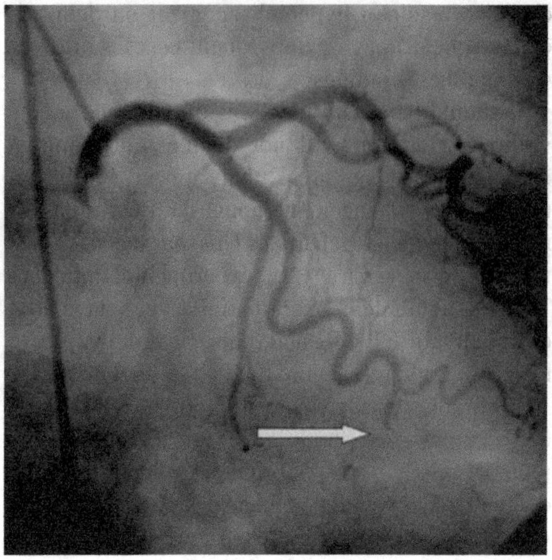

FIGURE 4.1. The arrow points to an occluded branch of the obtuse marginal on this still frame image from the patient's cardiac catheterization

CMR demonstration of delayed-enhancement was independently predictive of events beyond the standard clinical risk factors, or even the clinical model combined with angiographically significant coronary stenosis.[2] Therefore, the detection of even small infarctions conveys important prognostic information.

For optimum performance of the delayed-enhancement technique, the correct inversion time must be chosen. Selection of the correct inversion time can be performed with guidance from a preliminary TI scout view,[3] or simply through trial and error. An experienced examiner can often estimate the correct inversion time, with only a few iterations.

Note that choosing an incorrect inversion time that is too early will result in a significant portion of the myocardium being below the zero-crossing point, and thus demonstrate increased signal predominantly within the central portion of the myocardium.

The correct inversion time is characterized by near-complete absence of signal within the myocardium.[4, 5] An inversion time that is slightly too long will show only minimal degradation of image quality and is preferable to an inversion time that is too short. However, an inversion time that is far longer than the ideal will also demonstrate increased signal within the myocardium, and have a diminished sensitivity for the detection of infarction. For further reading regarding the correct performance of delayed-enhancement imaging, please refer to the section on delayed-enhancement imaging in Chapter 1, viability imaging

References

1. Wagner A, et al. Contrast-enhanced MRI and routine single photon emission computed tomography (SPECT) perfusion imaging for detection of subendocardial myocardial infarcts: an imaging study. Lancet. 2003;361(9355):374–379.
2. Kwong RY, et al. Impact of unrecognized myocardial scar detected by cardiac magnetic resonance imaging on event-free survival in patients presenting with signs or symptoms of coronary artery disease. Circulation. 2006;113(23):2733–2743.
3. Gupta A, et al. Myocardial infarction: optimization of inversion times at delayed contrast-enhanced MR imaging. Radiology. 2004;233(3):921–926.
4. Kim RJ, Shah DJ, Judd RM. How we perform delayed enhancement imaging. J Cardiovasc Magn Reson. 2003;5(3):505–514.
5. Simonetti OP, et al. An improved MR imaging technique for the visualization of myocardial infarction. Radiology. 2001;218(1):215–223.

Teaching File Case 5

32-year-old female with sarcoidosis, rule out cardiac involvement

Category: Technical/Viability

Findings

The left ventricular cavity is normal in size. The left ventricular wall thickness and motion appear normal. The right ventricle is likewise normal in appearance.

Evaluation of the valvular structures demonstrates mild tricuspid regurgitation.

Delayed enhanced images show no evidence of abnormal myocardial hyperenhancement to suggest presence of cardiac sarcoidosis. Single-shot delayed-enhancement images are seen as the first three images of the third row. The high-resolution segmented IR-FLASH images are seen in the last three images of the third row, as well as the entire fourth row.

Diagnosis

No evidence of cardiac sarcoid. Normal inversion-recovery delayed-enhancement images.

A TI scout series is noted in the fourth image of the second row. These images represent a series of inversion-recovery SSFP images acquired sequentially with progressively longer inversion times. These allow an estimation of the appropriate inversion time to produce nulling of the myocardium.[1] The next image in this row demonstrates an inversion recovery image obtained with an inversion time of 220 ms, and is clearly obtained too early. Note the extensive high signal throughout the myocardium due to the fact that the myocardial signal has not yet recovered above the zero crossing line.[2]

The next image (far right image of the second row) is obtained with an inversion time of 250 ms, and has only minimal residual intramyocardial signal, and is clearly closer to the correct time. The series of single shot images seen in the third row were obtained with an inversion time of 280 ms, as were the high-resolution segmented images. This was the inversion time that resulted in the best myocardial nulling.

In general, it is preferable to have an inversion time that is slightly too long than one that is too short.

References

1. Gupta A, et al. Myocardial infarction: optimization of inversion times at delayed contrast-enhanced MR imaging. Radiology. 2004;233(3):921–926.
2. Kim RJ, Shah DJ, Judd RM. How we perform delayed enhancement imaging. J Cardiovasc Magn Reson. 2003;5(3):505–514.

Teaching File Case 6

40-year-old male with known recent MI, evaluate extent

Category: Viability

Findings

The short-axis images demonstrate a mildly dilated LV cavity, which measures 5.9 cm in diameter. There is severe hypokinesia of the inferolateral wall at the basal and mid-ventricular levels, with milder hypokinesia of the anterolateral wall at the base. A small outpouching of the inferior wall at the base is noted, but its walls appear to demonstrate contractility. The global LVEF is mildly reduced at 47%. The right ventricle is normal in size and function.

Evaluation of the valvular structures reveals that the mitral and aortic valves are normal in appearance. Trace tricuspid regurgitation is noted.

Short-axis delayed-enhancement images in the third row demonstrate a transmural infarct of the inferolateral wall at the base. This involves only a portion of the inferolateral wall at the midventricular level, and the apical level shows minimal involvement. The T2-weighted images in the fourth row show high signal consistent with edema that involves the areas of infarction noted on the DE-MR images, but also involves additional portions of the inferior and lateral walls at the basal and midventricular levels.

Diagnosis

Acute inferolateral infarction in the territory of the circumflex coronary artery. A small diverticulum of the inferior wall at the base is incidentally noted.

The delayed-enhancement sequence can demonstrate areas of acute and chronic infarction with great precision, as previously described.[1] However, other entities including myocarditis, sarcoid, Fabry disease, and others can also demonstrate hyperenhancement.[2, 3] Delayed-enhancement due to coronary artery disease, fortunately, usually demonstrates characteristic findings that allow differentiation from these other causes: 1) It has a subendocardial component. 2) It follows a vascular territory. 3) It maybe associated with wall thinning and/or dyskinesia. 4) Acute infarcts may demonstrate wall thickening and/or the presence of a no-reflow zone.[4] Other cases will demonstrate these findings.

For general clinical reporting, we use the 17-segment model recommended by the American Heart Association. This model divides the basal and mid-cavity levels into 6 segments each, an apical level into 4 segments and the true apex into 1 segment. For each segment, left ventricular systolic function is graded visually using a 5-point scale ranging from normal wall motion to dyskinesis. LV ejection fraction is also provided, and is usually estimated from visual inspection of all the short- and long-axis views. However, for most of the cases given in this Teaching File, the LVEF has been confirmed using quantitative measurement by planimetry.

The delayed-enhancement images are also interpreted using a 5-point scale. For each segment the area or transmural extent of hyperenhanced tissue is graded visually. It is important that the delayed enhancement images are interpreted with the cine images immediately adjacent. The cine images can provide a reference of the diastolic wall thickness of each region. This will be helpful if delayed enhancement imaging is performed before there is significant contrast washout from the LV cavity, and there is difficulty in differentiating the bright signal from the LV cavity from hyperenhanced myocardium. An example of this phenomenon is shown in Chapter 2, Figure 2.4. For further discussion regarding the interpretation of delayed-enhancement and cine MR, see Chapter 2.

Both acute and chronic infarctions will demonstrate hyperenhancement, and therefore the delayed-enhancement sequence does not distinguish between the two. Other findings such as wall thinning and lack of edema indicate chronicity, while edema, increased wall thickness, and no-reflow zones may be seen with acute infarctions (see Chapter 3, Figure 3.5). T2-weighted imaging can also be useful in making this distinction.[5] Areas of acute infarction will demonstrate high signal on these T2-weighted images due to the edema associated with the injury, while chronic infarctions lacking edema will not. In fact, this sensitivity of T2-weighted imaging to the presence of edema has been reported to be useful for the depiction of areas of reversible injury (signifying myocardium at risk) adjacent to the areas of infarction on images obtained up to 48 hours after the acute event.[6] In this instance, the area of high signal on DE-MR represents the region of infarcted myocardium and the area of high signal on T2-weighted contains this infarcted region as well as the edematous (injured but viable) myocardium. The difference between the two represents the area at ischemic risk.

The small outpouching seen along the inferior wall is felt to represent a congenital diverticulum.[7] Note the lack of enhancement, indicating that it does not represent a scar with aneurysm formation. In addition, it is essentially obliterated in systole, indicating that it has muscular walls, and does not represent an aneurysm. Recent reports suggest that this entity may be more common than often thought, occurring in 2.2% of a series of patients studied with CT.[8] In that series they were noted to most often involve the basal inferior wall at the septal insertion site (as in the present case).

References

1. Elliott MD, Kim RJ. Late gadolinium cardiovascular magnetic resonance in the assessment of myocardial viability. Coron Artery Dis. 2005;16(6):365–372.
2. Edelman RR. Contrast-enhanced MR imaging of the heart: overview of the literature. Radiology. 2004;232(3):653–668.
3. Mahrholdt H, et al. Delayed enhancement cardiovascular magnetic resonance assessment of non-ischaemic cardiomyopathies. Eur Heart J. 2005;26(15):1461–1474.
4. Albert TS, Kim RJ, Judd RM. Assessment of no-reflow regions using cardiac MRI. Basic Res Cardiol. 2006;101(5):383–390.
5. Abdel-Aty H., et al. Delayed enhancement and T2-weighted cardiovascular magnetic resonance imaging differentiate acute from chronic myocardial infarction. Circulation. 2004;109(20):2411–2416.
6. Aletras AH, et al. Retrospective determination of the area at risk for reperfused acute myocardial infarction with T2-weighted cardiac magnetic resonance imaging: histopathological and displacement encoding with stimulated echoes (DENSE) functional validations. Circulation. 2006;113(15):1865–1870.
7. Ohlow MA. Congenital Left Ventricular Aneurysms and Diverticula: Definition, Pathophysiology, Clinical Relevance and Treatment. Cardiology. 2006;106(2):63–72.
8. Srichai MB, et al. Ventricular diverticula on cardiac CT: more common than previously thought. AJR Am J Roentgenol. 2007;189(1):204–208.

Teaching File Case 7

58-year-old male with known coronary artery disease

Category: Viability

Findings

The left ventricular cavity is dilated, and poor systolic function is noted. Evaluation of the myocardium demonstrates minimal thinning of the anterior wall at the mid-ventricular level and in the apex. Evaluation of the regional wall motion indicates the presence of hypokinesia of the basal anterior wall and anterolateral wall, progressing to dyskinesia of the true apex. Hypokinesia of the septum is noted beginning at the mid-ventricular level and progressing to severe hypokinesia at the apex.

The left ventricular ejection fraction is approximately 32%.

The right ventricle is and within normal limits in size and function.

Evaluation of the valvular structures demonstrates no significant mitral or tricuspid regurgitation. The aortic valve is trileaflet and normal in appearance. Mild dilatation of the left atrium is noted.

Delayed-enhancement images with the standard high-resolution segmented image acquisition are demonstrated in the bottom 2 rows. These demonstrate a focal transmural anterior segment infarct at the base, as well as subendocardial infarction of the anterior and anterolateral walls beginning at the basal level and extending to the apex. In addition, involvement of the inferolateral wall is noted beginning in the distal mid-ventricular level. The degree of transmurality is approximately 50% of the anterior and anterolateral segments in the basal and mid-ventricular levels, progressing to 75% as one proceeds to the apex, and is virtually 100% in the true apex.

The fourth image of the fourth row is a 3-D volumetric image acquisition in the 2-chamber plane. This also demonstrates well the area of infarction.

Diagnosis

Extensive anterior and anterolateral infarction is evident, with involvement of the true apex and a minimal portion of the apical inferior wall.

Delayed-enhancement MR, in combination with cine imaging, allows identification of myocardial stunning following acute myocardial infarction, or hibernating myocardium in the setting of chronic ischemic heart disease. In the latter situation, it then follows that delayed-enhancement imaging can be performed before coronary revascularization procedures to predict the likelihood that there will be functional recovery after revascularization. Specifically, there is an inverse relationship between the transmural extent of hyperenhancement, and the likelihood of wall motion recovery following revascularization. (For a graphic representation of this correlation, please refer to Chapter 3, Figure 3.3. For instance, myocardial regions that demonstrate little or no evidence of hyperenhancement (i.e. infarction) have high likelihood of recovery, whereas regions with transmural hyperenhancement have virtually no chance of recovery. Likewise, regions with intermediate levels of hyperenhancement (around 50%) have moderate chances of recovery. However, in this situation, it is important to remember that both myocardial viability and functional improvement are a continuum, and not simply a binary—yes or no—function. Thus, since it most closely reflects reality, it is better to consider these regions as all having a high chance for an intermediate amount of improvement rather than 50% likely to have complete recovery and the other 50%, no improvement whatsoever.[1–5]

References

1. Kim RJ, et al. The use of contrast-enhanced magnetic resonance imaging to identify reversible myocardial dysfunction. N Engl J Med. 2000;343(20):445–1453.
2. Bello D, et al. Gadolinium cardiovascular magnetic resonance predicts reversible myocardial dysfunction and remodeling in patients with heart failure undergoing beta-blocker therapy. Circulation. 2003;108(16):1945–1953.
3. Elliott MD, Kim RJ. Late gadolinium cardiovascular magnetic resonance in the assessment of myocardial viability. Coron Artery Dis. 2005;16(6):365–372.
4. Choi KM, et al. Transmural extent of acute myocardial infarction predicts long-term improvement in contractile function. Circulation. 2001;104(10):1101–1107.
5. Kim RJ, et al. Relationship of MRI delayed contrast enhancement to irreversible injury, infarct age, and contractile function. Circulation. 1999;100(19):1992–2002.

Teaching File Case 8

56-year-old male with recent myocardial infarction

Category: Viability

History

Assess for viability.

Findings

The left ventricular cavity is at the upper limits of normal in size. Akinesia of the anterior wall at the basal level is noted, progressing to dyskinesia at the mid-ventricular and apical levels. This involves portions of the anterior septum, and anterior lateral wall. A small focus of hypokinesia is seen in the inferior wall at the apex as well.

The right ventricle is normal in size and function.

The mitral and aortic valves are unremarkable. A trace amount of tricuspid regurgitation is noted.

Perfusion images obtained at rest demonstrates an anterior wall perfusion defect, along with a small area inferior wall of tracer defect in the apical region.

Delayed-enhancement images demonstrate extensive transmural infarction of the anterior wall beginning at the basal level, and extending to the apex. Involvement of the inferior wall at the apex is noted, with extensive infarction of the entire apex.

A dark focus is noted within the enhanced region in the mid-ventricular images. This can be appreciated on the 2-chamber delayed-enhancement view is well.

Diagnosis

Acute anterior wall infarction, with a no-reflow zone. A small inferior apical infarction is noted as well. Little residual viability is present in the anterior wall.

A no-reflow zone is evident on delayed-enhancement imaging as a dark region surrounded by hyperenhancing myocardium.[1, 2] This imaging abnormality reflects the impaired diffusion of the gadolinium tracer into the central core of the infarction. This finding is related to extensive microvascular obstruction produced by myocardial infarction that not only results in myocyte death, but also in extensive microvascular destruction with endothelial cell death as well. Thus, contrast diffuses into the periphery of the infarct resulting in its hyperenhancement, but is delayed in reaching the central core of the infarct.

The extent of the no-reflow zone in any given circumstance will depend on the time when imaging is initiated relative to the time of contrast administration.

This is related to the fact that these areas of microvascular obstruction will eventually fill in on delayed-enhancement imaging if the imaging is delayed sufficiently. For example, the no-reflow zone would be significantly larger and more apparent on images obtained at 5 minutes post contrast administration than at 35 minutes post contrast administration, relating to the delayed diffusion into the area of infarction by the contrast agent. To see a series of sequential image acquisitions demonstrating this process, please refer to Chapter 3, Figure 3.4.

The presence of microvascular obstruction has been shown to correlate with a significantly increased risk of adverse outcomes from myocardial infarction, including adverse remodeling, diminished systolic function, and arrhythmia.[3–6] The likelihood of microvascular obstruction for a given size infarction is related more closely to the transmurality of the infarction rather than its global extent.[7]

The imaging finding of a no-reflow zone is time dependent, not only within an exam, but depending on when the exam is performed relative to the infarction. That is, a patient may have a no-reflow zone seen during the first week after infarction that will become progressively more inconspicuous over the subsequent 8 weeks, and will usually disappear after that time.[7] The first-pass perfusion abnormality, however, will often persist at the site of the prior infarct, even after the no-reflow zone evident on delayed enhancement imaging resolves, indicating residual microvascular impairment.

References

1. Mahrholdt H, et al. Assessment of myocardial viability by cardiovascular magnetic resonance imaging. Eur Heart J. 2002;23(8):602–619.
2. Wagner A, et al. MR imaging of myocardial perfusion and viability. Magn Reson Imaging Clin N Am. 2003;11(1):49–66.
3. Wu KC, et al. Prognostic significance of microvascular obstruction by magnetic resonance imaging in patients with acute myocardial infarction. Circulation. 1998;97(8):765–772.
4. Wu KC, et al. Quantification and time course of microvascular obstruction by contrast-enhanced echocardiography and magnetic resonance imaging following acute myocardial infarction and reperfusion. J Am Coll Cardiol. 1998; 32(6):1756–1764.
5. Hombach V, et al. Sequelae of acute myocardial infarction regarding cardiac structure and function and their prognostic significance as assessed by magnetic resonance imaging. Eur Heart J. 2005;26(6): 549–557.
6. Gerber BL, et al. Microvascular obstruction and left ventricular remodeling early after acute myocardial infarction. Circulation. 2000;101(23):2734–2741.
7. Albert TS, Kim RJ, Judd RM. Assessment of no-reflow regions using cardiac MRI. Basic Res Cardiol. 2006;101(5):383–390.

Teaching File Case 9

48-year-old male with chest pain

Category: Stress test

History

EKG and enzymes are negative. He had a negative myocardial perfusion SPECT study.

Findings

Short-axis cines are seen in the top row. The first three images are spatially matched to the locations obtained for the perfusion images, which are seen in the first three images of the second and third row. The perfusion study is performed with adenosine stress, using 140 ug/kg/min administered for 3 minutes prior to contrast administration. The stress imaging study is performed first, and is displayed in the second row. The resting study is performed 10–15 minutes later, at rest, without adenosine stress, and is displayed in the third row. This is the format used throughout this teaching file.

In the perfusion images, note the progressive transit of the first pass of contrast –initially, the right ventricular cavity is seen to fill, then the left ventricular cavity, and then the myocardium opacifies. Note that the myocardium fills from the "outside in"; that is, from the epicardium to the endocardium.

Standard 3-chamber, 4-chamber, and 2-chamber views are seen in the remainder of the second row.

The still frame images noted on the right side of the third row are T2-weighted images obtained to evaluate for edema as may be seen with acute ischemic injury with or without infarction. These are negative in this case.

Single-shot delayed-enhancement images are noted in the fourth row, obtained with short and long inversion time in multiple planes. The images with a "short" inversion time are similar in appearance to the standard delayed-enhancement images, while the "long" inversion time (TI or inversion time of 550–700 msec) images show the myocardium as having medium signal intensity with a light grey appearance.

In the fifth row, the first three delayed-enhancement images that are displayed are spatially matched to the locations of the cine images and the stress/rest perfusion images. Other delayed-enhancement images are demonstrated as well.

This study was negative for ischemia. The cine images demonstrate normal left ventricular cavity size and wall motion. The right ventricle is unremarkable as well.

The stress and rest perfusion images demonstrate no perfusion deficit. A perfusion deficit would appear as a dark region extending from the subendocardium into the myocardium, and persisting for a minimum of 4 to 5 heartbeats. In addition, the deficit will usually follow a coronary artery territory, and should be more apparent on the stress images than the resting images in order to signify inducible ischemia.

Artifacts will have a similar appearance on stress and rest images. A common artifact seen on perfusion images is the subendocardial dark-rim artifact, thought to be in part the result of susceptibility effects during the passage of contrast, as it is noted to diminish in intensity with subsequent cycles. Low spatial resolution and respiratory motion may also contribute to this artifact. This is usually limited to the immediate subendocardial region, and is often more prominent along the septum. It is present on both the stress and rest images, and does not extend into the myocardium.

To eliminate respiratory motion during the critical phase of contrast passage through the myocardium, it is advisable to monitor the acquisition of the perfusion images in real-time at the scanner console, and to instruct the patient to hold their breath when the contrast is observed in the RV cavity. If real-time monitoring is not available, the patient should be instructed to breath-hold after a 5–6 second delay following the start of the contrast infusion.

Artifacts likely related to the use of parallel image acceleration are noted on both the stress and rest images, manifested as vertical bands through the central and lateral myocardium. They are present on both the stress and rest images, and have a characteristic appearance.

Perfusion deficits associated with infarction will be recognized by the apparent match in location between the perfusion deficit, and the area of abnormal delayed-enhancement. They may or may not be less apparent on the rest study depending on the degree to which they hyperenhance.

The frequent finding of hyperenhancement of areas of prior infarction and the resultant decrease in sensitivity for visualization of a perfusion deficit is one reason why stress perfusion should be performed prior to resting perfusion imaging.

An additional RF artifact is seen on all of the standard delayed-enhancement images, causing a straight line of high signal dots across the image, in the phase-encode direction.

Diagnosis

Normal adenosine stress perfusion imaging study without evidence of ischemia. Artifacts are noted, but do not significantly limit the study.

Adenosine has advantages over Persantine, in that it has a more rapid onset and offset of action.

Its half-life is approximately 10 seconds. Contraindications to its use include a history of asthma, severe bronchospasm, or heart block.

Adenosine stress is useful in the detection of epicardial coronary artery disease in that it produces a four or five-fold increase in flow in the territory supplied by a normal epicardial coronary artery. However, in the territory supplied by a stenotic vessel that cannot dilate in response to adenosine differential flow will be observed, which will result in a dark region on the perfusion images, signifying a perfusion deficit.

The perfusion imaging sequence used in these examples is a Siemens turbo-FLASH T1-weighted acquisition with a preceding saturation pulse in order to diminish the residual transverse magnetization and to accentuate T1 weighting. The imaging sequence and the preceding saturation pulse result in an imaging time of 150 to 160 ms per slice, which means that 4 slices will take approximately 640 ms. The R-R interval is approximately 640 ms at a heart rate of approximately 95 beats per minute. Therefore, when the heart rate is higher than 95, the operator will usually needed to decrease the number of slices to 3/ cycle. It is important, however, to position the slices to ensure comprehensive LV coverage.

General Electric uses a notched interleaved saturation perfusion sequence, and acquires 6 to 8 slices, with each slice obtained at every other heartbeat.[1]

Perfusion imaging has been well validated in various comparative studies with SPECT imaging. Most studies have demonstrated slight superiority of MR perfusion imaging versus SPECT,[2] and clearly MR is superior in the detection of infarcts.[3–6]

Research studies have emphasized quantitative analysis of the perfusion upslope curves, but visual analysis of the image data is most often used in the clinical setting. Stress and rest perfusion images are scored for perfusion defects in 16 segments (segment 17 at the apex usually is not visualized). Then, a systematic stepwise approach is used to determine the presence or absence of coronary artery disease. Importantly, we use an interpretation algorithm (Chapter 2, Figure 2.5) that includes data from delayed enhancement imaging to improve the accuracy of detecting coronary artery disease over that of perfusion imaging alone. Using this interpretation algorithm, a CMR stress test is deemed "positive for CAD" if myocardial infarction is present on DE-MRI OR if perfusion defects are present during stress imaging, but absent at rest ("reversible" defect) in the absence of infarction. Conversely, the test is deemed "negative for CAD" if no abnormalities are found (e.g. no MI and no stress/rest perfusion defects) OR if perfusion defects are seen at both stress and rest imaging ("matched" defect) in the absence of infarction. In the latter, matched defects are regarded as artifacts and not suggestive of CAD. When both DE-MRI and stress perfusion MRI are abnormal, the test is scored positive for ischemia if the perfusion defect is larger than the area of infarction. For further discussion of the interpretation algorithm, please refer to Chapter 2.

The interpretation algorithm is based on two simple principles. First, with perfusion MRI and DE-MRI, there are two independent methods to obtain information regarding the presence or absence of myocardial infarction (MI). Thus, one method could be used to confirm the results of the other. Second, DE-MRI image quality (e.g. signal-to-noise ratio) is far better than perfusion MRI since it is less demanding in terms of scanner hardware (DE-MRI images can be built up over several seconds rather than in 0.1 seconds as is required for first-pass perfusion). Thus, DE-MRI should be more accurate for the diagnosis of MI, and the presence of infarction on DE-MRI favors the diagnosis of CAD, irrespective of the perfusion MRI results. Conceptually, it then follows that perfusion defects that have similar intensity and extent during both stress and rest ("matched" defect) but do not have infarction on DE-MRI are artifactual and should not be considered positive for CAD (with rare exceptions). Concerning this latter point, it is important to recognize that the interpretation of stress/rest perfusion MRI is NOT analogous to stress/rest radionuclide imaging. For instance, "matched" defects on perfusion MRI are more far likely to represent artifact than prior myocardial infarction. Additionally, infarcted regions—particularly those that are large and transmural—often appear "reversible" on perfusion MRI. This is because infarcted regions will accumulate the contrast given during the stress perfusion imaging stage, and during rest perfusion imaging, (10–15 minutes later), these regions may not show a perfusion defect (hypointensity) since delayed "hyperenhancement" to some degree is already present.

References

1. Slavin GS, et al. First-pass myocardial perfusion MR imaging with interleaved notched saturation: feasibility study. Radiology. 2001;219(1):258–263.
2. Ishida N, et al. Noninfarcted myocardium: correlation between dynamic first-pass contrast-enhanced myocardial MR imaging and quantitative coronary angiography. Radiology. 2003;229(1):209–216.
3. Klem I., et al. Improved detection of coronary artery disease by stress perfusion cardiovascular magnetic resonance with the use of delayed enhancement infarction imaging. J Am Coll Cardiol. 2006;47(8):1630–1638.
4. Wagner A, et al. MR imaging of myocardial perfusion and viability. Magn Reson Imaging Clin N Am. 2003;11(1):49–66.
5. Wagner A, et al. Contrast-enhanced MRI and routine single photon emission computed tomography (SPECT) perfusion imaging for detection of subendocardial myocardial infarcts: an imaging study. Lancet. 2003;361(9355):374–379.
6. Lee DC, et al. Magnetic resonance versus radionuclide pharmacological stress perfusion imaging for flow-limiting stenoses of varying severity. Circulation. 2004;110(1):58–65.

Teaching File Case 10

65-year-old female with recurrent chest pain

Category: Stress test

History

She also has a history of hypertension.

Findings

The short-axis views demonstrate mild concentric left ventricular hypertrophy, with preserved left ventricular global and regional wall motion. The left ventricular ejection fraction is greater than 55%.

The right ventricle is normal in size and function.

Evaluation of the valvular structures suggests the presence of mitral valve prolapse. Mild mitral regurgitation is noted.

Perfusion images demonstrate a focal area of diminished perfusion in the inferior wall on the stress images that shows significant improvement on the resting images.

3-D volumetric delayed-enhancement images show no evidence of infarction in this region. The patient had difficulty with breath holding, and therefore the standard segmented delayed-enhancement inversion recovery images were not obtained.

Diagnosis

Inferior wall inducible ischemia secondary to right coronary artery disease, without evidence of prior infarction.

In this case, a true perfusion deficit is quite apparent. However, in other cases, the finding may be more equivocal or difficult to distinguish from subendocardial dark-rim artifact.[1] Clues to the correct diagnosis of a true perfusion deficit include 1) persistence for at least 4 or 5 heartbeats, 2) extension of the dark signal intensity region into the myocardium and not simply the subendocardium, and 3) clear-cut evidence of change between the stress and rest images.[2] In addition, the deficit should follow a vascular territory. This latter distinction can sometimes be difficult in cases of postoperative evaluation.

Comparison with the delayed-enhancement images is also critical in order to distinguish regions of prior infarction with residual microvascular disease from areas of inducible ischemia. In this case, 3-D images were used for this purpose. No evidence of prior infarction is noted, and therefore the perfusion defect noted signifies the presence of ischemia.

References

1. Di Bella EV, Parker DL, Sinusas AJ. On the dark rim artifact in dynamic contrast-enhanced MRI myocardial perfusion studies. Magn Reson Med. 2005;54(5):1295–1299.
2. Klem I, et al. Improved detection of coronary artery disease by stress perfusion cardiovascular magnetic resonance with the use of delayed-enhancement infarction imaging. J Am Coll Cardiol. 2006;47(8): 1630–1638.

Teaching File Case 11

54-year-old white male, status—post recent MI

Category: Viability

History

Echo shows low ejection fraction.

Findings

The left ventricular cavity is mildly dilated. Wall motion analysis indicates akinesia progressing to dyskinesia of the anterior wall as one proceeds from the mid-ventricular level to the apex. No significant thinning is noted, but no thickening during systole is apparent, either.

Perfusion images demonstrate a large nonperfused region along the anterior wall of the left ventricle.

Postcontrast images demonstrate nonenhancing mural thrombus lining a large aneurysm of the anterior wall, best appreciated on the pre- and postcontrast 2-chamber views seen in the second row.

Evaluation of the valvular structures demonstrates fusion of the noncoronary and the right coronary cusps with impaired valvular opening and insignificant aortic stenosis. Trace aortic insufficiency is also apparent.

Delayed-enhancement imaging demonstrates that on images with a short inversion time, a large infarction that is essentially transmural is noted in the anterior wall from the base to the apex, becoming progressively more circumferential near the apex. Evidence of a large mural thrombus is noted, but since it is below the zero-crossing line on short inversion recovery images, it appears high in signal. This appearance can be confusing. However, single-shot inversion recovery images with a long inversion time (first, third, and fifth images of the fourth row) demonstrate clearly that the thrombus is low in signal intensity, confirming its nonvascular nature.

Diagnosis

Anterior infarction with aneurysm formation and secondary mural thrombus.

This represents a true ventricular aneurysm, secondary to a large anterior wall infarction. It is complicated by extensive mural thrombus formation. It involves the anterior wall, as is most common with this form of aneurysm. It has a wide "mouth," and layers of myocardium remain, consistent with this diagnosis.[1]

Interestingly, the large thrombus was not seen on echo. Several studies have demonstrated the superiority of contrast-enhanced MR imaging as compared to echo for the detection of ventricular thrombi. It is estimated that echo may fail to detect from 50 to 60% of thrombi that are detected with MR.[2]

Thrombus can be difficult to detect without contrast, but are quite evident after contrast administration. In our experience, the delayed-enhancement sequence with a long inversion time is the most sensitive for the detection of thrombus.[3] On this sequence, only thrombus and fluid remain low in signal intensity when an inversion time of 550–700 msec is used.

References

1. Konen E, et al. True versus false left ventricular aneurysm: differentiation with MR imaging–initial experience. Radiology. 2005;236(1):65–70.
2. Srichai MB, et al. Clinical, imaging, and pathological characteristics of left ventricular thrombus: a comparison of contrast-enhanced magnetic resonance imaging, transthoracic echocardiography, and transesophageal echocardiography with surgical or pathological validation. Am Heart J. 2006;152(1):75–84.
3. Bruder O, et al. [Detection and characterization of left ventricular thrombi by MRI compared to transthoracic echocardiography]. Rofo. 2005;177(3): 344–349.

Teaching File Case 12

23-year-old male with a diagnosis of spondyloepiphyseal dysplasia

Category: Technical/VEC

History

The study is performed to evaluate the aortic valve. The patient is on hemodialysis.

Findings

The left ventricle is noted to demonstrate concentric hypertrophy. The regional and global systolic function is normal.

The right ventricle is normal in size and function.

Evaluation of valvular structures demonstrates severe aortic stenosis, with a markedly diminished opening that is measured at approximately 0.54 sq cm. The patient is small in size, and the aortic root is noted to be small in size as well, measuring approximately 2 cm in diameter. Velocity-encoded flow phase contrast images are seen as the fourth through sixth images of the third row. The phase-reconstructed images (fourth and sixth images) demonstrate that apparent signal reversal is noted in the systolic images of the fourth image that is not present on the sixth image. This represents aliasing. The fourth image, which demonstrates aliasing was obtained with a peak velocity (or Venc) of 300cm/sec while the fourth image is obtained with a Venc of 500 cm/sec. The measured peak velocity was 440 cm/sec, consistent with a gradient of 80 mmHg. The mitral valve is unremarkable in appearance.

The MR angiogram demonstrates that the aorta is small in size but is commensurate with the patient's small body habitus.

Delayed-enhancement imaging demonstrates a small focus of hyperenhancement in the inferior wall at the basal level.

A dialysis access catheter is noted in place in the superior vena cava, and extends into the right atrium. Delayed-enhancement imaging demonstrates a small amount of pericatheter thrombus.

Diagnosis

Severe aortic stenosis is demonstrated. Several different mucopolysaccharidoses can result in aortic valve pathology,[1] but a definite association with spondyloepiphyseal dysplasia has not been reported.

There are two techniques for the CMR quantification of aortic stenosis: direct planimetry of the valve area, and phase contrast velocity-encoded imaging.

Recent papers have demonstrated an excellent correlation between measurements of the cross-sectional area of the aortic valve opening on transesophageal echo with planimetry using small field-of-view SSFP cine images. Therefore, it may compete with transesophageal echo for quantification of aortic stenosis.[2] Further information about the utility of CMR for the evaluation of aortic stenosis may be found in Chapter 4.

MR imaging also has the additional advantage of providing a more comprehensive assessment of the global systolic function, as well as providing information regarding the presence or absence of myocardial scarring.[3]

This case is included here as it demonstrates the use of phase contrast velocity-encoded flow imaging. In this form of imaging, velocity encoding phase shifts result from the sequential application of bipolar magnetic field gradients, which are composed of two lobes with opposite polarities. These opposed gradients will produce a phase shift with the first pulse that will be reversed by the second pulse. Therefore, stationary spins will acquire equal and opposite phases in the two gradients, and will have no net phase at the end of the sequence. However, flowing spins will acquire a net phase change, which will be dependent on their velocity in the direction of the flow-encoding gradients. Gradients can be varied in amplitude or duration to sensitize the pulse sequence to fast or slow flow. The Venc is the maximum velocity-encoded by the sequence and is selected by the operator.[4, 5]

The maximum value or Venc selected should just exceed the anticipated velocities to be measured. Aliasing occurs when the maximum velocity sampled exceeds the upper limit imposed by the chosen Venc, resulting in apparent velocity reversal. To avoid aliasing the velocity threshold must be correctly selected. However, care must be taken not to set the Venc too high as a maximum velocity that is much higher than the peak velocity will result in increased noise and reduced precision.

Aliasing will result in artifactual reduction of the measured flow, in direct proportion to the extent of aliasing, and therefore accurate flow measurements require its recognition. It is recognized in the velocity images where the voxels of assumed peak velocities have an inverted signal intensity compared with that of surrounding voxels. In the present case, aliasing is noted on the fourth image series of the third row.

With sequences currently available, phase contrast measurement can be performed in a breath hold. Both the magnitude and phase images are often reviewed. Magnitude and phase images of a bicuspid aortic valve may be seen in Chapter 1, Figure 1.9. For further discussion of velocity-encoded flow-sensitive sequences, please refer to Chapter 1.

These sequences are typically used in two situations—quantification of gradients across stenotic valves, and for measurement of flow. The peak gradient across a stenotic valve can be calculated using the Bernouilli equation – $\Delta P = 4 V^2$ where velocity V is in meters per second, and the gradient is given in mm Hg. On most scanners, the velocities are given in cm/sec, and must be converted to m/sec for the calculation.

References

1. Mohan UR, et al. Cardiovascular changes in children with mucopolysaccharide disorders. Acta Paediatr. 2002;91(7):799–804.
2. Kupfahl C, et al. Evaluation of aortic stenosis by cardiovascular magnetic resonance imaging: comparison with established routine clinical techniques. Heart. 2004;90(8):893–901.
3. Elliott MD, Kim RJ. Late gadolinium cardiovascular magnetic resonance in the assessment of myocardial viability. Coron Artery Dis. 2005;16(6): 365–372.
4. Lotz J, et al. Cardiovascular flow measurement with phase-contrast MR imaging: basic facts and implementation. Radiographics. 2002;22(3): 651–671.
5. Glockner, J.F., D.L. Johnston, and K.P. McGee, Evaluation of cardiac valvular disease with MR imaging: qualitative and quantitative techniques. Radiographics. 2003;23(1):e9.

Teaching File Case 13

33-year-old male with fatigability and shortness of breath

Category: Technical/VEC

History

A murmur was noted on physical exam.

Findings

The left ventricular cavity is mildly dilated, but has normal wall thickness and normal systolic function. The right ventricle is normal in appearance. The left atrium is unremarkable, as is the right atrium.

Evaluation of the valvular structures demonstrates a bicuspid aortic valve with an eccentric jet of aortic insufficiency manifested as a thin region of dark signal intensity emanating from the valve leaflets, and extending into the LV cavity.

Velocity-encoded measurements demonstrate that there is mild aortic stenosis, and a regurgitant fraction of approximately 33%.

Delayed-enhancement imaging shows no evidence of prior infarction.

Diagnosis

The patient has a bicuspid aortic valve, which has become insufficient. The patient was known to have a bicuspid valve for many years, but has only become symptomatic lately, likely due to the superimposed insufficiency.

Many case of aortic insufficiency are of unclear etiology.[1] Degenerative change in a bicuspid valve is one of the more common identifiable causes of AI.

This case demonstrates the utility of MR imaging in the quantification of aortic insufficiency as well as the assessment of left ventricular function. The same velocity-encoded phase contrast sequences that are used to calculate gradients can also be used to measure flow.[2–4] However, care must be taken in the use of velocity-encoded imaging for the evaluation of flow when there is significant turbulence producing spin dephasing, such as in aortic or mitral insufficiency. In instances such as the present case, a more reliable means of determining the regurgitant volume entails measurement of the antegrade flow through the pulmonic valve, which is subtracted from the antegrade flow through the aortic valve; the difference represents the aortic regurgitant volume, presuming there is no pulmonic insufficiency. For further discussion on the use of velocity-encoded flow-sensitive sequences for the quantification of regurgitant valvular lesions, please also see Chapter 4.

References

1. Roberts WC, et al. Causes of pure aortic regurgitation in patients having isolated aortic valve replacement at a single US tertiary hospital (1993 to 2005). Circulation. 2006;114(5):422–429.
2. Buonocore MH, Bogren H. Factors influencing the accuracy and precision of velocity-encoded phase imaging. Magn Reson Med. 1992;26(1):141–154.
3. Glockner, J.F., D.L. Johnston, and K.P. McGee, Evaluation of cardiac valvular disease with MR imaging: qualitative and quantitative techniques. Radiographics. 2003; 23(1):e9.
4. Gelfand EV, et al. Severity of mitral and aortic regurgitation as assessed by cardiovascular magnetic resonance: optimizing correlation with Doppler echocardiography. J Cardiovasc Magn Reson. 2006;8(3): 503–507.

Teaching File Case 14

20-year-old female with a history of Ehlers-Danlos syndrome

Category: Technical/Angiography

History

The study is performed to exclude an aneurysm.

Findings

MR angiography was performed using the large field-of-view afforded by a state of the art 1.5 Tesla magnet. A 450mm field-of-view was used, which in this small patient allowed comprehensive chest, abdomen, and pelvis MR angiography with one injection.

No focal aneurysm is seen. The great vessel origins are normal in appearance. Volume rendered and color volume rendered images are demonstrated, along with maximum intensity projection images.

The fourth image of the second row is a VIBE sequence, which is a heavily T1-weighted fat-saturated 3-D volumetric acquisition. It is obtained in the axial plane in the present instance.

Diagnosis

Normal magnetic resonance angiogram.

MR angiography is performed using thin section T1-weighted imaging during the arterial passage of contrast administration. Synchronization of the image acquisition with the arterial passage of contrast is most often performed by using fluoroscopic monitoring of the contrast passage, with scan initiation triggered after visualization in the appropriate region.[1,2] This will be shown in subsequent cases.

Multiple thin slices are obtained in a 3-D volumetric technique, and are then assembled into maximum intensity projection images, as well as volume rendered images. Multi-planar review of the obtained images is also performed, in order to visualize the vessels in cross-section and to study their walls.

Images in the present case were acquired in the coronal plane, as information was desired about the subclavian and pelvic vessels as well as the aorta. It should be noted that the plane of imaging is freely selectable with MR angiography, but by convention, the studies are usually performed in either the sagittal or coronal plane.

The slice resolution, the slice thickness, and the volume of coverage are all selectable parameters. Increasing slice resolution will increase imaging time, as will diminishing slice thickness for a given volume of acquisition. To see a graphical representation of these trade-offs, please refer to Chapter 6, Figure 6.2. Therefore, in situations where breath holding would be required such as in chest and abdomen MR angiography, the duration of the acquisition becomes the limiting factor. A breath-hold exceeding 25 seconds becomes problematic for most patients, and imaging should generally be completed within this time frame.

MR angiography has been well validated in a variety of vascular regions, most notably for evaluation of renal artery stenosis where it compares very favorably with digital subtraction angiography.[3,4] It is also been well accepted for abdominal, pelvic, and lower extremity runoff imaging for comprehensive multistation evaluation of the peripheral vasculature in patients likely to require revascularization. It has advantages over conventional catheter and CT angiography in that no radiation or potentially nephrotoxic contrast is required. The examination can be performed in 30 minutes. No arterial puncture is required.[5,6]

References

1. Earls JP, et al. Breath-hold single-dose gadolinium-enhanced three-dimensional MR aortography: usefulness of a timing examination and MR power injector. Radiology. 1996;201(3):705–710.
2. Hany TF, et al. Optimization of contrast timing for breath-hold three-dimensional MR angiography. J Magn Reson Imaging. 1997;7(3):551–556.
3. Hany TF, et al. Evaluation of the aortoiliac and renal arteries: comparison of breath-hold, contrast-enhanced, three-dimensional MR angiography with conventional catheter angiography. Radiology. 1997;204(2): 357–362.
4. Yucel EK, C.L. Dumoulin, and A.C. Waltman, MR angiography of lower-ex tremity arterial disease: preliminary experience. J Magn Reson Imaging. 1992; 2(3):303–309.
5. Fenchel M., et al. Whole-body MR angiography using a novel 32-receiving-channel MR system with surface coil technology: first clinical experience. J Magn Reson Imaging. 2005;21(5):596–603.
6. Steffens JC, et al. Bolus-chasing contrast-enhanced 3D MRA of the lower extremity. Comparison with intraarterial DSA. Acta Radiol. 2003;44(2):185–192.

Teaching File Case 15

56-year-old male with lower leg pain

Category: Technical/Angiography

Findings

The vasculature is unremarkable. In the upper row, a time-resolved imaging sequence at the lower leg station is displayed first. The second image series are MR fluoroscopic images used to trigger the acquisition. Rotating maximum intensity projection (MIP) images of the abdomen-pelvis station comprise the next 2 images. A still and rotating series of images of the upper legs are then shown, and the final image of the upper row is a rotating MIP display of the lower leg vessels. The second row of images represents sequential imaging from the abdomen/pelvis to the upper legs to the lower legs.

Diagnosis

This is a normal MR angiographic imaging study.

This study is performed with T1-weighted 3-D volumetric acquisitions of the abdomen, pelvis, and lower extremities. Initial noncontrast image acquisitions are obtained, which will serve as mask images for later subtraction. Subsequently, contrast is administered, at a slow rate in order to promote arterial opacification and to minimize venous contamination. Usually, 40 cc of contrast are administered, at approximately 1.4 cc/sec for the first 20 cc, and at 0.5 cc/sec for the remainder. Image acquisitions in the upper stations must be obtained rapidly in order to minimize the likelihood of venous contamination at the level of the lower leg.

The image acquisitions have to be synchronized to the arterial passage of contrast. There are two main strategies for performing this. The first is the use of a timing bolus, where 2 cc of gadolinium are administered, and sequential one per second images of the abdomen are obtained. The time delay for optimal opacification is then calculated, and imaging planned to coincide with the contrast passage.

The second technique involves continuous MR fluoroscopic visualization of the abdomen station, with triggering upon visualization of contrast entering the abdominal aorta. This technique is usually preferred, as variations in cardiac output, venous filling, and IV functioning are automatically taken into account. This technique was used in this case.[1, 2]

Peripheral MR runoff angiography performs well in comparison with conventional catheter angiography, and in some reports, is superior for the detection of small crural runoff vessels. The main limitation is the frequent finding of venous contamination that can vary from the level of a nuisance that minimally degrades image quality to a finding that significantly compromises image interpretation. Various strategies for minimizing venous contamination have been developed.

The first involves the use of inflated blood pressure cuffs about the thighs, which are inflated to a level of approximately 50 mmHg.[3] These must remain in place throughout the study, as any alteration would result in subtraction artifacts if there is any change between the mask images and the contrast-enhanced images. This technique has been shown to be reproducible and to slow arterial transit, and delay venous filling. However, bypass grafts must be handled cautiously, and some patients do not tolerate the cuff inflation well.

The second technique involves a hybrid methodology in which dedicated imaging of the lower leg is performed as the initial imaging segment of the study. The abdomen/pelvis and upper leg stations are subsequently performed in the usual way. This technique has 2 main implementations.

In the first implementation, a timing bolus is performed at the level of the knees, and 15 cc of contrast are injected at 1cc/sec along with 25 cc of flush at 1 cc/sec. Standard angiographic data sets are acquired. Two acquisitions are obtained to allow for any side-to-side variation in the rate of arterial filling.[4]

In the second technique, lower resolution time-resolved images are obtained without a timing bolus. In this instance, 8 cc of contrast are administered at 1 cc/sec with flush administered at the same rate. The injection and the image acquisition start simultaneously. The lower resolution angiographic data set is acquired in 9 seconds, and repeated acquisitions are obtained for a total of 12 to 15 acquisitions. An initial scout exam is also obtained to allow subtraction of the subsequent data sets. This technique allows for assessment of the rapidity of filling, and is robust, in that venous contamination never obscures arterial opacification.

A time-resolved sequence of the lower leg station comprises the first image set of this exam. Subsequently, runoff angiography is performed in the standard fashion, with fluoroscopic triggering of the abdominal station. This is acquired in approximately 13 seconds. The table is then moved to the upper leg level, and imaging of the upper leg stations performed which takes approximately 18 seconds. Additional imaging of the lower legs is then performed at higher resolution. This takes approximately 23 seconds.

The resulting images can be displayed as rotating MIP data sets as shown here. Alternatively, still frame images can also be generated as seen in the second row.

Although the maximum intensity projection images allow a quick assessment of patency and anatomy, review of the source images in a multiplanar format at a dedicated workstation is strongly suggested. The maximum intensity projection algorithm can result in obscuration of filling defects and subtle lesions. To see an example of this pitfall of MIP imaging, please refer to Chapter 6, Figure 6.3. In addition, recognition of stent artifact frequently requires review of the source images. Incidental findings noted in other areas are also best detected on review of source images.

References

1. Hany TF, et al. Optimization of contrast timing for breath-hold three-dimensional MR angiography. J Magn Reson Imaging. 1997;7(3):551–556.
2. Wilman AH, et al. Fluoroscopically triggered contrast-enhanced three-dimensional MR angiography with elliptical centric view order: application to the renal arteries. Radiology. 1997;205(1):137–146.
3. Zhang HL, et al. Decreased venous contamination on 3D gadolinium-enhanced bolus chase peripheral mr angiography using thigh compression. AJR Am J Roentgenol. 2004;183(4):1041–1047.
4. Pereles FS, et al. Accuracy of stepping-table lower extremity MR angiography with dual-level bolus timing and separate calf acquisition: hybrid peripheral MR angiography. Radiology. 2006;240(1):283–290.

Teaching File Case 16

53-year-old man with hypertension, rule out renal artery stenosis

Category: Angiography

Findings

The angiographic images demonstrate that there are two right renal arteries that are small in size but are patent without narrowing. There is an approximately 75% stenosis of the left renal artery, which is single. The volume-rendered images also demonstrate these findings. The sagittal view demonstrates well a minimal deformity of the celiac axis, without narrowing. A moderate right common iliac narrowing is also apparent. Note the fifth image series, which consist of images obtained as a small bolus of contrast is administered.

Diagnosis

Left renal artery stenosis. Two right renal arteries. Median arcuate ligament impression on the celiac axis.

Renal artery imaging with MR has been shown to have excellent sensitivity and specificity for the detection of significant renal arterial narrowing. It is comparable to DSA in its accuracy, but does not require an arterial puncture or nephrotoxic contrast. It has largely replaced other imaging tests for the diagnosis of renal artery stenosis.

The MR angiographic data set is acquired in the coronal plane, using heavily T1-weighted spoiled gradient echo images. Present scanner technology allows for near isotropic in-plane resolution of approximately 1 to 1.5 mm. High resolution imaging is necessary, given that the normal diameter of the renal arteries ranges from approximately 5 to 8 mm, and detection of stenosis requires the ability to detect very small changes in caliber.[1]

The scans must be acquired during the arterial phase of contrast passage, and therefore the scan acquisition has to be synchronized to this phase of contrast transit. This can be performed with a timing bolus, where a small amount (2cc) of contrast is given and sequential axial images are obtained through the abdominal aorta at the level of the renal arteries until the contrast bolus is visualized. The appropriate scan delay is then calculated.[2] This was the technique used in this case.

The second means of synchronizing the image acquisition with the contrast passage is the use of fluoroscopic triggering wherein multiple coronal images are obtained as the contrast is administered, with triggering performed when the abdominal aorta is clearly visualized.[3] Both techniques work well.

One drawback of using the timing bolus technique is the subsequent presence of the administered contrast within the collecting systems, which can obscure some of the hilar portions of the renal vessels.

Accessory renal arteries are found in approximately 25–30% of patients, and are particularly important in the evaluation of prospective renal donors.[4]

The median arcuate ligament of the diaphragm is noted to sometimes produce kinking of the celiac axis on images obtained at end-expiration. Often, repeating the images in inspiration will demonstrate significant resolution of this finding.[5]

References

1. Leung DA, et al. MR angiography of the renal arteries. Radiol Clin North Am. 002;40(4):847–85.
2. Earls JP, et al. Breath-hold single-dose gadolinium-enhanced three-dimensional MR aortography: usefulness of a timing examination and MR power injector. Radiology. 1996;01(3):705–70.
3. Wilman AH, et al. Fluoroscopically triggered contrast-enhanced three-dimensional MR angiography with elliptical centric view order: application to the renal arteries. Radiology. 1997;05(1): 137–146.
4. Israel GM, et al. Comprehensive MR imaging in the preoperative evaluation of living donor candidates for laparoscopic nephrectomy: initial experience. Radiology. 2002;225(2):427–432.
5. Lee VS, et al. Celiac artery compression by the median arcuate ligament: a pitfall of end-expiratory MR imaging. Radiology. 2003;228(2):437–442.

Teaching File Case 17

59-year-old male with atrial fibrillation

Category: Technical/Angio

History

A pre-ablation pulmonary vein MR angiogram is requested.

Findings

The morphologic images obtained prior to the angiographic data set allow accurate positioning of the imaging slab for MR angiography. They also provide an overview of the pulmonary venous anatomy. These are dark-blood and bright-blood images as seen in the first 4 images of the upper right. Dark-blood imaging is performed with HASTE (half-Fourier acquisition turbo-spin echo) imaging, and bright-blood imaging is performed with steady-state free precession (SSFP or true FISP) imaging. These take approximately 45 seconds per each 30-image data set acquired.

The imaging volume should include the entire left atrium, and slice positioning is most often performed in either the axial or a modified axial plane. Other imaging planes may also be used, but attention must be paid to the spatial resolution along the axis in question.

Subsequently, after acquisition of the angiographic data set, maximum intensity projections can be created, along with volumetric imaging. Trimming of the images so as to optimally display the left atrium requires attention to the detail, so as not to trim away important structures. The result can be very helpful in understanding the sometimes complex anatomy.[1–3]

In the present example, 4 discrete pulmonary veins are seen entering the left atrium. The right middle lobe pulmonary vein joins the right upper lobe pulmonary vein, which is the most common pattern in our experience. The right lower lobe pulmonary vein, left upper, and left lower lobe pulmonary veins all have separate entrances into the left atrium.

The left atrial appendage is also well visualized.

The imaging can be performed with ECG gating, but given that many of these patients have significant arrhythmia, some centers perform this imaging without ECG triggering. The present exam was performed without ECG triggering.

Review of the morphologic imaging obtained at the beginning of the exam is important to establish the position of the esophagus relative to the left atrium and the pulmonary veins. Passage of the esophagus adjacent to the ostia of the pulmonary veins should be noted, as the esophagus may be injured during the radiofrequency ablation procedure.[4] In addition, creation of atrial-esophageal fistulae has been reported, with devastating consequences. In the present case, the esophagus is observed to pass in proximity to the ostium of the right lower lobe pulmonary vein.

Diagnosis

Normal pulmonary venous anatomy. The esophagus extends adjacent to the ostium of the right lower lobe pulmonary vein.

References

1. Vonken EP, et al. Contrast-enhanced MRA and 3D visualization of pulmonary venous anatomy to assist radiofrequency catheter ablation. J Cardiovasc Magn Reson. 2003;5(4):545–551.
2. Pilleul F, Merchant N. MRI of the pulmonary veins: comparison between 3D MR angiography and T1-weighted spin echo. J Comput Assist Tomogr. 2000;24(5):683–687.
3. Hauser TH, et al. A method for the determination of proximal pulmonary vein size using contrast-enhanced magnetic resonance angiography. J Cardiovasc Magn Reson. 2004;6(4):927–936.
4. Cury RC, et al. Relationship of the esophagus and aorta to the left atrium and pulmonary veins: implications for catheter ablation of atrial fibrillation. Heart Rhythm. 2005;2(12):1317–1323.

Teaching File Case 18

50-year-old male who has had recurrent embolic events with clots noted in the femoral and popliteal arteries bilaterally on different occasions

Category: Angio

History

The study is requested to evaluate for a possible aortic source.

Findings

The abdominal aortogram was unremarkable and showed no evidence of aneurysm. The thoracic aortogram is included here. The volume rendered images demonstrate no irregularity or plaque. No obvious aneurysm is seen.

Review of the source images in multiple planes demonstrates the presence of a small thrombus in the left atrium near the orifice of the left atrial appendage. This is best appreciated on the thin section reconstructions where it appears as a focus of low signal intensity and is dark on the post-contrast images.

Diagnosis

A small adherent thrombus is seen in the roof of the left atrium closely adjacent to the opening to the left atrial appendage.

Although the patient did not have a history of sustained atrial fibrillation, the clinicians caring for the patient felt it likely that he had intermittent paroxysmal atrial fibrillation, which predisposed him to the development of this thrombus.

The study illustrates the necessity for reviewing not only the volume rendered and maximum intensity projection full volume images, but the source images as well. Due to the technique used in the creation of maximum intensity projection images, filling defects such as thrombi can be easily missed if they are enclosed in high signal intensity material. Therefore, review of the source images in thin section (submaximal volume) mode is required to exclude filling defects.

The use of MR in the detection of left atrial and left atrial appendage thrombi has been the subject of two conflicting reports. One suggested an excellent sensitivity for the detection of thrombi, while the other suggested that thrombi were missed with an alarming frequency.[1, 2] However, a positive finding such as the present example is unlikely to represent artifact, and mandates appropriate therapy.

References

1. Mohrs OK, et al. Thrombus detection in the left atrial appendage using contrast-enhanced MRI: a pilot study. AJR Am J Roentgenol. 2006;186(1):198–205.
2. Ohyama H, Mizushige K, Hosomi N. Magnetic resonance imaging of left atrial thrombus. Heart. 2002;88(3):233.

Teaching File Case 19

71-year-old male with a history of chest pain and recent myocardial infarction

Category: Stress test

History

An MR stress test was requested.

Findings

The left ventricular cavity size is mildly dilated. The overall wall thickness is normal, but a focal area of thinning is seen in the inferior wall of the basal level. Regional wall motion analysis indicates that the inferior wall is akinetic, from the basal level to the mid-ventricular level. This is noted initially on the short-axis views and is confirmed on the 2-chamber view. The remainder of the left ventricular myocardium demonstrates normal wall motion.

The right ventricle is normal in size and function.

Evaluation of the valvular structures demonstrates mild mitral and tricuspid regurgitation. No significant aortic stenosis or insufficiency is seen.

The perfusion images demonstrate a focal area of diminished perfusion in the inferior wall at the basal and mid-ventricular levels, as well as at the apical level. The resting images in the third row demonstrate that this same region appears to show hyperenhancement prior to the administration of the second bolus of contrast.

Delayed-enhancement images demonstrate a large area of nearly transmural infarction involving the inferior wall, with involvement of the inferior portions of the septum and inferolateral walls at the basal level. The remainder of the myocardium appears viable.

Diagnosis

Infarction of the inferior wall at the basal and mid-ventricular levels, with involvement of the inferior septum and inferolateral walls.

The perfusion deficit noted corresponds with the area of prior infarction, except for perhaps a small focus at the apex. Therefore, there is minimal ischemia, with the perfusion deficit noted representing postinfarction microvasculature impairment.

Perfusion deficits may persist in regions affected previously by large areas of infarction, particularly when the infarction is nearly transmural as in the present example. Therefore, perfusion image analysis requires comparison not only with the resting perfusion images, but also with the delayed-enhancement images to ascertain which perfusion deficits represent infarctions and which perfusion deficits represent true ischemic myocardium that remains viable but at risk.[1–3]

Although the saturation-recovery FLASH perfusion sequence (as used throughout this teaching file) has been shown to be clinically useful, other options including True-Fisp saturation recovery perfusion sequences are the subject of research.[4]

References

1. Hunold, P., T. Schlosser, and J. Barkhausen, Magnetic resonance cardiac perfusion imaging-a clinical perspective. Eur Radiol. 2006;
2. Barkhausen, J., et al. Imaging of myocardial perfusion with magnetic resonance. J Magn Reson Imaging. 2004;19(6):750–7.
3. Arai, A.E., Magnetic resonance first-pass myocardial perfusion imaging. Top Magn Reson Imaging. 2000; 11(6):383–98.
4. Fenchel M., et al. Multislice first-pass myocardial perfusion imaging: Comparison of saturation recovery (SR)-TrueFISP-two-dimensional (2D) and SR-TurboFLASH-2D pulse sequences. J Magn Reson Imaging. 2004;19(5):555–63.

Teaching File Case 20

34-year-old male with a history of two prior cardiac surgeries

Category: Congenital

Findings

The left ventricular cavity is at the upper limits of normal in size. The wall thickness is also at the upper limits of normal in size, measuring 1.2 cm. The global and regional wall motion is normal. The left ventricular ejection fraction is greater than 60%.

The right ventricular size and function is unremarkable.

The most prominent finding is an abnormal aortic valve, with turbulence seen both in systole as well as diastole. Velocity-encoded measurements indicate a gradient of 55 mmHg in systole, and also demonstrate a 15% regurgitant fraction. The right coronary cusp is noted to be essentially immobile. The left and noncoronary cusps demonstrate mobility, and there is a suggestion that the noncoronary leaflet is flail. (The non-coronary cusp abuts the inter-atrial septum, while the left cusp can be recognized by its proximity to the left atrial appendage).

The mitral and tricuspid valves are unremarkable in appearance.

Delayed-enhancement imaging is normal except for a small focus at the left ventricular apex. No other scar formation is seen.

MR angiographic images of the aorta demonstrate that there is an outwardly convex bulge in the ascending portion of the aorta, and the aorta has a maximum diameter 4.5 cm.

Diagnosis

By history, this patient had undergone prior valvuloplasty of a bicuspid aortic valve. The noncoronary cusp is now flail, and there is immobility of the right coronary cusp, with extensive aortic stenosis noted. Aortic insufficiency is evident as well.[1,2] The 15% regurgitant fraction was calculated from the velocity-encoded phase contrast images, and may underestimate the regurgitant fraction due to loss of signal secondary to spin dephasing. A more accurate value can be obtained from comparison of the antegrade flow volumes through the aortic root and the proximal pulmonary artery. The difference between these measurements represents the regurgitant volume.

Bicuspid aortic valve is the most common congenital cardiac abnormality.[3, 4] It is estimated to occur in between 1 and 2% of the population. Associated cardiac defects are seen in approximately 20% of such patients, including coarctation of the aorta, which is the most common coexisting abnormality. Patent ductus arteriosus and ventricular septal defects are also associated. A left dominant coronary circulation is more common in patients with bicuspid aortic valve, with an incidence of 30 to 50% in this population.

Bicuspid aortic valves typically have a "fish-mouth" appearance, resulting from fusion of one of the commisures, with two rather than three valve leaflets present, although a third raphe may be seen. This case is atypical, likely the result of prior surgery, with prior commissurotomy having been performed. The prior commissurotomy likely separated the left and non- coronary cusp, but with resultant flail appearance of the non- coronary cusp.

Bicuspid aortic valve is associated with the development of aneurysmal dilatation of the ascending aorta. This is seen even in the absence of a significant eccentric jet, suggesting that a dysplasia of the formation of the media of the aortic wall may be responsible.

The etiology of the small apical scar is uncertain, but may be related to the patient's prior surgery.

References

1. Krombach GA, et al. Cine MR imaging of heart valve dysfunction with segmented true fast imaging with steady state free precession. J Magn Reson Imaging. 2004;19(1):59–67.
2. Rao V, et al. Aortic valve repair for adult congenital heart disease: A 22-year experience. Circulation. 2000;102(19 Suppl 3):III40–43.
3. Yener N, et al. Bicuspid aortic valve. Ann Thorac Cardiovasc Surg. 2002;8(5):264–267.
4. Zeppilli P, et al. Bicuspid aortic valve: an innocent finding or a potentially life-threatening anomaly whose complications may be elicited by sports activity? J Cardiovasc Med (Hagerstown). 2006;7(4): 282–287.

Teaching File Case 21

69-year-old male with unstable angina

Category: Stress test

Findings

Cine images demonstrate that the left ventricle is normal in size and overall function. The regional wall motion is normal throughout, except for a small region of hypokinesia in the anterior septum at the basal level. Minimal thinning in this region is suspected as well.

The right ventricle is normal in size and function.

Evaluation of the valvular structures demonstrates no significant regurgitant lesion.

Adenosine stress perfusion imaging demonstrates an extensive perfusion deficit in the anteroseptal and anterior wall at the basal and mid-ventricular levels, with extension to involve the anterior septum and anterior wall of the apical region as well. This area appears normal at rest.

Delayed-enhancement images demonstrate a very tiny area of infarction in the anteroseptal wall at the basal level, and the remainder of the myocardium is entirely viable.

Diagnosis

Anteroseptal and anterior wall ischemia. Tiny area of myocardial infarction in the anterior septum.

The above-demonstrated example represents a comprehensive approach to the noninvasive diagnosis of coronary artery disease.

A recent study using this protocol demonstrated that the combination of perfusion imaging and delayed-enhancement cardiac MR imaging had a sensitivity of 89%, a specificity of 87%, as well as an accuracy of 88% for the diagnosis of coronary artery disease signified by the presence of a greater than 70% stenotic lesion. The combination of delayed-enhancement imaging with perfusion imaging resulted in significant improvement over the performance of perfusion imaging alone which had a sensitivity of 84%, but a specificity of only 58%. The exceptionally high specificity of delayed-enhancement imaging was largely responsible for this improved performance.[1] In the present example, it can be clearly seen that the perfusion deficit is significantly larger than the small area of infarction, indicating significant inducible ischemia.

Importantly, only visual interpretation was performed in that study. No cumbersome analytic tools were used other than simple visual evaluation. Therefore, the study could be performed and interpreted rapidly. The interpretation algorithm is shown in Chapter 2, Figure 2.5.

Another group also evaluating the use of first pass perfusion MR imaging along with delayed-enhancement imaging demonstrated similar findings. That group also demonstrated that the combination of stress first pass perfusion and delayed-enhancement MR imaging had a sensitivity of 87% with a specificity of 89% and accuracy of 88% compared with coronary angiography in the detection of coronary artery narrowing greater than 70%.[2]

References

1. Klem I, et al. Improved detection of coronary artery disease by stress perfusion cardiovascular magnetic resonance with the use of delayed-enhancement infarction imaging. J Am Coll Cardiol. 2006;47(8):1630–1638.
2. Cury RC, et al. Diagnostic performance of stress perfusion and delayed-enhancement MR imaging in patients with coronary artery disease. Radiology. 2006;240(1):39–45.

Teaching File Case 22

27-year-old male with end-stage renal disease on hemodialysis

Category: Pericardium

History

He has persistent jugular venous distention despite adequate dialysis.

Findings

The left ventricular cavity is mildly dilated, and mildly reduced global systolic function is evident. The left ventricular ejection fraction is 47%. The right ventricle demonstrates mild dilatation as well, with mildly reduced function.

Evaluation of the valvular structures demonstrates mild mitral regurgitation and mild tricuspid regurgitation. The aortic valve is trileaflet and normal in appearance.

The most striking finding is diffuse thickening of the pericardium, with evidence of complex fluid within the pericardial sac. In addition, a rounded mass lesion is seen superior to the left ventricle on the short-axis views at the basal and mid-ventricular levels. This measures approximately 2.2 cm in diameter. Images with a long inversion time demonstrate that this is low in signal intensity, consistent with thrombus.

The 4-chamber view demonstrates a septal bounce, a finding often associated with constrictive pericarditis. In addition, real-time images seen as the first two images of the second row demonstrate septal flattening/inversion on the first few images after a deep inspiration.

Diagnosis

Dialysis-asociated hemorrhagic pericarditis with intrapericardial thrombus apparent, and with resultant effusive/constrictive physiology.[1, 2]

Uremia is a common cause of pericarditis. It often results in a hemorrhagic effusion, and the frequency of its development is related to the adequacy of dialysis. Patients on chronic dialysis may also develop pericarditis with effusions, which may be worsened if they are excessively anticoagulated for hemodialysis.

In this case there is a complex pericardial effusion with signal characteristics of proteinaceous fluid and blood. A focal thrombus is seen just superior to the LV.

The pericardium is thickened, and there is evidence of constrictive physiology with minimally impaired diastolic filling and a paradoxical septal bounce.[2–4] A septal bounce, or "shivering septum" has been reported to be present in up to 85% of patients with constrictive pericarditis. Real-time imaging provides a more direct method of visualizing the altered physiology. Imaging during a deep inspiration shows that there is abnormal ventricular interdependence such that augmentation of RV filling results in right-to-left septal displacement. This finding has been reported to be present in patients with constrictive pericarditis but absent in those with restrictive cardiomyopathy.[5] To see still frame images demonstrating this pathophysiology, please refer to Chapter 5, Figure 5.3. For further reading regarding pericardial disease, see also Chapter 5.

References

1. Glockner JF, Imaging of pericardial disease. Magn Reson Imaging Clin N Am. 2003;11(1):149–162, vii.
2. Srichai MB, Axel L. Magnetic resonance imaging in the management of pericardial disease. Curr Treat Options Cardiovasc Med. 2005;7(6):449–457.
3. Lima JA, Desai MY. Cardiovascular magnetic resonance imaging: current and emerging applications. J Am Coll Cardiol. 2004;44(6):1164–1171.
4. Arata MA, Reddy GP, Higgins CB. Organized pericardial hematomas: magnetic resonance imaging. J Cardiovasc Magn Reson. 2000;2(1):1–6.
5. Francone M, et al. Assessment of ventricular coupling with real-time cine MRI and its value to dfferentiate constrictive pericarditis from restrictive cardiomyopathy. Eur Radiol. 2006;16(4):944–951.

Teaching File Case 23

51-year-old male with a history of prior myocardial infarction, status–post PCI of the right coronary artery, sent for evaluation of ischemia and viability

Category: Stress test

Findings

The LV is normal in size and function with a left ventricular ejection fraction of 55%. The myocardial thickness is at the upper limits of normal measuring 1.2cm.

The wall motion appears normal throughout. The valvular structures are unremarkable.

The perfusion images demonstrate an area of diminished perfusion in the inferior basal wall on the stress images that is less apparent on the resting images. This finding is fairly subtle however.

Delayed-enhancement images demonstrate a very tiny subendocardial infarction of the inferoseptum at the basal level. The remainder of the myocardium is viable throughout.

Diagnosis

Ischemia is noted in the inferior wall (RCA territory), with a tiny area of infarction seen. However, the perfusion deficit far exceeds the region of the infarction, indicating residual inducible ischemia.[1–3]

Correlation of the perfusion images with the delayed-enhancement images is necessary to correctly determine which perfusion deficits are due to ischemia and which are due to infarction.[4] Therefore, it is quite helpful to have images displayed as they are in the present format, which allows easy comparison of various sequences obtained at the same spatial location. That is, the short-axis cine images in the top row are obtained at the same spatial locations as the corresponding stress (second row) and rest (third row) perfusion images. The delayed-enhancement images are also spatially matched to the cine and perfusion images. This facilitates comparison of suspected wall-motion abnormalities with perfusion defects and suspected infarctions. This comparison with the cine images is also useful in cases where there is difficulty discriminating the blood pool from an area of suspected subendocardial hyperenhancement.

References

1. Klem I, et al. Improved detection of coronary artery disease by stress perfusion cardiovascular magnetic resonance with the use of delayed-enhancement infarction imaging. J Am Coll Cardiol. 2006;47(8):1630–1638.
2. Mahrholdt H, et al. Left ventricular wall motion abnormalities as well as reduced wall thickness can cause false positive results of routine SPECT perfusion imaging for detection of myocardial infarction. Eur Heart J. 2005;26(20):2127–2135.
3. Barkhausen J, et al. Imaging of myocardial perfusion with magnetic resonance. J Magn Reson Imaging. 2004;19(6):750–757.
4. Arai AE. Magnetic resonance first-pass myocardial perfusion imaging. Top Magn Reson Imaging. 2000;11(6):383–398.

Teaching File Case 24

46-year-old female with chest pain

Category: Cardiomyopathy

History

She has a history of mild, well-controlled hypertension.

Findings

Concentric hypertrophy of the left ventricle is noted. This is quite profound, with measurements of approximately 2 cm in the anterior and posterior wall. The left ventricular cavity size is within normal limits. The ejection fraction is at the high end of normal, owing to the near obliteration of the cavity during systole. It measures approximately 70%. The left ventricular mass is measured 385 grams.

The right ventricular wall thickness is increased as well.

Evaluation of the valvular structures demonstrates that minimal systolic anterior motion of the mitral valve is apparent, with mild mitral regurgitation, and turbulence is seen in the left ventricular outflow tract extending through the aortic valve. However, phase contrast velocity-encoded images of the aortic valve demonstrated that it is trileaflet in appearance, and shows no significant stenosis. A very mild degree of aortic insufficiency is noted; less than 5%.

Images through the long axis of the aorta demonstrate a dissection flap, with a small jet of flow seen to extend through the proximal dissection flap just distal to the left subclavian artery. This is best appreciated on the fourth image of the second row.

Delayed-enhancement (DE) imaging subsequently performed was degraded by respiratory motion on the high-resolution static images. The single-shot DE images demonstrate diffuse abnormal enhancement in the left ventricular myocardium, with particular involvement of the anterior wall in a patchy, diffuse pattern.

Diagnosis

Hypertrophic cardiomyopathy (HCM). This is the most common genetic cardiac abnormality, with a prevalence of 1/500.

Extensive hypertrophy is apparent. Given the left ventricular outflow tract obstruction, this likely represents the variant of HCM known as hypertrophic obstructive cardiomyopathy. This is the most common pattern in the United States, with approximately 2/3 of patients with HCM demonstrating a pattern of hypertrophy with asymmetric septal involvement.[1]

Delayed-enhancement imaging has been reported to be abnormal in approximately 80% of patients with hypertrophic cardiomyopathy. The most common pattern of involvement is focal hyperenhancement of the RV insertion sites upon the septum as shown in Chapter 3, Figure 3.8, but diffuse enhancement such as evident in the present example has also been reported.[2–4]

Early reports suggest that there is likely a correlation between the degree of hyperenhancement, the degree of baseline ventricular myocardial thickening, and the degree of impairment of systolic function. The greater the baseline thickening in the myocardium, the greater impairment of systolic function, and the more likely the region will demonstrate hyperenhancement.[3]

Additionally, cardiac MRI may prove helpful in risk stratification, as patients with hypertrophic cardiomyopathy are known to be at risk for sudden death. In fact, hypertrophic cardiomyopathy is the most common cause of sudden cardiac death in patients under of 35 years of age. Initial reports suggest that the likelihood of progressive disease is associated with progressively greater degrees of hyperenhancement. For further discussion regarding the use of CMR in the evaluation of HCM, please refer to Chapter 3.

A type B aortic dissection is also apparent, beginning distal to the left subclavian artery, and extending into the abdomen. The relationship of this finding to the hypertrophic cardiomyopathy is uncertain. The MR imaging appearance is characteristic. The flap is clearly visualized on both cine and static images. An MR angiogram was subsequently performed, which allowed clear depiction of the branch vessels, and their respective origins from the true and false lumens.

References

1. Soler R, et al. Magnetic resonance imaging of primary cardiomyopathies. J Comput Assist Tomogr. 2003; 27(5):724–734.
2. Moon JC, et al. Toward clinical risk assessment in hypertrophic cardiomyopathy with gadolinium cardiovascular magnetic resonance. J Am Coll Cardiol. 2003;41(9):1561–1567.
3. Choudhury L, et al. Myocardial scarring in asymptomatic or mildly symptomatic patients with hypertrophic cardiomyopathy. J Am Coll Cardiol. 2002;40(12): 2156–2164.
4. Bogaert J, et al. Original report. Late myocardial enhancement in hypertrophic cardiomyopathy with contrast-enhanced MR imaging. AJR Am J Roentgenol. 2003;180(4):981–985.

Teaching File Case 25

51-year-old male with chest pain

Category: Stress test

Findings

Short-axis views demonstrate that the left ventricular thickness is at the upper limits of normal. The left ventricular cavity size is normal. The wall motion is normal throughout.

The right ventricle is normal in size and function.

Evaluation of the valvular structures shows that the patient has a mild degree of mitral regurgitation. The aortic valve is competent and normal in appearance. A trace amount of tricuspid insufficiency is noted.

Perfusion imaging demonstrates a well-defined perfusion defect in the anterolateral wall extending from the basal levels to the apical level. The resting images show no artifact to explain this finding.

Delayed-enhancement images show no evidence of infarction in this region.

Diagnosis

Anterolateral ischemia from base to apex as described. No evidence of prior infarction.

MR perfusion imaging has been shown to compare favorably with SPECT imaging for the detection of epicardial coronary artery disease.[1,2] In addition, the viability imaging obtained with MR is clearly superior to that of SPECT imaging.[3] Simultaneous evaluation of the valvular structures and functional capacity of the myocardium is also a significant advantage of MR imaging.

References

1. Fenchel M, et al. Detection of regional myocardial perfusion deficit using rest and stress perfusion MRI: a feasibility study. AJR Am J Roentgenol. 2005;185(3):627–635.
2. Sakuma H, et al. Diagnostic accuracy of stress first-pass contrast-enhanced myocardial perfusion MRI compared with stress myocardial perfusion scintigraphy. AJR Am J Roentgenol. 2005;185(1):95–102.
3. Wagner A, et al. Contrast-enhanced MRI and routine single photon emission computed tomography (SPECT) perfusion imaging for detection of subendocardial myocardial infarcts: an imaging study. Lancet. 2003;361(9355):374–379.

Teaching File Case 26

34-year-old male with long-standing hypertension

Category: Aorta

History

He now presents with chest pain.

Findings

The left ventricular cavity size is within normal limits. Mild, concentric hypertrophy is apparent. The overall left ventricular function is within normal limits, but hypokinesia of the inferior wall is evident, extending from the base to the mid-ventricular level.

The right ventricle is normal in size and function.

Evaluation of the valvular structures demonstrates that no significant mitral regurgitation is noted.

Marked dilatation of the aortic root is noted, and is associated with mild aortic insufficiency.

Note is made of a moderate-sized pericardial effusion. In addition, the pericardial fluid is noted to be complex in nature, and is not simple fluid. Notice the swirling pattern seen, indicating the likely presence of complex fluid or blood within the pericardial sac.

Evaluation of the proximal aorta on the 3-chamber views indicates the presence of a small flap along the anterior margin of the aorta, closely adjacent to the orifice of the right coronary artery. This same flap is also appreciated on the "candy-cane" view of the ascending aorta and great vessels.

Delayed-enhancement views show no evidence of an infarction or thrombus.

Diagnosis

Localized dissection of the immediately supravalvular portion of the ascending aorta, extending to involve the orifice of the right coronary artery, with resultant ischemia of the right coronary artery territory resulting in hypokinesia of the inferior wall.

The dissection extends in a transmural fashion, which results in the development of hemopericardium.

The patient underwent emergent repair, which was successful, and which confirmed the above findings.

Dissection of the aorta is frequently associated with long-standing hypertension, or less commonly may be associated with a connective tissue abnormality such as Marfans syndrome or Ehlers-Danlos syndrome (type IV).

The Stanford dissection classification scheme is now the most widely adopted, and results in 2 distinct classes: Type A dissections begin in the ascending aorta, and proceed for a variable distance distally. Type B dissections begin in the descending aorta, usually immediately distal to the left subclavian artery, and proceed distally without involvement of the ascending aorta. These are usually treated medically, while the type A dissections are usually treated surgically.[1–5] Further discussion regarding the use of CMR in the evaluation of aortic dissection may be found in Chapter 7.

Rupture into the pericardium (as seen in this case) is an ominous finding, often associated with the sudden development of cardiac tamponade and death. Thus, the presence of hemopericardium should alert one to the need for urgent surgery.

References

1. Matsunaga N, et al. Magnetic resonance imaging features of aortic diseases. Top Magn Reson Imaging. 2003;14(3):253–266.
2. Geisinger MA, et al. Thoracic aortic dissections: magnetic resonance imaging. Radiology. 1985;155(2): 407–412.

3. Sabik JF, et al. Long-term effectiveness of operations for ascending aortic dissections. J Thorac Cardiovasc Surg. 2000;119(5):946–962.
4. Westaby S, Katsumata T, Freitas E. Aortic valve conservation in acute type A dissection. Ann Thorac Surg. 1997;64(4):1108–1112.
5. Srichai MB, et al. Acute dissection of the descending aorta: noncommunicating versus communicating forms. Ann Thorac Surg. 2004;77(6):2012–2020; discussion 2020.

Teaching File Case 27

16-year-old female with a history of prior therapy for a congenital lesion

Category: Congenital

Findings

The left ventricular chamber size and function appear normal.

The right ventricle also appears normal in size and function. No wall motion abnormalities are seen.

On the 2-chamber view, turbulent flow is noted in the proximal descending aorta. A dedicated image through this region confirms turbulent flow. A subsequently performed MR angiogram confirms an area of focal narrowing in the proximal descending aorta just distal to the left subclavian artery. Subsequently obtained velocity-encoded images demonstrate a gradient of 20mm Hg. through this region.

Also noted is the presence of a bicuspid aortic valve. Velocity-encoded images demonstrate a gradient of 12mm Hg.

Diagnosis

Coarctation of the aorta, with associated bicuspid aortic valve.

In this entity, an abnormal constriction is present in the proximal descending aorta, usually just distal to the origin of the left subclavian artery. This disorder ranges in severity from a severe infantile form that presents at the time of ductal closure and may be associated with extensive tubular hypoplasia of the aortic arch, to an abnormality that may be detected incidentally at the time of a school physical when diminished pulses in the patient's legs are noted. Upper extremity hypertension is frequently noted in these patients. In fact, the hypertension may persist even after complete correction of the coarctation.

Dilated intercostal vessels are commonly seen, as collaterals develop to supply the distal descending aorta. They may produce characteristic rib notching due to pressure erosion along the undersurface of the upper ribs. Phase-contrast imaging can be used to evaluate the degree and significance of collateral flow.[1]

Coarctation of the aorta is associated with a bicuspid aortic valve in approximately 50–75% of cases. Other left-sided obstructive lesions including tubular hypoplasia of the aorta, subaortic stenosis, and abnormalities of the mitral valve are also associated. Noncardiac associated lesions include berry aneurysms in the cerebral circulation.

Coarctation is said to occur in approximately 25% of patients with Turners syndrome.

Late complications of coarctation include recoarctation, aneurysm formation at the site of prior repair, ascending aorta dilatation, and aortic valve abnormalities (stenosis and regurgitation). Hypertension is also frequently seen, even in those with apparently successful repair. Long-term survival is significantly affected by age at operation, with the best survival rates noted in those who underwent repair between 1 and 5 years of age.[2–5] Further review of the use of CMR in the evaluation of congenital heart disease may be found in Chapter 4.

References

1. Pujadas S, et al. Phase contrast MR imaging to measure changes in collateral blood flow after stenting of recurrent aortic coarctation: initial experience. J Magn Reson Imaging. 2006;24(1):72–76.
2. Roos-Hesselink JW, et al. Aortic valve and aortic arch pathology after coarctation repair. Heart. 2003;89(9):1074–1077.
3. Braverman AC, et al. The bicuspid aortic valve. Curr Probl Cardiol. 2005;30(9):470–522.
4. Webb G, Treatment of coarctation and late complications in the adult. Semin Thorac Cardiovasc Surg. 2005;17(2):139–142.
5. Prisant LM, et al. Coarctation of the aorta: a secondary cause of hypertension. J Clin Hypertens (Greenwich). 2004;6(6):347–350, 352.

Teaching File Case 28

51-year-old male with known coronary artery disease, now with chest pain

Category: Stress test

Findings

A stress/rest myocardial MR perfusion study was performed. The short-axis views demonstrate anterior hypokinesia, which is mild at the basal level, but severe in the mid-ventricular level, and accompanied by wall thinning beginning at the mid-ventricular level and extending to the apex. Anteroseptal and inferoseptal involvement is also seen at the mid-ventricular level, with dyskinesia noted in the mid and apical segments.

The right ventricle is normal in size and function.

Evaluation of the valvular structures demonstrates mild tricuspid regurgitation. No significant mitral regurgitation is seen. The aortic valve appears normal.

The perfusion images demonstrate a large region of diminished perfusion involving the anterior wall as well as the anteroseptum beginning at the basal level, and extending to the apex. In addition, a more focal nearly transmural perfusion deficit is seen involving the inferior wall from the basal level to the mid-ventricular level.

The delayed-enhancement images demonstrate extensive infarction of the anterior wall, the anteroseptal and inferoseptal walls at the basal and mid-ventricular levels, with nearly circumferential involvement infarction of the apex. The inferior wall demonstrates only a small infarction at the basal level, and the area of inducible ischemia appears to far exceed the area of infarction.

Diagnosis

Extensive prior anterior, anteroseptal and inferoseptal infarction. A small inferior infarction is noted, but significant inducible inferior ischemia is noted.

MR imaging has been shown to have excellent sensitivity in detecting the presence of multivessel disease. In fact, in one series from Japan, detection of two and three-vessel disease was accomplished with a higher sensitivity than that of one vessel disease.[1]

The sequencing of image acquisition is clearly important, but often not sufficiently emphasized in the literature. Specifically, one can easily imagine that had contrast been administered for rest perfusion prior to the stress study, the intensity of the perfusion deficit in the inferior wall might have been masked. In addition, the area of prior infarction in the anterior, anteroseptal and inferoseptal walls would likely have taken up significant contrast, and masked the intensity of the perfusion deficit in this region. Therefore, it can be seen that there are significant advantages to performing the stress images first followed by the resting images.[2]

The ability of MR to detect multivessel disease represents a significant advantage over nuclear imaging, which may have diminished accuracy in this setting.

References

1. Ishida N, et al. Noninfarcted myocardium: correlation between dynamic first-pass contrast-enhanced myocardial MR imaging and quantitative coronary angiography. Radiology. 2003;229(1):209–216.
2. Klem I, et al. Improved detection of coronary artery disease by stress perfusion cardiovascular magnetic resonance with the use of delayed-enhancement infarction imaging. J Am Coll Cardiol. 2006;47(8): 1630–1638.

Teaching File Case 29

33-year-old female with multifocal pneumonia and a new murmur

Category: Valve disease

Findings

The short-axis views demonstrate that the left ventricular size and function appear normal. The wall thickness is normal as well.

Evaluation of the right ventricle demonstrates a lobulated soft tissue mass that moves into and out of the plane of imaging in the first three images of the top row. This same structure can be seen on the middle two images of the second row which are obtained in the long axis of the right ventricle. A pedunculated soft tissue density is seen attached to the chordae tendinae of the tricuspid valve. Tricuspid regurgitation is apparent, with an eccentric jet noted on the 4-chamber views.

Images obtained following the administration of IV contrast material demonstrate that the lesion in question does not show contrast enhancement. It is uniformly low in signal intensity. No other areas of signal abnormality are seen.

Extracardiac findings include the presence of airspace disease at the right lung base associated with a small right pleural effusion.

Diagnosis

Pedunculated vegetation affecting the tricuspid valve apparatus in a patient with acute bacterial endocarditis. Septic pulmonary emboli are evident in the right lower lobe.

MR imaging, with its excellent contrast resolution and high spatial resolution imaging of valvular structures may be useful in the evaluation of endocarditis. Although transesophageal echocardiography is currently considered the gold standard for evaluation of valvular vegetations, MR imaging is often diagnostic.[1–4]

Valvular vegetations can be recognized on MR imaging by their intimate association with the valves, and by their uniform low signal intensity following the administration of contrast, much like thrombus. In fact, histologically, vegetations usually represent an admixture of fibrin and inflammatory cells.

The differential diagnosis for a mobile intracavitary mass would include a myxoma, or possibly a bland thrombus. However, myxomas usually demonstrate heterogenous enhancement. Bland thrombus was unlikely in this case, given the patient's positive blood cultures and septic pulmonary emboli.

References

1. Pollak Y, Comeau CR, Wolff SD. Staphylococcus aureus endocarditis of the aortic valve diagnosed on MR imaging. AJR Am J Roentgenol. 2002;179(6):1647.
2. Caduff JH, Hernandez RJ, Ludomirsky A. MR visualization of aortic valve vegetations. J Comput Assist Tomogr. 1996;20(4):613–615.
3. Akins EW, et al. Perivalvular pseudoaneurysm complicating bacterial endocarditis: MR detection in five cases. AJR Am J Roentgenol. 1991;156(6):1155–1158.
4. Sachdev M, Peterson GE, Jollis JG. Imaging techniques for diagnosis of infective endocarditis. Infect Dis Clin North Am. 2002;16(2):319–337, ix.

Teaching File Case 30

The patient has a history of prior surgery in childhood

Category: Congenital

Findings

The left ventricle is at the upper limits of normal in size, and appears slightly elongated in the vertical axis. The right ventricle is enlarged, and moderately trabeculated. In addition, ballooning of the right ventricular outflow tract is noted, with aneurysmal dilatation apparent. In addition, the pulmonary valve is not visualized, and the velocity-encoded images demonstrate extensive pulmonic regurgitation.

Also noted is mild aortic insufficiency on the velocity-encoded images.

MR angiographic images confirm the ballooning aneurysmal dilatation of the RV outflow tract, and demonstrate branch pulmonary artery stenosis on the left. Velocity-encoded images through this region are also obtained and confirm the suspected left pulmonary artery stenosis at its origin.

Delayed-enhancement imaging demonstrates enhancement of the right ventricular outflow tract at the site of the patient's prior surgery.

Diagnosis

Tetralogy of Fallot, post-op, with free pulmonic insufficiency.

The patient had Tetralogy of Fallot diagnosed in infancy, and subsequently underwent surgical correction involving resection of the stenotic outflow tract and pulmonary valve. No pulmonary valve replacement was performed at that time. As a result, extensive pulmonic insufficiency is seen. Also, aneurysmal dilatation of the right ventricular outflow tract secondary to the prior surgery is apparent.

Tetralogy of Fallot comprises four findings seen in combination: overriding of the aorta, ventricular septal defect, right ventricular infundibular and/or pulmonary valve stenosis, and right ventricular hypertrophy, which is related to the above. The common embryologic abnormality underlying this disorder is under-development of the RV infundibulum, resulting in malalignment of the upper portion of the ventricular septum, associated with abnormal rotation of the conotruncal region, resulting in overriding of the aorta, encroachment on the pulmonary outflow tract, and a malalignment VSD. The right ventricular hypertrophy is secondary to the right ventricular obstruction.[1–3]

Branch pulmonary artery stenosis is often seen in patients with Tetralogy.

Approximately 15–25% of patients with Tetralogy will also develop some degree of aortic insufficiency in adulthood.[4]

The differential diagnosis is quite limited. The findings of absence of the pulmonic valve along with obvious postsurgical changes in the right ventricular outflow tract would be most commonly associated with prior surgical relief of obstruction of the right ventricular outflow. The overriding of the aortic characteristic of Tetralogy of Fallot is not particularly apparent in this case. However, mild aortic insufficiency is apparent as can be seen with this disorder.

RV outflow tract aneurysm and pulmonic regurgitation are both independently associated with impaired RV function and diminished RVEF.[5]

Note that MR imaging can provide angiographic and functional imaging of the RV, as well as the pulmonary arteries, and can provide accurate data regarding the regurgitant fraction as well as the gradient induced by the PA stenosis. Further review of the use of CMR in the evaluation of congenital heart disease may be found in Chapter 4.

References

1. Brickner ME, Hillis LD, Lange RA. Congenital heart disease in adults. First of two parts. N Engl J Med. 2000;342(4):256–263.
2. Brickner ME, Hillis LD, Lange RA. Congenital heart disease in adults. Second of two parts. N Engl J Med. 2000;342(5):334–342.
3. Anderson RH, Weinberg PM. The clinical anatomy of Tetralogy of Fallot. Cardiol Young. 2005;15(Suppl 1): 38–47.
4. Bhat AH, Smith CJ, Hawker RE. Late aortic root dilatation in Tetralogy of Fallot may be prevented by early repair in infancy. Pediatr Cardiol. 2004;25(6): 654–659.
5. Geva T, et al. Factors associated with impaired clinical status in long-term survivors of tetralogy of Fallot repair evaluated by magnetic resonance imaging. J Am Coll Cardiol. 2004;43(6):1068–1074.

Teaching File Case 31

61-year-old male, status–post myocardial infarction, with multivessel coronary artery disease noted at cardiac catheterization

Category: Viability

History

The study is requested to evaluate for viability in the various segments, as multivessel revascularization is contemplated.

Findings

The left ventricular cavity is enlarged and measured approximately 6 cm in diastole. Evaluation of the regional wall motion demonstrates that at the basal level, the anterior and anteroseptal walls show preserved function. The inferior, inferoseptal, and inferolateral walls demonstrate severe hypokinesia/akinesia. The anterolateral wall demonstrates mild hypokinesia.

At the mid-ventricular level, the anterior wall becomes hypokinetic, but the anteroseptal and inferoseptal segments demonstrate normal contractility. The inferior wall is slightly thicker at the mid-ventricular level, and shows improved contractility. The lateral wall is severely hypokinetic.

At the apical level, the anterior wall is noted to be thinned and dyskinetic, with dyskinesia extending to the true apex. The inferior wall distally demonstrates normal contractility, as do the apical septal and lateral walls. Left ventricular ejection fraction was measured at 27%.

The right ventricular size and function are normal.

Evaluation of the valvular structures demonstrates that an eccentric jet of mild to moderate mitral regurgitation is noted, and the left atrium is minimally enlarged. The tricuspid and aortic valves are unremarkable.

Resting perfusion images demonstrate an area of perfusion deficit in the lateral wall.

Delayed-enhancement imaging demonstrates subendocardial hyperenhancement involving the anterior wall beginning at the basal level, and extending nearly to the apex. The degree of transmurality is less than 50% throughout, and is approximately 25% at the basal level and approaches 50% at the mid-ventricular level. The anterior septum is viable throughout.

The inferior wall demonstrates thinning, but only very minimal subendocardial hyperenhancement at the basal and apical levels. A focus of more extensively transmural hyperenhancement is seen in the mid ventricular inferior wall, but this is quite small.

Transmural infarction is seen in the lateral wall at the basal and mid-ventricular levels. The apical lateral wall appears unremarkable.

Enhanced images with a long inversion time show no evidence of thrombus.

Diagnosis

Significant residual viability is noted. Specifically, although the anterior wall appears thinned and akinetic, as does much of the inferior wall, significant residual viability is noted in both regions. Surgical revascularization of all three coronary vessels was performed.

This case demonstrates again the utility of MR imaging for the determination of myocardial viability. It is important to note that in the setting of chronic ischemic disease, the myocardium may be dysfunctional and even thinned from ischemia as well as infarction. The distinction between the two is of critical importance as patients with viable myocardium who are not revascularized actually fare worse than those with non-viable myocardium.[1] The process whereby chronic low-grade ischemia results in down-regulation of myocardial function and thinning of the myocardium such that the reduced metabolic demands of the myocardium better match the impaired supply is termed "hibernation." Repetitive low-grade episodic ischemia (also termed repetitive stunning) likely results in a similar process. Myocardial viability imaging using the delayed-enhancement enhancement sequence provides the best currently available means of distinguishing viable but thinned and/or dysfunctional myocardium (no enhancement) from non-viable, infarcted myocardium (enhancement present). Importantly, CMR can also demonstrate the relative proportion of infarcted and viable myocardium across the ventricular wall, and thereby estimate the likelihood of functional recovery following revascularization. For further discussion regarding the use of delayed-enhancement imaging in the evaluation of myocardial viability in the setting of chronic coronary arery disease, see also Chapter 3.

The resting perfusion images showed a focal perfusion deficit in the lateral wall location corresponding with the area of prior transmural infarction. This demonstrates that perfusion imaging whether at stress or rest may reflect microvascular impairment secondary to prior infarction with scar formation.[2,3]

This form of microvascular obstruction should be differentiated in the observer's mind from the microvascular obstruction typified by the no-reflow zone seen on delayed-enhancement imaging. In the instance of perfusion imaging, this reflects differential transit of contrast on a first pass perfusion technique. Areas of persistent microcirculatory damage from prior infarction whether acute or chronic may demonstrate such an appearance.[3]

A no-reflow zone as demonstrated by delayed-enhancement imaging refers specifically to a focus of dark nonenhancing myocardium contained within hyperenhanced myocardium, a finding typically seen in acute transmural infarctions. Its apparent size diminishes during the examination, as contrast diffuses into the lesion. Sequential imaging at five-minute intervals beginning at 5 minutes after contrast administration will demonstrate the process of gradual delayed-enhancement as the contrast diffuses slowly into the necrotic core of the infarct.[4] Other cases in this teaching file will demonstrate this finding.

The no-reflow phenomenon observed on delayed-enhancement imaging is a transient phenomenon in a larger sense as well, in that it is commonly seen in acute infarctions within the first week after the event, but gradually disappears and is usually not seen by 8 weeks after the infarction.

References

1. Allman KC, et al. Myocardial viability testing and impact of revascularization on prognosis in patients with coronary artery disease and left ventricular dysfunction: a meta-analysis. J Am Coll Cardiol. 2002;39(7):1151–1158.
2. Hombach V, et al. Sequelae of acute myocardial infarction regarding cardiac structure and function and their prognostic significance as assessed by magnetic resonance imaging. Eur Heart J. 2005;26(6): 549–557.
3. Arai AE. Magnetic resonance first-pass myocardial perfusion imaging. Top Magn Reson Imaging. 2000;11(6):383–398.
4. Wagner A., et al. MR imaging of myocardial perfusion and viability. Magn Reson Imaging Clin N Am. 2003;11(1):49–66.

Teaching File Case 32

29-year-old male with a history of syncope and an abnormality noted on ECG

Category: Cardiomyopathy

Findings

The left ventricle is minimally elongated in the vertical axis. The septum is noted to be dyskinetic from the basilar level to the apex. The anterior, anterolateral, inferolateral and inferior walls of the left ventricle demonstrate minimally reduced wall motion.

The right ventricle is noted to be enlarged, and demonstrates poor contractility. Prominent trabeculations are also apparent.

Evaluation of the valvular structures demonstrates that no mitral or aortic insufficiency is seen. Mild tricuspid insufficiency is noted. The pulmonic valve is unremarkable in appearance.

Delayed enhancement imaging demonstrates transmural enhancement of the antero-septum at the basal and midventricular levels, with preservation of the apical septum. In addition, extensive enhancement of the right ventricular free wall is noted. A small focus of possible enhancement is noted in the lateral wall of the left ventricle as seen in the fourth image of the third row.

Diagnosis

ARVD. The ECG abnormality noted was an epsilon wave. Electrophysiology testing confirmed the diagnosis.

This disorder should probably be properly termed ARVC, as this represents a distinct cardiomyopathy likely related to mutations in the genes coding for desmosomal proteins.[1–3] It is most often inherited is an autosomal dominant trait, with variable penetrance. This then results in apoptosis of the right ventricular cardiomyocytes, with resultant fibrosis and fatty replacement. Approximately 15% of cases demonstrate left ventricular involvement.

The diagnosis is made on a combination of clinical, electrophysiological, and imaging findings including right ventricular dilatation, and poor function. The presence of fat in the right ventricular free wall was formerly often a subject of investigation by MR imaging, but has been found to be a frequent source of misdiagnosis.[4,5] It is not a criterion for the diagnosis.

At most experienced centers, evaluation of the cine images for impaired contractility and for the presence of areas of focal dyskinesia of the right ventricle is most often used to suspect the diagnosis. Delayed-enhancement imaging is not a part of the Task Force criteria for diagnosis. However, in a report of a small series of 12 patients, DE-MR was found to be quite helpful in confirming the presence of right ventricular fibrosis.[6] Approximately two-thirds of the affected patients demonstrated right ventricular enhancement, while none of the normal patients demonstrated such right ventricular enhancement.

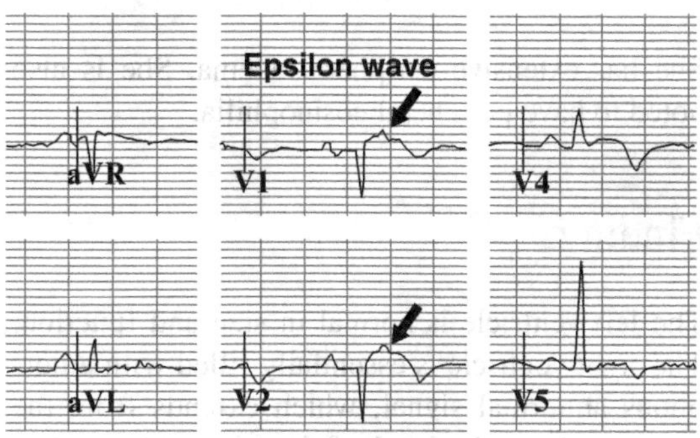

FIGURE 32.1. The arrows denote an epsilon wave in leads V1 and V2 in this patient's ECG

In addition, patients demonstrating abnormal delayed-enhancement on MR imaging were more likely to demonstrate inducibility of their tachyarrhythmia on electrophysiologic testing.[6]

The pattern of enhancement in this case is similar to that seen with sarcoidosis. However, sarcoidosis would not be expected to produce the global right ventricular dysfunction and extensive right ventricular trabeculation noted in this exam. Myocarditis could also conceivably result in this appearance, but again, would not usually be expected to produce the extensive abnormality noted in the right ventricle.

References

1. Syrris P, et al. Arrhythmogenic right ventricular dysplasia/cardiomyopathy associated with mutations in the desmosomal gene desmocollin-2. Am J Hum Genet. 2006;79(5):978–984.
2. Lahtinen AM, et al. Plakophilin-2 missense mutations in arrhythmogenic right ventricular cardiomyopathy. Int J Cardiol. 2007.
3. Moric-Janiszewska E, Markiewicz-Loskot G. Review on the genetics of arrhythmogenic right ventricular dysplasia. Europace. 2007;9(5):259–266.
4. Bluemke DA, et al. MR Imaging of arrhythmogenic right ventricular cardiomyopathy: morphologic findings and interobserver reliability. Cardiology. 2003;99(3):153–162.
5. Bomma C, et al. Misdiagnosis of arrhythmogenic right ventricular dysplasia/cardiomyopathy. J Cardiovasc Electrophysiol. 2004;15(3):300–306.
6. Tandri H, et al. Noninvasive detection of myocardial fibrosis in arrhythmogenic right ventricular cardiomyopathy using delayed-enhancement magnetic resonance imaging. J Am Coll Cardiol. 2005;45(1): 98–103.

Teaching File Case 33

54-year-old female with signs of right heart failure

Category: Cardiomyopathy

History

She has extensive peripheral edema. She is also noted to have peripheral eosinophilia.

Findings

The left ventricle is normal in size and function. The right ventricle is essentially filled with amorphous abnormal signal, which extends from the apex nearly to the level of the tricuspid annulus, and superiorly into the right ventricular outflow tract almost to the level of the pulmonary valve. Marked dilatation of the right atrium is apparent. The fifth image of the second row is a right ventricular 2-chamber view and demonstrates the extensive impact of this abnormal soft tissue material filling much of the right ventricular cavity and extending into the right ventricular outflow tract. Note the extensive distention of the inferior vena cava.

Bulging of the interatrial septum is apparent. The mitral valve is normal in appearance. Extensive tricuspid regurgitation is noted. The aortic valve is unremarkable in appearance.

Perfusion images obtained during the dynamic administration of contrast are shown in the third row, and demonstrate a large area of nonenhancing material occupying much of the right ventricular cavity. Marginal enhancement is noted along the endocardial surface adjacent to this filling defect.

Postcontrast VIBE images demonstrate extensive low signal in the region of abnormality. Large bilateral pleural effusions are evident along with a small pericardial effusion. Extensive subcutaneous edema is noted, along with dilatation of the inferior vena cava.

Cine imaging obtained following administration of contrast in the fifth row demonstrates extensive impairment of contractility of the right ventricle associated with the extensive nonenhancing filling defect.

Delayed-enhancement images noted in the fourth row demonstrate that on images obtained with a long inversion time, abundant thrombus can be appreciated in the right ventricular cavity. Images obtained with a short inversion time demonstrate extensive endocardial enhancement adjacent to this thrombus, involving much of the right ventricular subendocardium.

Diagnosis

Loeffler's endocarditis (eosinophilic endomyocardial fibrosis).

This disorder usually results from cardiac involvement in the setting of idiopathic hypereosinophilia syndrome (IHES). Criteria for the diagnosis include persistent eosinophilia in excess of 1500/cc for >6 months duration, with multisystem involvement, and absence of known causes of eosinophilia.

It is said to be more common in men, and usually presents with easy fatigability along with nonproductive cough and dyspnea. Congestive heart failure often leads to the diagnosis of cardiac involvement. The most significant complications of IHES include nervous system and cardiac involvement. Heart disease is the major cause of morbidity and mortality.

This disorder results in extensive infiltration of the ventricular endocardium by eosinophils, with subsequent degranulation, and arteriolar necrosis with resultant endocardial fibrosis. This is responsible for the diffuse endocardial RV enhancement noted in this case. The intensive inflammatory changes result in superimposed thrombus formation, which subsequently occupies much of the ventricular cavity. Marked impairment of diastolic filling of the ventricles is noted, with a resultant severe restrictive cardiomyopathy.[1–3]

Current treatment involves not only the use of high doses of steroids, but also the administration of hydroxyurea as well as other potent immunosuppressives. Occasionally, surgery may be necessary to relieve the obstruction produced by the mass-like thrombus and endocardial fibrosis. This is considered a palliative therapy however. New therapies including the use of imatanib have been reported and may prove helpful.[4]

References

1. Salanitri GC. Endomyocardial fibrosis and intracardiac thrombus occurring in idiopathic hypereosinophilic syndrome. AJR Am J Roentgenol. 2005;184(5):1432–1433.
2. Bishop GG, Bergin JD, Kramer CM. Hypereosinophilic syndrome and restrictive cardiomyopathy due to apical thrombi. Circulation. 2001;104(2):E3–E4.
3. Puvaneswary M, Joshua F, Ratnarajah S. Idiopathic hypereosinophilic syndrome: magnetic resonance imaging findings in endomyocardial fibrosis. Australas Radiol. 2001;45(4):524–527.
4. Rotoli B, et al. Rapid reversion of Loeffler's endocarditis by imatinib in early stage clonal hypereosinophilic syndrome. Leuk Lymphoma. 2004;45(12): 2503–2507.

Teaching File Case 34

37-year-old male with long standing sarcoidosis

Category: Pulm HTN

Findings

Cine images demonstrate that the left ventricle is within normal limits in size. The left ventricular systolic function is globally depressed, and the left ventricular ejection fraction is measured at 34%.

Paradoxical septal motion early in diastole is noted.

The right ventricle is dilated, and thick-walled, and demonstrates reduced systolic function as well.

Moderately severe tricuspid regurgitation is apparent, with marked dilatation of the right atrium. The pulmonic valve appears to be competent. The aortic and mitral valves are unremarkable in appearance.

Delayed-enhancement images obtained with the standard segmented technique (first 4 images of the second row of images) demonstrate extensive hyperenhancement of the right ventricular insertion sites upon the septum, extending from the basal to the apical levels. In addition, the single shot images demonstrate apparent enhancement of the midwall of the septum, likely artifactual given the lack of enhancement seen on the high resolution delayed-enhancement images.

Real-time images demonstrate persistent displacement of the septum from right-to-left independent of the phase of respiration.

Diagnosis

Severe pulmonary hypertension, secondary to extensive underlying pulmonary parenchymal disease. Right heart catheterization confirmed severe pulmonary hypertension.

Although the patient has a history of sarcoidosis, the findings described are felt to be secondary to the extensive pulmonary hypertension induced by the lung disease, and not from primary cardiac sarcoid. Hyperenhancement of the RV insertion sites upon the septum has been reported with pulmonary hypertension, and the pattern described is characteristic, with involvement in the present case extending from the basal to nearly the apical levels.[1]

The real time images demonstrate septal displacement to the left that is independent of the phase of inspiration, a finding that has been associated with cor pulmonale.[2]

References

1. Blyth KG, et al. Contrast enhanced-cardiovascular magnetic resonance imaging in patients with pulmonary hypertension. Eur Heart J. 2005;26(19):1993–1999.
2. Francone M, et al. Real-time cine MRI of ventricular septal motion: a novel approach to assess ventricular coupling. J Magn Reson Imaging. 2005;21(3):305–309.

Teaching File Case 35

Status-post surgical treatment for left lower leg claudication

Category: Angiography

History

Now with right lower leg claudication.

Findings

The abdominal aorta is normal in contour and caliber. The renal arteries are patent bilaterally. Wedge-like peripheral defects are noted involving the periphery of the kidneys bilaterally, consistent with areas of prior scarring.

The iliac bifurcations are unremarkable. A short segment weblike narrowing is seen in the left external iliac artery just distal to the bifurcation, and is felt to be mild in degree.

The left common femoral artery is patent, and supplies a left femoral-popliteal bypass graft. This is anastomosed to the left popliteal artery at the adductor canal and is widely patent.

On the right, the superficial femoral artery is occluded at its origin. Reconstitution of the popliteal artery at the adductor canal via collaterals is apparent.

The standard runoff images demonstrate venous contamination on the left, but clear visualization of the right lower leg demonstrates a widely patent tibioperoneal trunk and posterior tibial artery. Extensive disease is noted in the anterior tibial artery on the right which is occluded in the midportion of the calf.

On the left, the posterior tibial artery is also well developed and widely patent. The anterior tibial artery demonstrates multisegmental plaque, but is patent to the level of the ankle and supplies the dorsalis pedis. The peroneal artery is patent to the distal aspect of the lower leg. The time-resolved images are helpful in demonstrating these findings free of venous contamination.

Diagnosis

Patent left femoral bypass graft, with occlusion of the right SFA. Runoff occurs via the posterior tibial arteries bilaterally, with patency of a diseased anterior tibial artery noted on the left.

These findings in the lower legs are more apparent on the time-resolved images, which demonstrate the left lower leg free of venous contamination.

Various strategies have been employed to eliminate venous contamination in peripheral MR runoff angiography. There are basically two modifications of the standard bolus-chase technique which are designed to decrease venous contamination.

First, blood pressure cuffs can be applied to the thighs, and inflated to approximately 50 mmHg. This will diminish the arterial transit speed, and delay or diminish venous return. Standard multistation bolus chase angiography is then performed.[1]

The second technique is termed a hybrid technique, and entails performance of MR angiography in the lower legs in a dedicated fashion prior to the bolus chase injection. The hybrid technique can be performed with standard angiographic imaging using a timing bolus centered on the popliteal artery, with subsequent injection of 15 cc of gadolinium at 1 cc/sec followed by 25 cc of saline flush at the same rate, with 2 angio acquisitions of the lower legs. Standard imaging is then performed of the abdomen-pelvis and upper legs. Recent articles indicate that this technique has a very high success rate in imaging the lower legs without venous contamination.[2]

The second way to perform a hybrid technique is with time-resolved imaging as performed in this case. In this technique, sequential angiographic data sets with a higher temporal resolution of approximately 8 seconds per acquisition are performed. This is accomplished by minimally diminishing the image resolution in the readout and phase directions, while maintaining a slice thickness of approximately 1.5 mm. Sequential acquisitions are obtained as 8 cc of contrast are administered at 1 cc/sec, with saline flush administered at the same rate. Using this technique, images free of venous contamination can uniformly be obtained as seen in the present example.

References

1. Zhang HL, et al. Decreased venous contamination on 3D gadolinium-enhanced bolus chase peripheral mr angiography using thigh compression. AJR Am J Roentgenol. 2004;183(4):1041–1047.
2. Pereles FS, et al. Accuracy of stepping-table lower extremity MR angiography with dual-level bolus timing and separate calf acquisition: hybrid peripheral MR angiography. Radiology. 2006;240(1):283–290.

Teaching File Case 36

14-year-old male in for follow-up of known asymptomatic abnormality

Category: Congenital

Findings

Analysis of the ventricular chambers indicates that ventricular inversion is apparent, with the posterior ventricle representing a morphologic right ventricle. The left ventricle is anterior in location, and is smooth-walled. The right ventricle is posteriorly located and is the systemic ventricle. It appears heavily trabeculated, and demonstrates mildly decreased systolic function.

The aorta is seen to originate in an abnormal anterior location from this right ventricle. Additionally, the outflow tract leading to the aorta has a right ventricular configuration, with an infundibulum apparent. In addition, there is no evidence of fibrous continuity between the systemic ventricular arteriovenous and atrioventricular valves as is usually the case.

The morphologic left ventricle fills the pulmonic valve. No evidence of outflow tract obstruction is seen, no evidence of septal defect is apparent. The tricuspid valve (which is left-sided and fills the systemic ventricle) appears normal with no significant regurgitation.

Delayed-enhancement imaging shows no evidence of significant scar formation.

Diagnosis

L-loop transposition of the great vessels.

This represents a case of L-TGA, also known as congenitally corrected transposition of the great vessels. In this entity, the systemic venous return flows into the right atrium, and then passes through the mitral valve into an anteriorly located

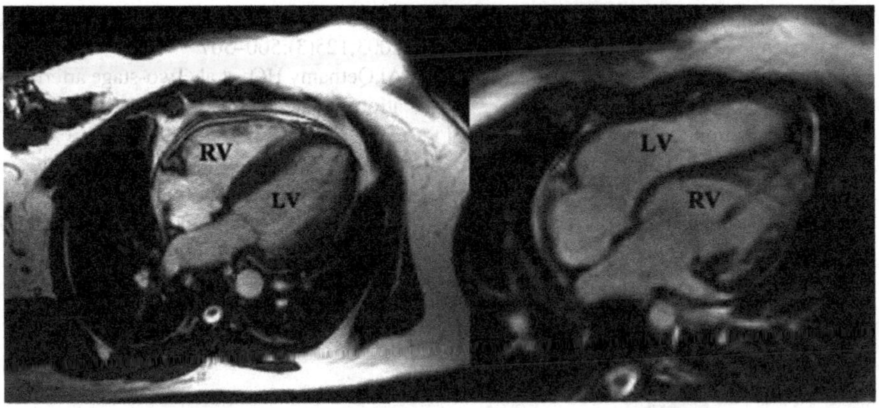

FIGURE 36.1. Still frame 4-chamber cine images demonstrate the ventricular arrangements characteristic of D-Loop and L-Loop anatomy

morphologic left ventricle. The left ventricle then fills the pulmonary artery. Therefore, although the left ventricle fills the pulmonary artery (transposition), since the right atrium empties into the left ventricle, the net result is that the systemic venous return is pumped into the pulmonary circulation. Therefore, the circulation is said to be corrected. By extension, the pulmonary venous return fills the left atrium, and subsequently passes through the tricuspid valve into the systemic morphologic right ventricle, from which it is then pumped into the aorta.[1]

Recognition of the morphologic right ventricle is based on several findings, including its heavier trabeculation, the presence of a papillary muscle originating along the septum, a trileaflet atrioventricular valve, and the presence of an infundibulum with separation of the AV and VA valves.

The left ventricle is recognized by a smooth-walled appearance, with absence of a septal papillary muscle. A two leaflet (mitral) valve is evident. Fibrous continuity is usually present between the aortic and mitral valves.

Looping of the heart may be determined from an analysis of the ventricular inflows: in a D-loop (the normal arrangement) the inflow to the morphologic right ventricle lies to the right of the inflow to the left ventricle; in an L-loop, the inflow to the RV lies to the left of the inflow to the LV.

In actuality, the so-called corrected transposition infrequently results in complete correction of all congenital abnormalities. These patients frequently (~80%) have Ebstein's malformation of the malpositioned tricuspid valve, and often have complex congenital heart disease. Complete correction without coexisting abnormality (as in this case) is distinctly uncommon, probably occurring in less than 5% of cases.

Long-term, even patients as fortunate as this patient have difficulties related to the right ventricle assuming the systemic workload. Over time, this is not usually well tolerated, and diminished life expectancy is the rule.[2, 3]

Surgical correction is possible but rarely performed because of the associated high mortality rate. When contemplated, the repair must occur in stages, as the LV will not support the pressures and resistance of the systemic circuit without adequate "training." This is usually accomplished with pulmonary artery banding, followed later by a "double-switch" procedure wherein the great arteries are switched (as in the Jatene procedure for the usual transposition) along with an atrial switch procedure to re-route the atrial connections (Mustard or Senning procedure).[4–6] Further review of the use of CMR in the evaluation of congenital heart disease may be found in Chapter 4.

References

1. Guit GL, et al. Levotransposition of the aorta: identification of segmental cardiac anatomy using MR imaging. Radiology. 1986;161(3):673–679.

2. Ohuchi H, et al. Comparison of the right and left ventricle as a systemic ventricle during exercise in patients with congenital heart disease. Am Heart J. 1999;137(6):1185–1194.
3. Warnes CA. Transposition of the great arteries. Circulation. 2006;114(24):2699–2709.
4. Devaney EJ, et al. Combined arterial switch and Senning operation for congenitally corrected transposition of the great arteries: patient selection and intermediate results. J Thorac Cardiovasc Surg. 2003;125(3):500–507.
5. Al Qethamy HO, et al. Two-stage arterial switch operation: is late ever too late? Asian Cardiovasc Thorac Ann. 2002;10(3):235–239.
6. Duncan BW, et al. Results of the double switch operation for congenitally corrected transposition of the great arteries. Eur J Cardiothorac Surg. 2003;24(1):11–19; discussion 19–20.

Teaching File Case 37

56-year-old male with nonspecific chest pain

Category: Coronary MRA

Findings

An adenosine stress rest cardiac MRI was performed. This demonstrates that the initial cine images show no wall motion abnormality. The left ventricle is normal in size and wall thickness. The global and regional wall motion is normal.

The right ventricle is normal in size and function and wall thickness.

Adenosine stress and subsequent rest perfusion imaging shows no evidence of inducible ischemia.

Whole heart coronary MR angiography was performed and is depicted in the images of the third row. The initial image represents the navigator tracking of the diaphragmatic position. The whole heart coronary MR angiogram is noted as the second image of the third row. Subsequent maximum intensity projections performed from this dataset are seen in the remainder of the third row. These demonstrate aneurysmal dilatation of the right coronary artery throughout its length, achieving a maximum diameter of approximately 9 mm along the margin of the heart.

The most distal portion of the RCA is normal in diameter. There appears to be a small amount of nonocclusive mural thrombus within the distal portion of the aneurysmally dilated RCA.

The proximal and midportion of the left anterior descending coronary artery also appear dilated, to a maximum diameter of approximately 6 to 7 mm.

Diagnosis

No evidence of inducible ischemia. Aneurysmal dilatation of the right coronary artery, with less extensive dilatation of the left coronary artery (see Figure 37.1).

A coronary artery aneurysm is defined as an area of dilatation resulting in a diameter 1.5 times the diameter of normal adjacent segments. These are uncommon lesions, which have been diagnosed with increased frequency since the development of coronary arteriography, as well as noninvasive imaging techniques. The overall incidence is approximately 1.5–5%, with a male predominance. The right coronary artery is preferentially affected. Atherosclerosis is felt to account for approximately 50% of coronary artery aneurysms in adults.[1–3] Kawasaki's disease is a frequent cause in children.[4] Complications include thrombosis and

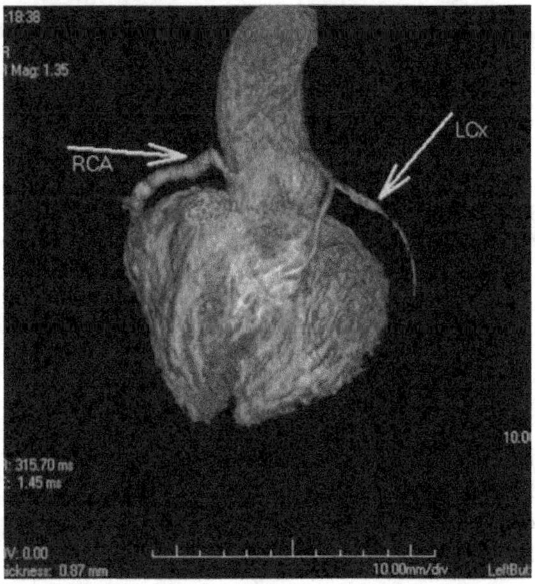

FIGURE 37.1. A volume-rendered 3D image from the whole heart coronary MR angiogram demonstrates aneurysmal dilatation of the right coronary artery and milder ectasia of the left circumflex coronary artery

distal embolization, as well as rupture and vasospasm. Surgery is often advised based on the extent of dilatation and coexisting ischemic symptoms. Antiplatelet therapy is performed for those cases not referred for surgery.

The addition of coronary MR angiography to the standard stress and rest perfusion imaging study represents a "one-stop shop" approach to the detection of coronary artery disease.[5,6] Physiologic information obtained from the adenosine stress and rest perfusion imaging can be combined with the anatomic information provided by direct coronary artery visualization using the whole heart technique.

The addition of dynamic diaphragmatic navigator tracking has improved the performance of coronary MR angiography. These studies can now be performed in 10 minutes or less on a routine basis, and do not require extensive operator interaction for the acquisition of a diagnostic study. Recent literature suggests that compared to the standard thin slab 2 dimensional and 3 dimensional imaging techniques, this whole heart 3-D technique has improved robustness and accuracy comparable to previously published data regarding coronary MR angiography.[7–9] For further discussion regarding coronary MRA, please refer to Chapter 2.

References

1. Syed, M. and M. Lesch, Coronary artery aneurysm: a review. Prog Cardiovasc Dis. 1997;40(1):77–84.
2. Pahlavan, P.S. and F. Niroomand, Coronary artery aneurysm: a review. Clin Cardiol. 2006;29(10):439–43.
3. Swaye, P.S., et al. Aneurysmal coronary artery disease. Circulation. 1983;67(1):134–8.
4. Suzuki, A., et al. Coronary arterial lesions of Kawasaki disease: cardiac catheterization findings of 1100 cases. Pediatr Cardiol. 1986;7(1):3–9.
5. Viswamitra, S., et al. Magnetic resonance imaging in myocardial ischemia. Curr Opin Cardiol, 2004;19(5):510–6.
6. Kramer, C.M., Integrated approach to ischemic heart disease. The one-stop shop. Cardiol Clin, 1998;16(2): 267–76.
7. Prakken, N.H., et al. 3D MR coronary angiography: optimization of the technique and preliminary results. Int J Cardiovasc Imaging. 2006.
8. Sakuma, H., et al. Detection of coronary artery stenosis with whole-heart coronary magnetic resonance angiography. J Am Coll Cardiol. 2006;48(10): 1946–50.
9. Sakuma, H., et al. Assessment of coronary arteries with total study time of less than 30 minutes by using whole-heart coronary MR angiography. Radiology. 2005;237(1):316–21.

Teaching File Case 38

48 year old female who is status–post left iliac fossa renal transplant, now with rising blood pressure, and mild decrease in GFR

Category: Angiography

Findings

There is a mild degree of narrowing of the right common iliac artery and eccentric plaque along the right lateral margin of the terminal aorta. Two areas of mild eccentric narrowing are noted along the margins of the left common iliac artery.

The main finding is the presence of two transplant renal arteries supplying the left iliac fossa transplant. The upper artery is widely patent. The more inferior artery demonstrates a kink just distal to its origin, resulting in a moderately severe degree of narrowing. Review of the color volume rendered images demonstrates a subtle discrepancy in perfusion of the lower one-half of the left kidney, with diminished image intensity apparent.

Diagnosis

A moderately severe stenosis is produced by a kink in the more inferior of two transplant renal arteries. This was confirmed at angiography.

MR angiographic evaluation of the renal arteries has been widely reported.[1–3] The sensitivity and specificity are comparable to catheter digital subtraction angiography.[4] More importantly, the study can be performed without an arterial puncture, or potentially nephrotoxic contrast.

Surveillance of iliac fossa renal transplants for the development of transplant renal artery stenosis is often performed using Doppler ultrasonography.[5] However, in equivocal circumstances, or when direct vascular imaging is desired, MR angiography has advantages over more invasive techniques.[6]

References

1. Leung DA, Hany TF, Debatin JF. Three-dimensional contrast-enhanced magnetic resonance angiography of the abdominal arterial system. Cardiovasc Intervent Radiol. Jan-Feb 1998;21(1):1–10.
2. Dellegrottaglie S, Sanz J, Rajagopalan S. Technology insight: Clinical role of magnetic resonance angiography in the diagnosis and management of renal artery stenosis. Nat Clin Pract Cardiovasc Med. Jun 2006;3(6):329–338.
3. Prince MR. Renal MR angiography: a comprehensive approach. J Magn Reson Imaging. May-Jun 1998;8(3):511–516.
4. Schoenberg SO, Rieger J, Weber CH, et al. High-spatial-resolution MR angiography of renal arteries with integrated parallel acquisitions: comparison with digital subtraction angiography and US. Radiology. May 2005;235(2):687–698.
5. Leung DA, Hoffmann U, Pfammatter T, et al. Magnetic resonance angiography versus duplex sonography for diagnosing renovascular disease. Hypertension. Feb 1999;33(2):726–731.
6. Knopp MV, Floemer F, Schoenberg SO, von Tengg-Kobligk H, Bock M, van Kaick G. Non-invasive assessment of renal artery stenosis: current concepts and future directions in magnetic resonance angiography. J Comput Assist Tomogr. Nov 1999;23 Suppl 1:S111–117.

Teaching File Case 39

42-year-old male with a heart murmur

Category: Congenital

History

Echocardiography was nondiagnostic.

Findings

The left ventricular cavity size and wall thickness appear normal, as does the regional and global left ventricular function. The right ventricle is normal as well.

The 3-chamber view demonstrates turbulence in the region of aortic valve, with apparent thickening of the valve leaflets. A small field-of-view cine image through the aortic valve demonstrates a bicuspid configuration of the valve. Although three commisures appear to be present, the valve is bicuspid.

The accompanying MR angiogram demonstrates no evidence of coarctation or other significant abnormality.

Velocity encoding images demonstrate no aliasing at a velocity of 200 cm/sec.

Diagnosis

This represents a case of bicuspid aortic valve, the most common congenital cardiac abnormality.[1, 2]

It is estimated that approximately 1% of the population has a congenitally bicuspid aortic valve. Occasionally, as is seen in this case, three apparent commisures are present, but the valve is functionally bicuspid.[3]

The abnormal valve morphology results in turbulent flow, as well as eccentric jets, which over time promote valve degeneration and may contribute to aortic root dilatation (which may develop even without flow abnormalities in patients with a bicuspid aortic valve). Eventually, significant stenosis usually develops, often by the fourth or fifth decade. Not infrequently, insufficiency will develop as well.

MR imaging has been shown to demonstrate accuracy equal to that of transesophageal echocardiography in planimetry of the aortic valve, and for estimation of aortic stenosis severity. Velocity-encoded images can be obtained in order to demonstrate the peak velocity of the stenotic jet and thereby the gradient.[4] In the present case, no significant gradient was present, despite the significant turbulence noted on cine imaging.

References

1. Zeppilli, P., et al. Bicuspid aortic valve: an innocent finding or a potentially life-threatening anomaly whose complications may be elicited by sports activity? J Cardiovasc Med (Hagerstown). 2006;7(4):282–7.
2. Braverman, A.C., et al. The bicuspid aortic valve. Curr Probl Cardiol. 2005;30(9):470–522.
3. Roberts, W.C. and J.M. Ko, Frequency by decades of unicuspid, bicuspid, and tricuspid aortic valves in adults having isolated aortic valve replacement for aortic stenosis, with or without associated aortic regurgitation. Circulation. 2005;111(7):920–5.
4. Waters, E.A., S.D. Caruthers, and S.A. Wickline, Correlation analysis of stenotic aortic valve flow patterns using phase contrast MRI. Ann Biomed Eng. 2005;33(7):878–87.

Teaching File Case 40

66-year-old male with hypertension, status–post prior bypass grafting to the left anterior descending and right coronary arteries

Category: Stress test

History

The study is performed for evaluation of chest pain.

Findings

Short-axis images demonstrate concentric left ventricular hypertrophy, consistent with the patient's history of hypertension.

The wall motion analysis indicates mild hypokinesia of the anteroseptum and anterior wall, with mild thinning of the anterior septum.

The right ventricle is normal in size and function. No significant mitral regurgitation is noted. Trace tricuspid regurgitation is noted, noting that the images are degraded somewhat by minimal breathing artifact.

Perfusion images obtained with adenosine stress are noted in the second row. A perfusion deficit is noted in a small segment of the anterior wall at the basal and mid-ventricular levels, and extends to the apex. A second defect is seen in the inferior wall, extending from the base to the apex as well. The rest images were not obtained as the patient requested early termination of the exam.

Delayed-enhancement images demonstrate subendocardial infarction involving the anterior septum and anterior wall at the basal and mid-ventricular levels. The remainder of the anterior wall is completely viable. A tiny focus of hyperenhancement is seen in the inferior wall at the mid-ventricular level.

Diagnosis

Two-vessel ischemia.

Subendocardial infarction is noted, but the degree of ischemia exceeds the region of infarction in the anterior wall. This finding is more pronounced in the inferior wall, where only a tiny infarct is noted, with a significant area of inducible ischemia. Significant residual viability is noted in both locations. This ability to detect multivessel disease is a distinct advantage of perfusion MR imaging relative to other modalities.[1] Although it is preferable to have both stress and rest perfusion images in order to exclude artifacts, the present study was felt to be diagnostic.

On the 3-chamber view, which is the far right image of the top row, extensive dark-band artifact is noted traversing the ascending aorta just above the aortic valve.[2] This obscures an area of significant abnormality that had been noted on prior imaging. The patient had a known pseudoaneurysm in this location, and the present study was performed for preoperative evaluation. This clearly demonstrates the impact artifacts can have on imaging, and the care that must be taken to exclude them from relevant areas of imaging.

References

1. Ishida, N., et al. Noninfarcted myocardium: correlation between dynamic first-pass contrast-enhanced myocardial MR imaging and quantitative coronary angiography. Radiology. 2003;229(1):209–16.
2. Li, W., et al. Dark flow artifacts with steady-state free precession cine MR technique: causes and implications for cardiac MR imaging. Radiology. 2004; 230(2):569–75.

Teaching File Case 41

66-year-old patient with recurrent bouts of heart failure

Category: Cardiomyopathy

Findings

Marked concentric left ventricular hypertrophy is apparent, with right ventricular thickening noted as well. The left ventricular ejection fraction it is reduced, but less extensively than the systolic dysfunction would suggest, due to the diminished end-diastolic volume noted.

Evaluation of the valvular structures demonstrates trace aortic insufficiency. No significant mitral tricuspid regurgitation is apparent.

The perfusion images demonstrate homogenous perfusion throughout.

Inversion recovery scout images (TI scouts) are demonstrated in the third row, after the perfusion images. These demonstrate that the blood pool and the myocardium are difficult to null at different time points, indicating extensive abnormality of the myocardium.

Images obtained with attempts made to null the myocardium show that diffuse subendocardial enhancement is apparent.

Diagnosis

Amyloidosis. This is the most common identifiable cause of restrictive cardiomyopathy in the United States. Cardiac involvement is the leading cause of death in patients with amyloidosis.

The finding of global concentric hypertrophy of the left and right ventricles, along with the markedly abnormal enhancement pattern described is quite characteristic of amyloidosis.

In this disorder, abnormal contrast kinetics are present, resulting in more rapid clearance of the contrast agent from the blood pool, and more extensive uptake by the myocardium. It is likely that profound expansion of the extracellular space induced by the infiltration by amyloid fibrils results in abnormal enhancement of the myocardium. Because of the altered contrast kinetics, and the rapid decrease in contrast within the blood pool with more extensive uptake of the myocardium, the myocardium and blood pool have similar null points on the inversion scout images, resulting in difficulty in achieving nulling of the myocardium separate from the blood pool. This pattern is characteristic of amyloidosis. Also, when nulling on delayed-enhancement imaging can be achieved, a pattern of diffuse subendocardial enhancement is often noted.[1,2]

References

1. Maceira, A.M., et al. Cardiovascular magnetic resonance in cardiac amyloidosis. Circulation. 2005; 111(2):186–93.
2. Sueyoshi, E., et al. Cardiac Amyloidosis: Typical Imaging Findings and Diffuse Myocardial Damage Demonstrated by Delayed Contrast-Enhanced MRI. Cardiovasc Intervent Radiol. 2006.

Teaching File Case 42

47-year-old female with left leg pain

Category: Angiography

Findings

The abdominal aorta is unremarkable in appearance. The renal arteries are patent as are the celiac axis and SMA. Both iliac arteries are unremarkable in appearance.

The upper leg station demonstrates abrupt cutoff of the left popliteal artery just at and above the left knee joint. The infraarticular popliteal artery is reconstituted.

The lower leg station confirms the popliteal artery obstruction.

The time-resolved imaging sequences (fifth image of the top row) confirm the left popliteal artery obstruction, although it is on the upper margin of the study.

Diagnosis

This represents a case of popliteal artery occlusion secondary to embolism.

Subsequent thrombolysis was performed, and confirmed the finding described. Thrombolysis resulted in complete removal of the clot, and no significant underlying stenosis was seen.

The differential diagnosis for popliteal artery occlusion would include atherosclerotic disease, although the patient's young age and the absence of other lesions argue against this diagnosis in this instance. Popliteal entrapment syndrome due to aberrant insertions of the medial head of the gastrocnemius muscle can also result in popliteal artery disease and occlusive changes, but is usually only apparent on dynamic imaging.[1–3]

Cystic adventitial disease can rarely result in popliteal artery occlusion, but the patients usually have a long history of intermittent claudication affecting the lower leg. In addition, review of the axial source images in this case does not show any cystic changes in the adventitia.[2]

Incidental note is made of an anomalous high origin of the right anterior tibial artery, which originates at or slightly above the level of the knee joint.

A cardiac MR was subsequently performed in this patient, and demonstrated no evidence of atrial or ventricular thrombi. The source of the patient's thrombus is uncertain at this time.

References

1. Wright, L.B., et al. Popliteal artery disease: diagnosis and treatment. Radiographics. 2004;24(2):467–79.
2. Elias, D.A., et al. Clinical evaluation and MR imaging features of popliteal artery entrapment and cystic adventitial disease. AJR Am J Roentgenol. 2003; 180(3):627–32.
3. Gozzi, M., et al. Peripheral arterial occlusive disease: role of MR angiography. Radiol Med (Torino). 2006; 111(2):225–37.

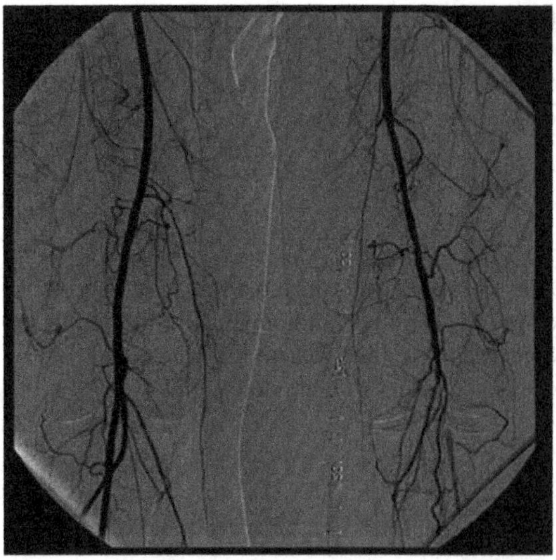

FIGURE 42.1. Conventional angiogram confirming clot in the popliteal artery

Teaching File Case 43

22-year-old female with a history of prior cardiac catheterization for electrophysiological studies that demonstrated easy passage of the catheter from the right atrium into the left atrium

Category: Congenital

History

The study was requested to evaluate for possible atrial septal defect.

Findings

Cine images demonstrate that the left ventricular size and function are within normal limits. The right ventricle also appears to be of normal size, making the diagnosis of atrial septal defect somewhat unlikely. The multiple 4-chamber views obtained demonstrate that no atrial septal defect is apparent. The HASTE images (dark-blood) seen in the second row demonstrate enlargement of the main pulmonary artery segment as well as the left main pulmonary artery. Turbulent flow is seen through the region of the pulmonic valve on the right ventricular outflow tract view seen as the far right image series of the second row. The far right image of the third row of images demonstrates the pulmonic valve in the axial plane.

Velocity-encoded images are seen in the bottom row. Note the aliasing seen on the initial velocity-encoded image with the velocity set at 150 cm/sec. The image without aliasing was obtained with a velocity of 250 cm/sec.

Diagnosis

Valvular pulmonic stenosis.

Characteristic imaging findings include the turbulent flow noted on the cine images through the valve plane. Also, dilatation of the main pulmonary artery is noted as well as preferential dilatation of the left pulmonary artery contrasted with the nondilated right pulmonary artery. This latter differential dilatation is due to the eccentric jet of turbulent flow which extends down the left pulmonary artery because of its in-line orientation, as opposed to the right pulmonary artery which takes a more right angle course from the main pulmonary artery.[1]

The degree of stenosis is quite mild, and is calculated by using Bernoulli's equation – Gradient (ΔP) = $4V^2$ where the velocity is given in meters/sec. In this case, the peak velocity was 200 cm/sec, which equals 2 m/sec. Therefore, in this case, the gradient measured 4 × 2 squared or 16 mmHg.[2]

No atrial septal defect was found. Rather, it is likely that the catheter traversed the foramen ovale more readily than usual because of the minimally elevated right heart pressures induced by the right ventricular outflow obstruction.

References

1. Brickner, M.E., L.D. Hillis, and R.A. Lange, Congenital heart disease in adults. First of two parts. N Engl J Med. 2000;342(4):256–63.
2. Lotz, J., et al. Cardiovascular flow measurement with phase-contrast MR imaging: basic facts and implementation. Radiographics. 2002;22(3):651–71.

Teaching File Case 44

18-year-old female with trauma from a motor vehicle accident, with equivocal chest CT findings

Category: Aorta

Findings

Images obtained in the oblique sagittal plane of the long axis of the aorta demonstrate a shelf-like filling defect within the proximal descending aorta approximately 2 cm distal to the origin of the left subclavian artery. This produces flow turbulence. It is well seen on the maximum intensity projection images of the MR angiogram as well as the volume rendered image. (The fifth and sixth images of the first row).

HASTE, SSFP, and VIBE morphologic images are seen in the first 3 series of the second row. These demonstrate a left pleural effusion. More importantly, they confirm the disruption of the anterior margin of the proximal descending aorta. The appearance is consistent with an intimal injury. Other cine images obtained demonstrate that the myocardial function is normal without evidence of cardiac contusion or other abnormality. Imaging of the aortic valve shows no disruption.

Interestingly, the fluoroscopic image used for triggering the MR angiogram (far right image of the third row) demonstrates the finding quite nicely.

Diagnosis

Traumatic rupture of the aorta with an intimal flap apparent. This produces the flow disturbance evident on the cine images obtained in the long axis of the aorta.

Imaging of the acute trauma patient is most often performed with computed tomography, due to its widespread availability and high degree of accuracy.[1] However, occasionally pulsatility artifact can impair visualization of an intimal flap on non-gated chest CT imaging. In addition, CT was likely equivocal in this case in part because there is little outward pseudoaneurysm formation, and very little mediastinal hematoma.

The use of MR imaging in this circumstance has been the subject of a few reports.[2–4] These reports indicate that it has excellent accuracy, and can be safely performed.

References

1. Macura KJ, Szarf G, Fishman EK, Bluemke DA. Role of computed tomography and magnetic resonance imaging in assessment of acute aortic syndromes. Semin Ultrasound CT MR. Aug 2003;24(4): 232–254.
2. Fattori R, Celletti F, Descovich B, et al. Evolution of post-traumatic aortic aneurysm in the subacute phase: magnetic resonance imaging follow-up as a support of the surgical timing. Eur J Cardiothorac Surg. May 1998;13(5):582–586; discussion 586–587.
3. Fattori R, Celletti F, Bertaccini P, et al. Delayed surgery of traumatic aortic rupture. Role of magnetic resonance imaging. Circulation. Dec 1 1996;94(11): 2865–2870.
4. Hughes JP, Ruttley MS, Musumeci F. Case report: traumatic aortic rupture: demonstration by magnetic resonance imaging. Br J Radiol. Dec 1994;67(804): 1264–1267.

Teaching File Case 45

49-year-old male with known coronary artery disease, status–post prior myocardial infarction

Category: Cardiomyopathy

History

Assess for viability.

Findings

The left ventricular cavity is dilated, and global systolic dysfunction is noted, with a left ventricular ejection fraction calculated at 16%. Wall motion analysis reveals that global hypokinesia is present, and the anterior wall from base to apex demonstrates akinesia progressing to dyskinesia in the apical region. Thinning of the anterior wall is also noted.

Relatively preserved contractility is noted in the inferior wall at the base, but this also diminishes as one proceeds to the apex.

The right ventricle demonstrates slightly better preserved systolic function. It is within normal limits in size.

Moderate mitral regurgitation is noted, and the left atrium is mildly dilated at 4.2 cm. Velocity-encoded images were obtained through the mitral valve, and clearly show the failure of coaptation.

The aortic valve is trileaflet. The tricuspid valve demonstrates mild insufficiency.

Pulmonary angiographic images demonstrate no evidence of vessel cutoff or filling defect.

Delayed-enhancement imaging demonstrates extensive infarction of the anterior wall extending to involve the anteroseptal and anterolateral walls beginning in the basal level and extending to the apex. The infarction seen in the anterior wall is essentially transmural beginning at the basal level, and extending to involve the apex. The only regions with significant preservation of viability are the inferior wall, the inferior septum, and a portion of the inferolateral wall at the base. At the true apex the inferior wall is also involved with near transmural infarction.

Delayed-enhancement images with a long inversion time demonstrate a tiny focus of low signal at the left ventricular apex best appreciated on the 4-chamber views of the long TI images. This represents a tiny adherent thrombus.

Diagnosis

Ischemic cardiomyopathy.

Extensive prior infarction is noted, with limited residual viability. The anterior wall is essentially completely nonviable from the basal level to the apex. Portions of the anterior margins of the lateral and septal walls are also involved.

Cardiac MRI provides the most accurate means of assessing the relative ratio of viable to infarcted myocardium, and therefore is the best modality to facilitate accurate surgical planning for possible reconstruction or revascularization.[1–4]

As noted in prior cases, MR evaluation usually provides a clear differentiation between the causes of a dilated cardiomyopathy. The first step in this algorithmic approach is to evaluate the DE-MR images for the presence of hyperenhancement. In the setting of a dilated cardiomyopathy if no delayed-enhancement is present, a non-ischemic etiology is extremely likely. If hyperenhancement is present, the pattern (CAD vs. non-CAD type) should be noted. In the present case, the pattern of enhancement as well as the regional heterogeneity of dysfunction is consistent with ischemic cardiomyopathy with extensive prior infarction. A cartoon representation of the pattern recognition approach using DE-MR may be seen in Chapter 3, Figure 3.14. For further reading regarding differential diagnosis of cardiomyopathies, please refer to Chapter 3.

References

1. Kim, R.J. and D.J. Shah, Fundamental concepts in myocardial viability assessment revisited: when knowing how much is "alive" is not enough. Heart, 2004;90(2):137–40.
2. Mahrholdt, H., et al. Relationship of contractile function to transmural extent of infarction in patients with chronic coronary artery disease. J Am Coll Cardiol. 2003;42(3):505–12.
3. Bello, D., et al. Gadolinium cardiovascular magnetic resonance predicts reversible myocardial dysfunction and remodeling in patients with heart failure undergoing beta-blocker therapy. Circulation. 2003;108(16):1945–53.
4. Choi, K.M., et al. Transmural extent of acute myocardial infarction predicts long-term improvement in contractile function. Circulation. 2001;104(10):1101–7.

Teaching File Case 46

46 year-old with arrhythmia

Category: Cardiomyopathy

Findings

The left ventricular cavity is noted to be mildly dilated, and demonstrates mild global hypokinesia. The left ventricular ejection fraction is depressed at 48%. Excessive trabeculation of the left ventricular apex is noted, with extensive involvement of the anterior wall. The thickness of the trabeculated portion of the myocardium is more than two times that of the adjacent compacted myocardium.

The right ventricle also demonstrates mildly depressed function.

Evaluation of the valves demonstrates a bicuspid aortic valve, with aliasing noted when the Venc is set at a velocity of 150 cm/sec, which is absent at 200 cm/sec. The gradient measured 13 mmHg.

Perfusion imaging does not demonstrate a convincing perfusion abnormality.

Delayed enhanced imaging shows no evidence of abnormal hyperenhancement. No thrombus is seen.

Diagnosis

Noncompaction of the myocardium.[1] A bicuspid aortic valve is noted, but is thought to be an incidental finding.

Strictly speaking, this does not represent isolated left ventricular noncompaction, as that entity by definition has no coexisting cardiac abnormalities. Nonetheless, the bicuspid valve is likely incidental in this case.[2]

Noncompaction is felt to represent a distinct cardiomyopathy, characterized by excessive thickening of the myocardial wall which presents a two-layered structure: a thin compacted epicardial layer and a much thicker noncompacted endocardial layer.[3] The endocardial layer consists of prominent trabeculations and deep intratrabecular spaces which are in continuity with the left ventricular cavity.[4] The extent of noncompaction should be quantified at the site of maximal wall thickness. In noncompaction, the ratio of noncompacted to compacted myocardium is greater than 2 to 1 as measured in systole.

There is known to be familial occurrence of isolated left ventricular noncompaction, although the hereditary pattern is uncertain.

The clinical course is variable, with early reports suggesting inevitable progression to dilated cardiomyopathy and heart failure. However, more recent reports suggest a more benign clinical course.[5, 6]

Coronary microcirculatory disturbances have also been reported, with abnormal perfusion evident even in remote segments not involved with the disorder.[7] Perfusion imaging in this case was normal, however.

References

1. McCrohon JA, Richmond DR, Pennell DJ, Mohiaddin RH. Images in cardiovascular medicine. Isolated noncompaction of the myocardium: a rarity or missed diagnosis? Circulation. Aug 6 2002;106(6):e22–23.
2. Cavusoglu Y, Ata N, Timuralp B, et al. Noncompaction of the ventricular myocardium: report of two cases with bicuspid aortic valve demonstrating poor prognosis and with prominent right ventricular involvement. Echocardiography. May 2003;20(4):379–383.
3. Koo BK, Choi D, Ha JW, Kang SM, Chung N, Cho SY. Isolated noncompaction of the ventricular myocardium: contrast echocardiographic findings and review of the literature. Echocardiography. Feb 2002;19(2):153–156.
4. Bax JJ, Atsma DE, Lamb HJ, et al. Noninvasive and invasive evaluation of noncompaction cardiomyopathy. J Cardiovasc Magn Reson. 2002;4(3):353–357.
5. Ali SK, Godman MJ. The variable clinical presentation of, and outcome for, noncompaction of the ventricular myocardium in infants and children, an under-diagnosed cardiomyopathy. Cardiol Young. Aug 2004;14(4):409–416.
6. Salemi VM, Rochitte CE, Lemos P, Benvenuti LA, Pita CG, Mady C. Long-term survival of a patient with isolated noncompaction of the ventricular myocardium. J Am Soc Echocardiogr. Mar 2006;19(3):354 e351–354 e353.
7. Soler R, Rodriguez E, Monserrat L, Alvarez N. MRI of subendocardial perfusion deficits in isolated left ventricular noncompaction. J Comput Assist Tomogr. May-Jun 2002;26(3):373–375.

Teaching File Case 47

68-year-old female with chest pain

Category: Cardiomyopathy

History

Cardiac enzyme levels were minimally elevated at presentation. Cardiac catheterization performed after admission demonstrated no significant coronary artery disease.

Findings

The left ventricular wall thickness is normal. The left ventricular cavity size is at the upper limits of normal. Wall motion analysis demonstrates apical akinesia/dyskinesia, with preservation of wall motion of the base. The right ventricle is normal in appearance and contractility.

The mitral and aortic valves are unremarkable in appearance. No significant regurgitation is seen.

Delayed-enhancement imaging shows no evidence of hyperenhancement to suggest the presence of infarction. No thrombus is seen.

Diagnosis

The findings described are consistent with the apical ballooning syndrome.

Pseudonyms include the broken heart syndrome, and the takotsubo syndrome. This disorder is most commonly seen in middle-aged-to-elderly females, with an average onset in the sixth-seventh decade. Minimal enzyme leak is commonly seen, but significant necrosis is not seen and the disorder usually resolves without sequelae. The etiology is unclear, although preceding emotional or physical stress is often found in this population. The appearance is consistent with a pathophysiologic mechanism of myocardial stunning which resolves. Catecholamine excess was initially considered a likely etiology, but many patients are found to have normal catecholamine levels. Given that most patients have a history of severe preceding stress, transient coronary spasm has been suspected to represent the underlying abnormality, but this remains speculative at this time.[1–3]

MR allows depiction of the wall motion abnormality intrinsic to the syndrome, and demonstrates that the abnormality noted does not relate to a specific vascular territory. Also, MR is helpful in excluding infarction or myocarditis, which are the main differential diagnostic considerations.

References

1. Sharkey SW, et al. Acute and reversible cardiomyopathy provoked by stress in women from the United States. Circulation. 2005;111(4):472–479.
2. Dec GW. Recognition of the apical ballooning syndrome in the United States. Circulation. 2005;111(4):388–390.
3. Fritz J, et al. Transient left ventricular apical ballooning: magnetic resonance imaging evaluation. J Comput Assist Tomogr. 2005;29(1):34–36.

Teaching File Case 48

48-year-old with back pain

Category: Angiography

History

No history of trauma.

Findings

MR angiographic images are obtained, and two different stations were examined. The thoracic aortogram was obtained second, but is displayed first. The volume rendered images seen in the top row demonstrate clearly the presence of a localized pseudoaneurysm originating along the posterior aspect of the proximal descending aorta. In addition, localized aneurysmal dilatation of the right subclavian artery at the level of the origin of the right vertebral artery is seen. An unusual appearance of the great vessel origins is noted, with a bovine origin of the left common carotid artery apparent.

The axial source images are represented in the far right image of the top row. In addition, axial HASTE and FISP images are seen in the first 2 images of the second row. These allow clear distinction of the presence of an intimal flap separating the pseudoaneurysm from the native aortic lumen.

Images of the abdominal aorta and iliac vessels are demonstrated in the bottom row of images. A localized dissection of the right common iliac artery is noted, extending to the level of the iliac bifurcation.

The left common iliac artery is aneurysmally dilated, but no dissection is seen. These findings are confirmed on the thin section axial source images seen in the third image of the bottom row.

Diagnosis

The patient has Ehlers-Danlos syndrome (type IV), with spontaneous aortic and right common iliac artery dissections apparent.

Localized pseudoaneurysm formation is apparent. Surgery can be potentially troublesome in these patients due to their difficulty with wound healing and stitch retention. This patient underwent endovascular treatment as will be seen in the subsequent case.

Ehlers-Danlos syndrome type IV results from abnormal procollagen III synthesis and can lead to arterial, intestinal, and uterine rupture. Cardiovascular complications are a frequent cause of significant morbidity and mortality in these patients.[1–3]

The finding of spontaneous dissections in the absence of trauma and in atypical locations soon should prompt a search for an underlying connective tissue abnormality. Mycotic aneurysms should also be considered in the differential diagnosis of such lesions.

References

1. Oderich GS, et al. The spectrum, management and clinical outcome of Ehlers-Danlos syndrome type IV: a 30-year experience. J Vasc Surg. 2005;42(1): 98–106.
2. Germain DP, Herrera-Guzman Y. Vascular Ehlers-Danlos syndrome. Ann Genet. 2004;47(1):1–9.
3. Pinto YM, et al. Ehlers-Danlos syndrome type IV. N Engl J Med. 2000;343(5):366–368.

Teaching File Case 49

Same patient as in Teaching File Case 48, now status–post therapy

Category: Angiography

Findings

The present images demonstrate that the localized pseudoaneurysms previously noted involving the proximal descending aorta and right common iliac artery are no longer apparent. The third image demonstrates that an endograft is seen in place in the proximal descending thoracic aorta, and excludes the pseudoaneurysm, which is now filled with thrombus. The stent is not visible on the MR images and does not cause significant artifact, as it is composed of nitinol.

The other findings previously noted including an unusual appearance of the innominate artery with a bovine origin of the left carotid, and the right subclavian and left iliac artery aneurysms are unchanged.

Diagnosis

The patient is status–post covered endograft therapy of the localized dissection of the proximal descending aorta.

The nitinol stent present produces minimal artifact, and is difficult to perceive on the maximum intensity projection images.[1, 2] Review of the axial source images allows better depiction of the presence of the stent. Stainless steel stents such as the Palmaz stent produce significantly more artifact and signal drop-out.

Covered endograft treatment of both traumatic and nontraumatic aortic dissection involving the thoracic aorta is a relatively new therapy. However, early series are encouraging in that these stents have been placed with few complications and a decreased morbidity when compared with the surgical alternative.[3, 4]

In patients with contraindications to open surgery such as the present patient, the endovascular technique has obvious appeal, and will likely become the standard of care.[5]

References

1. Melzer et al. Nitinol in magnetic resonance imaging. Minim Invasive Ther Allied Technol. 2004;13(4): 261–271.
2. Cejna M, et al. MR angiography vs CT angiography in the follow-up of nitinol stent grafts in endoluminally treated aortic aneurysms. Eur Radiol. 2002;12(10):2443–2450.
3. Weigel S, et al. Thoracic aortic stent graft: comparison of contrast-enhanced MR angiography and CT angiography in the follow-up: initial results. Eur Radiol. 2003;3(7):1628–1634.
4. Krohg-Sorensen K, et al. Acceptable short-term results after endovascular repair of diseases of the thoracic aorta in high risk patients. Eur J Cardiothorac Surg. 2003;24(3):379–387.
5. Destrieux-Garnier L, et al. Midterm results of endoluminal stent grafting of the thoracic aorta. Vascular. 2004;12(3):179–185.

Teaching File Case 50

74-year-old female with a history of prior bioprosthetic mitral valve replacement, now with suspected leak

Category: Valve disease

History

The clinical concern is for perivalvular vs. intravalvular leak.

Findings

The short-axis images demonstrate the presence of a prosthetic mitral valve, with the support struts seen to extend into the left ventricular cavity. The left ventricle is normal in size and wall thickness, except for a small area of thinning noted to involve the inferior wall at the basal level.

The global left ventricular ejection fraction is normal at 50%.

The 3-chamber view demonstrates clearly an eccentric jet of mitral regurgitation originating along the anterior septal corner of the prosthetic valve, within the valve ring. The regurgitant fraction is measured on velocity encoding images at approximately 35 to 40%. This determination is problematic because of extremely high velocity of the regurgitant jet. The left atrium is dilated to a diameter of 4.8 cm.

The right ventricle demonstrates normal contractility. Moderately severe tricuspid regurgitation is noted, with marked dilatation of the right atrium to a diameter of approximately 6 cm. Early diastolic paradoxical septal motion is noted, consistent with right ventricular volume overload.

Delayed-enhancement imaging demonstrates a small area of infarction in the inferior wall at the mid-ventricular level.

Diagnosis

This represents a case of degenerative change within a bioprosthetic mitral valve resulting in moderately severe mitral regurgitation. The leak is not perivalvular, but within the valve, which mandates its replacement.[1, 2]

The patient subsequently underwent revision of the mitral valve replacement, and placement of a tricuspid valve prosthesis was simultaneously performed.

MR imaging allows accurate placement of the imaging plane across the regurgitant jet, and therefore can allow very precise quantification of regurgitant fractions.[3] However, in cases such as the present example where there is a very high-velocity jet or where there is significant spin-dephasing, an alternative means of determining the regurgitant mitral volume is desirable. This can be accomplished by performing a flow measurement of the volume passing through the aortic valve, and comparing this volume with the volume measured by tracing the endocardial contours on successive cine images through the LV (sum of disks method). Presuming there is no aortic insufficiency, the difference represents the regurgitant volume. Alternatively, the antegrade flow volume through the aortic valve can be compared to the antegrade mitral flow volume; the difference represents the regurgitant volume. For further discussion regarding the assessment of regurgitant valvular lesions, please refer to Chapter 4.

References

1. Kumar AS, et al. Experience with homograft mitral valve replacement. J Heart Valve Dis. 1998;7(2):225–228.
2. Pflaumer A, et al. Quantification of periprosthetic valve leakage with multiple regurgitation jets by magnetic resonance imaging. Pediatr Cardiol. 2005;26(5):593–594.
3. Hasenkam JM, et al. Prosthetic heart valve evaluation by magnetic resonance imaging. Eur J Cardiothorac Surg. 1999;16(3):300–305.

Teaching File Case 51

35-year-old female from the ED with chest pain

Category: Stress test

History

Resting nuclear myocardial perfusion imaging was normal.

Findings

The cine images in the short-axis plane demonstrate inferior wall hypokinesia at the basal and mid-ventricular levels, with less severe involvement of the inferior wall in the apical region.

The right ventricle is normal in size and function. The valvular structures are unremarkable.

Stress and rest perfusion images are obtained in the second and third rows, in locations approximating those of the short-axis cine views. The adenosine stress images in the second row demonstrate an area of diminished perfusion involving the inferior wall at the basal and mid ventricular levels, with less severe involvement of the inferior wall in the apical region.

The resting images show significant improvement in the appearance of this region.

Delayed-enhancement images demonstrate no focal infarction in this region.

Diagnosis

Inducible ischemia in the inferior wall, consistent with significant epicardial coronary disease in the right coronary artery (RCA) territory.

Rest nuclear myocardial perfusion imaging has been shown to have good negative predictive value, although in this patient the study was falsely negative. The wall motion abnormality that is quite apparent on MR imaging was not apparent on perfusion imaging, likely due to the lower spatial resolution of that technique.

Kwong reported a series of patients that were studied with MR in the emergency department for evaluation of chest pain. He found that analysis of regional wall motion was quite helpful, and in fact was more sensitive than first pass perfusion abnormalities (these were performed at rest in his study) in the detection of ischemia.[1]

Subsequent papers from this same group have demonstrated that a stress MR perfusion study has excellent prognostic power. Specifically, in their series of 135 patients presenting to the ED with chest pain, adenosine stress perfusion imaging had 100% sensitivity for the detection of significant coronary artery disease, and no patient with a negative study had any evidence of coronary artery disease or an adverse event at one-year follow-up.[2]

References

1. Kwong RY, et al. Detecting acute coronary syndrome in the emergency department with cardiac magnetic resonance imaging. Circulation. 2003;107(4): 531–537.
2. Ingkanisorn WP, et al. Prognosis of negative adenosine stress magnetic resonance in patients presenting to an emergency department with chest pain. J Am Coll Cardiol. 2006;47(7):1427–1432.

Teaching File Case 52

41-year-old male with fevers and an abnormal chest radiograph

Category: Valve disease

Findings

Minimal respiratory motion artifact degrades the cine image quality somewhat.

The short-axis views demonstrate normal left ventricular size and function. The short-axis views of the right ventricle demonstrate a minimally irregular polypoid filling defect along the septal side of the right ventricular outflow tract, best appreciated on the second and third short-axis cine views. This same abnormality is seen in the second row of images immediately beneath the pulmonic valve on the short-axis and RV outflow tract views. This appears to have a linear filling defect attached to it, which extends through the pulmonary valve into the main pulmonary artery. Small field-of-view images of the pulmonic valve (fourth row, third image) demonstrate irregularity and thickening of its central margins.

Delayed-enhancement images subsequently obtained demonstrate that this same mobile filling defect is quite low in signal intensity on images obtained with a long inversion time (third row, fourth, fifth, and sixth images). Evaluation of the pulmonary parenchyma on the same images demonstrates multiple cavitary lung nodules of varying sizes.

Diagnosis

This represents a case of bacterial endocarditis affecting the right ventricular outflow tract, the pulmonary valve, and extending into the main pulmonary artery segment. Septic pulmonary emboli account for the cavitary pulmonary nodules noted.

Vegetations are usually medium in signal intensity on precontrast images, similar to adjacent myocardium. They are usually attached to the valves, and may be quite mobile. There may also be attached to the chordae. Delayed-enhancement images obtained with a long inversion time (greater than 500 ms) demonstrate that these have low signal intensity, similar to thrombus.

Myxomas can also present as mobile filling defects,[1,2] and may prolapse through AV valves, but differ from vegetations in several ways: myxomas are usually attached to the fossa ovalis, rather than valvular structures, and myxomas usually demonstrate heterogeneous enhancement on post-contrast delayed-enhancement images, whereas vegetations are quite low in signal on delayed-enhancement images obtained with a long inversion time.[3]

Right-sided endocarditis is most often a sequela of IV drug abuse. This was the case in the present example.

References

1. Restrepo CS, et al. CT and MR imaging findings of benign cardiac tumors. Curr Probl Diagn Radiol. 2005;34(1):12–21.
2. Luna A, et al. Evaluation of cardiac tumors with magnetic resonance imaging. Eur Radiol. 2005;15(7): 1446–1455.
3. Heitner JF, et al. The case of the disappearing myxoma. J Cardiovasc Magn Reson. 2005;7(5):841–843.

Teaching File Case 53

40-year-old male with occasional syncope

Category: Cardiomyopathy

Findings

The left ventricular wall thickness and cavity size appear normal. The right ventricle is enlarged, and demonstrates a global decrease in systolic function. In addition, focal areas of dyskinesia are noted along the free wall in the short-axis views, particularly near the outflow tract. Abnormal trabeculation is apparent throughout the right ventricle, and is particular notable at the apex.

The valvular function appears normal.

The static spin-echo images with and without fat saturation illustrate the difficulty in detecting with certainty the presence of fatty infiltration. Epicardial fat is present in abundance, and there may be a small amount of fat within the RV myocardium, but this is difficult to state with certainty.

The delayed-enhancement images are quite helpful, and demonstrate that on the single-shot inversion recovery SSFP as well as the high resolution static images extensive hyperenhancement is seen along the right ventricular free wall. Hyperenhancement is also noted along the RV side of the septum. On one short-axis image of the single-shot series, possible enhancement in the left ventricular wall is also apparent.

Diagnosis

The findings described are consistent with arrhythmogenic right ventricular dysplasia (ARVD).

This is a form of cardiomyopathy characterized by fibrofatty infiltration of the right ventricle associated with right ventricular dilatation and functional impairment. It is a familial disorder that most often presents with arrhythmias, and can lead to sudden death. The diagnosis is made using Task Force criteria that encompass MR, clinical, and ECG features.[1] Classic MR imaging findings are said to include right ventricular thinning and fatty infiltration. However, as in this case, these findings can be difficult to detect. Therefore, the cine imaging findings of altered contraction and microaneurysm formation along with abnormal trabeculation are very helpful. Most patients meeting task force criteria demonstrate RV dilatation and diminished systolic function, as noted in the present case. Excessive trabeculation is also frequently seen.[2,3]

Recent reports have emphasized that the diagnosis can be difficult to make, and that an over-reliance on the apparent presence of fatty infiltration on MR imaging is a frequent cause of misdiagnosis.[4] A better distinction between normals and patients with ARVD was recently reported using delayed-enhancement imaging. In one small series, RV hyperenhancement was reported in 2/3 of patients, and correlated with an increased likelihood of inducibility. No normal patients demonstrated RV enhancement.[5]

The differential diagnosis for right ventricular dilatation would include valvular disorders such as pulmonic or tricuspid insufficiency, as well as a shunt lesion such as an ASD. Anomalous pulmonary veins can also result in dilatation of the right ventricle. However, no evidence of valvular insufficiency is seen on this exam, and the abnormal systolic contraction would be unexplained by the presence of an ASD.

References

1. Kayser HW, et al. Diagnosis of arrhythmogenic right ventricular dysplasia: a review. Radiographics. 2002;22(3):639–648; discussion 649–650.
2. Tandri H, et al. Magnetic resonance imaging findings in patients meeting task force criteria for arrhythmogenic right ventricular dysplasia. J Cardiovasc Electrophysiol. 2003;14(5):476–482.
3. Bluemke DA, et al. MR Imaging of arrhythmogenic right ventricular cardiomyopathy: morphologic findings and interobserver reliability. Cardiology. 2003;99(3):153–162.
4. Bomma C, et al. Misdiagnosis of arrhythmogenic right ventricular dysplasia/cardiomyopathy. J Cardiovasc Electrophysiol. 2004;15(3):300–306.
5. Tandri H, et al. Noninvasive detection of myocardial fibrosis in arrhythmogenic right ventricular cardiomyopathy using delayed-enhancement magnetic resonance imaging. J Am Coll Cardiol. 2005;45(1):98–103.

Teaching File Case 54

59-year-old female, with known three-vessel coronary artery disease, being considered for surgery

Category: Viability

History

The patient also had an abnormal echo with a suggestion of prior infarct in the anterior wall.

Findings

The left ventricle is normal in wall thickness, and demonstrates minimal cavity dilatation. Thinning of the anterior wall is noted associated with hypokinesia in the mid-ventricular level, progressing to akinesia and finally dyskinesia at the apex. Focal outpouching of the inferoapical region is noted.

The left ventricular ejection fraction is 28%.

The right ventricle is normal in size and function.

Evaluation of the valvular structures demonstrates that mild aortic stenosis is apparent. The mitral valve is unremarkable.

Delayed-enhancement imaging demonstrates that no significant anterior wall infarction is noted, from the base to the apical region, with only a small area of infarction seen in the true apex. This small area is essentially transmural, and is associated with the aneurysmal outpouching previously described.

Diagnosis

Hibernating myocardium.[1]

Even though the anterior wall is thinned, and severely hypokinetic, it shows no enhancement, and therefore demonstrates significant residual viability. The absence of contrast enhancement is strong evidence that this region remains viable. Therefore, it should benefit from revascularization.[2, 3]

The focal transmural apical infarction may require ventricular reconstructive surgery to gain full benefit from any planned revascularization, as this area will likely not recover function.

It should be noted that this information is readily available with MR imaging, and may not be as well demonstrated by modalities that only show what is viable. Specifically, an imaging study that only demonstrates what is viable would not show the relationship between areas of infarcted myocardium and areas of residual viable myocardium, as well as their relative proportions. It is this ratio that is of crucial importance in determining the likelihood of wall motion recovery from revascularization.[4] It can be clearly seen that chronic ischemic disease can result in myocardial thinning, and yet the myocardium may remain viable.

Studies have shown that patients with ischemic myocardium who are treated medically do significantly worse than those who are revascularized. Conversely, patients without significant reversible ischemic disease who are treated surgically have a worse outcome than those treated medically. Therefore, it is critically important to make an accurate distinction between those patients with viable but ischemic myocardium and those with irreversibly scarred myocardium.

References

1. Bonow RO, Myocardial hibernation: a noninvasive physician's point of view. Ital Heart J. 2002;3(5):285–290.
2. Kim RJ, et al. The use of contrast-enhanced magnetic resonance imaging to identify reversible myocardial dysfunction. N Engl J Med. 2000;343(20):1445–1453.

3. Choi KM, et al. Transmural extent of acute myocardial infarction predicts long-term improvement in contractile function. Circulation. 2001;104(10): 1101–1107.

4. Kim RJ, Shah DJ. Fundamental concepts in myocardial viability assessment revisited: when knowing how much is "alive" is not enough. Heart. 2004;90(2): 137–140.

Teaching File Case 55

83-year-old female with an abnormal chest x-ray

Category: Mass

Findings

The left ventricle is normal in size and function. The right ventricle is likewise normal.

The first short-axis view seen as the first image of the first row demonstrates a lung mass extending along the left lower lobe pulmonary vein into the left atrium. This is also well seen on the 4-chamber and 3-chamber views (first two images of the second row).

Perfusion imaging is displayed in the third row and shows that the large lung mass demonstrates significant enhancement. A portion of the mass within the left atrium does not appear to show significant enhancement.

The HASTE and SSFP images (fifth and sixth images of the third row) demonstrate well the extent of tumor. The tumor is seen to extend in proximity to the aorta, and into the left hilum. A small left pleural effusion is noted as well.

Multiple single-shot inversion recovery images with a long inversion time and short inversion time are seen in the fourth row. 4-chamber views, short-axis views, and 2-chamber views are obtained. The images with a long inversion time are recognized by the light gray appearance of the myocardium. Note that the mass is predominantly of similar signal intensity to the myocardium. However, the component that extends into the left atrial cavity demonstrates low signal consistent with thrombus on images with a long inversion time. Similar findings are seen on the high-resolution segmented images in the bottom two rows.

Diagnosis

Lung cancer extending along the left lower lobe pulmonary vein to invade the left atrium. Coating thrombus is noted as well.

Metastatic disease is 20–40 times more common than primary cardiac malignancy. Cardiac metastases are found at autopsy in approximately 10–12% of patients dying of cancer.[1] However, clinical recognition is significantly less common. They are most often found in the setting of late-stage disease, and are rarely the presenting finding of a malignancy.

Metastases can reach the heart one of four routes: retrograde lymphatic spread, direct invasion, transvenous extension, or hematogenous dissemination.[2] The present examination demonstrates transvenous extension of a lung cancer along the left lower lobe pulmonary vein into the left atrium. Lesions spreading by a transvenous extension to the left atrium are usually lung carcinomas. Primary tumors that commonly spread via transvenous extension to the right atrium include renal cell carcinoma, hepatocellular carcinoma, and adrenal carcinoma.[2]

Cardiac MR imaging has assumed a primary role in imaging metastatic cardiac disease. Its multiplanar imaging capabilities allow visualization of the entire cardiac structure, without limitation by acoustic windows. The multiple sequences available with cardiac MR imaging provide superior tissue characterization when compared with CT examination.[3] Therefore, when metastatic cardiac disease is suspected, MR imaging is the preferred approach. The use of CMR for the evaluation of known or suspected cardiac masses is reviewed in Chapter 5.

References

1. Klatt EC, Heitz DR. Cardiac metastases. Cancer. 1990;65(6):1456–1459.
2. Chiles C, Woodard PK, Gutierrez FR, Link KM. Metastatic involvement of the heart and pericardium: CT and MR imaging. Radiographics. 2001;21(2):439–449.
3. Grizzard JD, Ang GB. Magnetic resonance imaging of pericardial disease and cardiac masses. Cardiol Clin. 2007;25(1):111–140.

Teaching File Case 56

Known peripheral vascular disease

Category: Angiography

History

The study is performed in follow-up.

Findings

Rotating maximum intensity projection images are seen in the first 3 images of the top row. The fourth image is a time-resolved image obtained at the lower leg level. The fifth image of the top row is a thin section coronal image through the abdomen and pelvis region.

Static images at each level are displayed in the bottom row.

The study demonstrates that no abdominal aneurysm is seen. There appears to be a focal stenosis of the proximal portion of the celiac axis. The SMA is widely patent. The right renal artery demonstrates a focal, moderately severe stenosis in its proximal portion.

In the iliac arteries, apparent focal signal dropout in the left common iliac artery is noted. Review of the source images indicates that this is due to the presence of an intra-arterial stent. Similar but less extensive signal dropout is noted in the right common iliac artery. This is also felt to be due to the presence of a stent, likely composed of nitinol. This results in less extensive stent artifact.

The right external iliac artery distal to the stent appears to be mildly diffusely narrowed.

A large caliber graft is seen to originate from the right common femoral artery, and bypasses an apparent SFA occlusion. The graft appears to be patent throughout, but a short segment area of signal dropout is noted in the distal portion of the bypass graft, just above the anastomosis to the native popliteal artery. Two apparent weblike stenoses are noted, but on review of the source images, these are felt to be due to the presence of a stent within the distal portion of the graft. A focal high-grade narrowing of the native popliteal artery just above the knee joint is seen. The popliteal artery is patent as it crosses the knee.

On the left, multisegmental plaque is noted in the SFA, which appears to be moderately narrowed in its proximal and mid portions. No occlusion is noted. The image quality in the midportion of the upper leg is somewhat diminished by the presence of venous contamination.

Continuing on the left, the popliteal artery is patent as it crosses the knee and supplies a well-developed anterior tibial artery. This forms the dorsalis pedis artery. The left posterior tibial artery is also patent as it extends to the ankle.

On the right, the popliteal artery below the knee is patent. The anterior tibial artery is the predominant supply to the right foot.

Diagnosis

Intra-arterial stents are seen in place in the iliac arteries bilaterally, as well as in the patient's SFA bypass graft. This was confirmed on review of prior x-ray images.

Stents can produce a confusing appearance on magnetic resonance angiographic images, depending on their composition.[1] Stainless steel stents, such as the Palmaz stent, result in more extensive signal loss then do the nitinol stents. A stent should be suspected when there is apparent abrupt vessel cutoff, without collaterals,[2, 3] and without patient symptoms. Review of the source images is essential in order to detect stent artifact.[4] Multiplanar review of the images is often quite helpful. Occasionally, correlation with radiography may be necessary for complete evaluation.

References

1. Maintz D, et al. In vitro evaluation of intravascular stent artifacts in three-dimensional MR angiography. Invest Radiol. 2001;36(4):218–224.
2. Hunink MG, et al. Revascularization for femoropopliteal disease. A decision and cost-effectiveness analysis. JAMA. 1995;274(2):165–171.
3. Leng GC, Davis M, Baker D. Bypass surgery for chronic lower limb ischaemia. Cochrane Database Syst Rev. 2000;3:CD002000.
4. Lenhart M, et al. Stent appearance at contrast-enhanced MR angiography: in vitro examination with 14 stents. Radiology. 2000;217(1):173–178.

Teaching File Case 57

17-year-old male followed for a persistent abnormality noted originally on echocardiography

Category: Aorta

Findings

The left ventricle is normal in size and systolic function. No regional wall motion abnormality is seen. The right ventricle is also normal in appearance.

The aortic valve is trileaflet. No aortic insufficiency is noted.

Dilatation of the aortic root is noted, with annular dilatation apparent. The diameter of the aortic root measured 5 cm. The MR angiogram demonstrates a "tulip bulb" shape of the proximal aorta.

Diagnosis

This patient has Marfan syndrome, with annulo-aortic ectasia apparent.

Marfan syndrome is a connective tissue disorder characterized by a tall, asthenic body habitus, with arachnodactyly frequently noted. Other associated anomalies include pectus excavatum deformity, scoliosis, and frequent dislocation of the lens. A high arched palate is often noted as well. It is caused by mutations in the FBN 1 gene on chromosome 15.[1]

Imaging findings include dural ectasia, which is fairly specific for this disorder. Annulo-aortic ectasia is also characteristic, and its presence on imaging should suggest the likely diagnosis of underlying Marfan syndrome.

Annulo-aortic ectasia is thought to be due to an abnormality of formation of a matrix protein resulting in aortic medial weakness and characteristic dilatation. As the dilatation progresses, the patient may develop coexisting aortic insufficiency.

The most common cause of death in Marfan syndrome is cardiovascular disease, with aortic dissection being a frequent terminal event. Surveillance with echocardiography and/or MR is helpful in assessing the degree of dilatation of the aortic root, and for planning elective surgery when the aortic root dilatation exceeds 5 cm.[2, 3]

References

1. Nollen GJ, Mulder BJ. What is new in the Marfan syndrome? Int J Cardiol. 2004;97(Suppl 1): 103–108.
2. Boyer JK, Gutierrez F, Braverman AC. Approach to the dilated aortic root. Curr Opin Cardiol. 2004;19(6):563–569.
3. Bethea BT, et al. Results of aortic valve-sparing operations: experience with remodeling and reimplantation procedures in 65 patients. Ann Thorac Surg. 2004;78(3):767–772; discussion 767–772.

Teaching File Case 58

80-year-old female with an abnormal echocardiogram

Category: Mass

Findings

A large soft tissue mass is seen to nearly fill the right atrium. It appears to be attached to the inferior wall of the right atrium near the eustachian valve. The lesion is mobile, and can be seen to abut against the tricuspid valve, but produces only mild obstruction. Bowing of the inter-atrial septum is noted.

Perfusion images (first 2 images of the second row) demonstrate that the lesion does not appear to show significant enhancement and is quite hypovascular. T1 weighed fat-suppressed images seen in the third and fourth images of the second row pre- and postcontrast demonstrate minimal enhancement of a central core of the lesion, but the lesion itself is predominantly low in signal intensity. It is high in signal intensity on the

HASTE and SSFP images seen as the fifth and sixth images of the second row.

Delayed-enhancement images obtained with long and short inversion times are seen in the third row. The long TI images demonstrate that the lesion is low in signal intensity with a central higher signal intensity core that is similar to myocardial signal.

Imaging of the remainder of the heart demonstrates that the left ventricular function is normal. Thickening of the anterior leaflet of the mitral valve is apparent, but no significant mitral regurgitation is noted. Mild aortic stenosis is noted. Mild aortic insufficiency is also seen. Velocity-encoded series were also obtained and demonstrated no significant gradient or regurgitation.

Diagnosis

Right atrial myxoma.

Atrial myxomas are more common on the left side, accounting for approximately 85 to 90% of cases.[1] In 10–15% of cases, the lesion originates either within the right atrium or protrudes through the fossa ovalis into the right atrium.[2, 3]

The differential diagnosis would include a large thrombus. In fact, the lesion described could easily represent abundant thrombus surrounding a small myxoma. However, in this case, the entire lesion was accounted for by the myxoma, and little coating thrombus was found at pathology. The lesion could not simply represent thrombus, as there is a central core of enhancement that would not be seen with a pure thrombus.

Formally myxomas were often noted to be low in signal intensity on the cine sequences that used gradient echo techniques.[4] However, with the SSFP cine sequence, the image contrast of which is dependent on the T2/T1 ratio, the signal intensity is often noted to be quite high as in the present example. This relates to the gelatinous composition of the lesion, with a high fluid component, resulting in high signal intensity on sequences with T2-weighting.[5] This also accounts for its apparent high signal on the standard inversion time delayed-enhancement sequences. Specifically, the predominantly gelatinous component of the lesion is far below the zero-crossing line, and therefore has a bright appearance with a surrounding dark rim. It has a dark appearance on images with a long inversion time.

Myxoma is the most common primary cardiac neoplasm, accounting for approximately 50% of cases. A significant female predominance is noted, in the range of 1.5 to 1 to as high as 3 to 1. Patients often report constitutional symptoms, and are also subject to embolic events. Resection is almost always curative.

References

1. Luna A, Ribes R, Caro P, Vida J, Erasmus JJ. Evaluation of cardiac tumors with magnetic resonance imaging. Eur Radiol. 2005;15(7):1446–1455.
2. Grebenc ML, Rosado-de-Christenson ML, Green CE, Burke AP, Galvin JR. Cardiac myxoma: imaging features in 83 patients. Radiographics. 2002;22(3): 673–689.
3. Araoz PA, Mulvagh SL, Tazelaar HD, Julsrud PR, Breen JF. CT and MR imaging of benign primary cardiac neoplasms with echocardiographic correlation. Radiographics. 2000;20(5):1303–1319.
4. Semelka RC, Shoenut JP, Wilson ME, Pellech AE, Patton JN. Cardiac masses: signal intensity features on spin-echo, gradient-echo, gadolinium-enhanced spin-echo, and TurboFLASH images. J Magn Reson Imaging. 1992;2(4):415–420.
5. Grizzard JD, Ang GB. Magnetic resonance imaging of pericardial disease and cardiac masses. Cardiol Clin. 2007;25(1):111–140.

Teaching File Case 59

64-year-old female with symptoms of right heart failure

Category: Pericardium

Findings

The left ventricular size and function are normal.

The right ventricular size is within normal limits, but its configuration is abnormal in that it has a tubular appearance. In addition, marked thickening of the pericardium over the right ventricular free wall is apparent. Normal epicardial fat is seen interposed between the right ventricular free wall and the thickened pericardium. Static images confirm the extensive pericardial thickening.

Images seen in the third row in the axial plane demonstrate marked distention of the inferior vena cava.

Delayed-enhancement images show no evidence of scar.

Review of the 4-chamber cine images demonstrates a "septal bounce," along with bi-atrial distention.

Diagnosis

Constrictive pericarditis.

The extensive pericardial thickening evident in this case results in impaired filling of the right ventricle, with an abnormal tubular configuration. As a result of the altered filling dynamics, early septal displacement from right-to-left is noted, resulting in the "shivering septum." This sign of constrictive pericarditis is present in approximately 85% of cases of constrictive pericarditis.[1]

Constrictive pericarditis in the past was most often due to tuberculosis. In the modern era, in developed countries, idiopathic/ presumed post viral etiologies are the most common cause. Uremia, prior surgery and radiation therapy are the most common identifiable causes.

MR is quite useful in distinguishing constrictive pericarditis from restrictive cardiomyopathy, conditions which can have very a similar clinical presentation.

Although CT is superior in detecting the frequently associated pericardial calcification, it cannot demonstrate the physiologic abnormalities that the MR exam can display with ease. It should also be remembered that pericardial calcification can be present without constriction, and constriction can be present without calcification. In addition, dynamic provocative maneuvers can be performed with MR imaging as will be discussed in other sections of this teaching file. Therefore, MR is considered the modality of choice for the evaluation of suspected constrictive pericarditis.[2, 3] The use of CMR in the evaluation of pericardial disease is reviewed in Chapter 5.

References

1. Giorgi B, et al. Clinically suspected constrictive pericarditis: MR imaging assessment of ventricular septal motion and configuration in patients and healthy subjects. Radiology. 2003;228(2):417–424.
2. Breen JF, Imaging of the pericardium. J Thorac Imaging. 2001;16(1):47–54.
3. Sechtem U, Tscholakoff D, Higgins CB. MRI of the abnormal pericardium. AJR Am J Roentgenol. 1986;147(2):245–252.

Teaching File Case 60

55-year-old male for evaluation of suspected peripheral vascular disease

Category: Angiography

Findings

The abdomen/pelvis station demonstrates absence of the right kidney. Mild aneurysmal dilatation of the infrarenal aorta is noted.

However, the most striking abnormality is the presence of early venous filling involving the right femoral vein, the right iliac vein, and the inferior vena cava.

Review of source images demonstrated an arteriovenous fistula likely arising from the right profunda femoris artery.

The right superficial femoral artery is patent proximally, with a focal high-grade stenosis in its proximal portion, and is occluded in its midportion with reconstitution of the popliteal artery at the adductor canal. The left SFA is occluded at its origin, and is reconstituted just above the adductor canal.

The right popliteal artery demonstrates a focal narrowing just below the joint line, and three-vessel runoff is apparent bilaterally.

Diagnosis

Right femoral arteriovenous fistula.

These are most often secondary to prior instrumentation, usually from a vascular catheterization procedure.[1] Less commonly, repetitive arterial punctures can promote arteriovenous fistula formation. This patient had undergone a prior cardiac catheterization.

There are recognized on MR angiography as on conventional angiography by the presence of early and inappropriate venous filling during the arterial phase of imaging. They may result in a "steal" phenomenon, as the venous circulation is a low resistance circuit, with resultant shunting of blood away from the arterial circuit.

Endovascular repair with covered stent-graft placement is emerging as a promising treatment modality.[2]

References

1. Kelm M, et al. Incidence and clinical outcome of iatrogenic femoral arteriovenous fistulas: implications for risk stratification and treatment. J Am Coll Cardiol. 2002;40(2):291–297.
2. Thalhammer C., et al. Postcatheterization pseudoaneurysms and arteriovenous fistulas: repair with percutaneous implantation of endovascular covered stents. Radiology. 2000;214(1):127–131.

Teaching File Case 61

Patient has a history of arrhythmia and recent stroke

Category: Congenital

Findings

Short-axis cine images in the top row demonstrate no abnormality of left ventricular size or function. The right ventricle is also normal in size and function.

The 4-chamber views seen in the second and third row demonstrate prominent movement of the interatrial septum, suspicious for interatrial septal aneurysm.

The far right images of the second row are perfusion images. Still frames from these perfusion images are seen in the bottom row of the still images. The perfusion images were obtained with the patient performing a Valsalva maneuver. The still frames clearly demonstrate abnormal high signal material traversing the interatrial septum from the right atrium to the left atrium. Signal intensity measurements confirm this.

The mitral and aortic valves are unremarkable in appearance. No vegetations are seen.

Delayed-enhancement images demonstrate a tiny focus of delayed-enhancement in the inferolateral wall and the basal level.

Diagnosis

The perfusion images demonstrated a small amount of contrast traversing the interatrial septum, consistent with a small patent foramen ovale. This is quite subtle, and required meticulous review of the source images on a frame-by-frame basis.

The MR diagnosis of patent foramen ovale is dependent upon the real-time demonstration of flow traversing the interatrial septum as the patient performs a provocative maneuver. Patient cooperation and correct timing are necessary for diagnosis. Only a single small series using this technique has been reported, but it appeared quite useful.[1] No large series has been reported on the accuracy of this technique, particularly relative to other techniques. When it is positive, it is quite helpful however.

The interatrial septum appears abnormal in this case and is suspicious for inter-atrial septal aneurysm. Inter-atrial septal aneurysm has been reported to have an increased incidence of associated patent foramen ovale.[2] Both PFO and interatrial septal aneurysm have been associated with an increased risk of stroke and TIAs, although this remains controversial.[3–5]

References

1. Mohrs OK, et al. Diagnosis of patent foramen ovale using contrast-enhanced dynamic MRI: a pilot study. AJR Am J Roentgenol. 2005;184(1):234–240.
2. Agmon Y, et al. Frequency of atrial septal aneurysms in patients with cerebral ischemic events. Circulation. 1999;99(15):1942–1944.
3. Steiner MM, et al. Patent foramen ovale size and embolic brain imaging findings among patients with ischemic stroke. Stroke. 1998;29(5):944–948.
4. Burger AJ, Sherman HB, Charlamb MJ. Low incidence of embolic strokes with atrial septal aneurysms: A prospective, long-term study. Am Heart J. 2000;1391 Pt 1):149–152.
5. Meissner I, et al. Patent foramen ovale: innocent or guilty? Evidence from a prospective population-based study. J Am Coll Cardiol. 2006;47(2):440–445.

Teaching File Case 62

45-year-old male who is status–post repair of a ventricular septal defect

Category: Coronary MRA

Findings

The left ventricle is normal in size and wall thickness. The regional wall motion is normal as well. The left ventricular ejection fraction is 65%.

The right ventricle is normal in size, thickness, and systolic function.

The aortic valve is noted to have 3 leaflets, however, the noncoronary cusp appears larger than the left and right coronary cusps. In addition there is partial fusion of the noncoronary and right coronary cusp. No aortic stenosis is noted, with normal aortic valve area by planimetry.

A small residual ventricular septal defect is noted in the immediate subvalvular portion of the left ventricular outflow tract, best appreciated on the far right image of the second row. A jet of turbulent flow can be seen extending inferiorly from the left ventricular outflow tract into the right ventricle.

The images seen in the third row are obtained from a whole heart coronary MR angiographic acquisition. The first image of the third row displays the navigator tracing monitoring the position of the diaphragm. The small bars at the top of the acquisition window demonstrate that the acquisitions are obtained during end expiration when the diaphragm is at its most superior position. This is felt to be the most reproducible position. Automated tracking of the diaphragm position is now available which allows adjustment of the acquisition window in case there are changes in the patient's respiratory pattern.

A whole heart MR angiographic data set is the second image of the third row, and demonstrates that the left circumflex coronary artery is noted to originate from the right coronary cusp, and travels posterior to the aortic root to assume its more normal location in the left A-V groove. The right coronary is small in size and is not visualized beyond its proximal portion. The left circumflex is dominant. The left anterior descending artery comes off in the normal fashion from the left coronary cusp. These images also demonstrate continuity between the left ventricular outflow tract and the right ventricle. Multi-planar maximum intensity projection images from the same acquisition are seen is the remaining images in the third row.

The delayed-enhancement images show no evidence of prior infarction.

Diagnosis

A small residual ventricular septal defect is noted as described. An anomalous left circumflex coronary artery is evident, originating from the right coronary cusp and extending in a retroaortic fashion. The aortic valve demonstrates abnormal morphology, but no significant stenosis is seen.

The whole heart coronary MR angiography technique has advantages relative to the standard thin slab coronary angiography in that the image acquisition can be more reliably planned, and comprehensive imaging of all 3 coronary arteries is accomplished with one acquisition.[1, 2] Improved navigator tracking of the diaphragmatic position, with real-time adjustment as needed for diaphragmatic drift makes this sequence more robust and the acquisitions shorter in duration than the thin slab technique.[3] Total imaging time for the MR angiogram acquisition was approximately 7 minutes. It can be performed following the administration of contrast, and therefore can be performed following the perfusion sequence while waiting for contrast washout prior to acquisition of the delayed enhancement images.

The anomaly depicted in this case, the left circumflex coronary artery originating from the right cusp, is one of the most common forms of anomalous coronary artery origin. It has a benign clinical course, and does not require surgical correction.[4,5] However, coronary artery anomalies in which the anomalous vessel extends from the opposite cusp and has an inter-arterial course are subject to vascular compromise and therefore represent potentially dangerous variants.[6] Those lesions are often repaired surgically.

References

1. Nehrke K, et al. Free-breathing whole-heart coronary MR angiography on a clinical scanner in four minutes. J Magn Reson Imaging. 2006.
2. Sakuma H, et al. Detection of coronary artery stenosis with whole-heart coronary magnetic resonance angiography. J Am Coll Cardiol. 2006;48(10):1946–1950.
3. Sakuma H, et al. Assessment of coronary arteries with total study time of less than 30 minutes by using whole-heart coronary MR angiography. Radiology. 2005;237(1):316–321.
4. Harikrishnan S, et al. Congenital coronary anomalies of origin and distribution in adults: a coronary arteriographic study. Indian Heart J. 2002;54(3):271–275.
5. Angelini P, Normal and anomalous coronary arteries: definitions and classification. Am Heart J. 1989;117(2):418–434.
6. Angelini P., Coronary artery anomalies: an entity in search of an identity. Circulation. 2007;115(10):1296–1305.

Teaching File Case 63

18-year-old female status–post recent pregnancy, with increasing shortness of breath and fatigue

Category: Valve disease

History

She recently emigrated from the Middle East. Physical exam demonstrates a continuous murmur and bounding pulses. The study is requested to rule out patent ductus arteriosus.

Findings

The left ventricle is noted to be dilated, with minimally reduced function. The right ventricle is normal in size and function. The left atrium is at the upper limits of normal in size.

Evaluation of valvular structures demonstrates moderate mitral regurgitation, as well as moderately severe aortic insufficiency. Measurements indicate the regurgitant fraction is 50%. Foreshortening of the chordae tendinae and of the papillary musculature is apparent, along with an area of mass-like fibrosis, best appreciated on the 2-chamber view. Relative immobility of the posterior leaflet of the mitral valve is apparent, and restricted movement of the anterior leaflet is also apparent.

The MR angiographic evaluation of the aorta demonstrates no evidence of patent ductus arteriosus.

Diagnosis

Rheumatic heart disease.

The combined involvement of the mitral and aortic valves, as well as the patient's history of recent immigration from the Middle East suggests the likely presence of rheumatic heart disease resulting in valvular insufficiency of the mitral and aortic valves. Rheumatic heart disease can present at an earlier age in individuals living in endemic areas when compared with the later onset typical in the United States.

Rheumatic disease has a predilection for involvement of the mitral and aortic valves, and usually the mitral valve disease is more severe than the aortic disease, as well as earlier in onset. This case is atypical in that the aortic disease predominates.[1,2]

MR measurements of the regurgitant volumes can provide accurate assessment, and can be used to follow patients in whom surgery is not urgently required. In the present case, the patient was scheduled for aortic and mitral valve replacement surgery.

References

1. Choi EY, et al. Detection of myocardial involvement of rheumatic heart disease with contrast-enhanced magnetic resonance imaging. Int J Cardiol. 2006.
2. Gentles TL, et al. Left ventricular mechanics during and after acute rheumatic fever: contractile dysfunction is closely related to valve regurgitation. J Am Coll Cardiol. 2001;37(1):201–207.

Teaching File Case 64

38-year-old female admitted for non-ST-segment elevation MI

Category: Stress test

History

She underwent angioplasty and stent placement in the left anterior descending (LAD) coronary artery. However, a few days later, she had recurrence of her chest pain. Enzymes are negative. A stress MR exam was requested.

Findings

Adenosine stress MRI was performed. The short-axis cine views are arranged in the top row, with stress images at the same locations in the second row. Adenosine was used to produce pharmacologic stress.

In the third row, perfusion images at rest are demonstrated.

Delayed-enhancement images are also obtained and are demonstrated in the fifth row, at spatially matched locations.

These images demonstrate that the left ventricular cavity size and wall thickness appear normal. The global systolic function is normal. No definite area of significant hypokinesia is noted.

The stress perfusion images in the second row demonstrate a focal perfusion deficit seen in the anterior portion of the septum in the second and third images of the perfusion sequence. This region has a normal appearance on the resting images.

Delayed-enhancement images in the same locations demonstrate that a small focus of hyperenhancement is seen in the second image of the fifth row, with the third image having a normal appearance.

The right ventricle appears normal in size and function. Evaluation of the valvular structures demonstrates borderline prolapse of the anterior leaflet of the mitral valve, but no significant mitral regurgitation is seen. The aortic valve is normal in appearance. No significant tricuspid regurgitation is seen.

Diagnosis

Anterior septal ischemia secondary to stent placement covering the septal perforator in this region, resulting in ischemia.

A tiny septal infarction is noted, but the region of ischemia is felt to exceed the area of the small infarction.

Perfusion imaging by MR has been extensively studied, often in a research setting where the protocols used are not always similar to those in clinical practice. However, in those studies, the physiological information obtained by MR has been well validated. Excellent correlation with PET studies has been noted,[1, 2] and studies of MR determination of myocardial perfusion reserve have shown excellent sensitivity and specificity for the detection of coronary artery disease.[3] However, many of the studies demonstrating the accuracy of MR perfusion imaging have not been clinically practical. In this regard, the study reported recently by Klem is notable for its real-world applicability.[4] That methodology is replicated throughout this teaching file. Importantly, only visual assessment is used, and comparison of the cine and delayed-enhancement images with the perfusion images provides complementary information that optimizes the diagnostic performance of CMR for the detection of CAD.

References

1. Ibrahim T, et al. Assessment of coronary flow reserve: comparison between contrast-enhanced magnetic resonance imaging and positron emission tomography. J Am Coll Cardiol. 2002;39(5):864–870.
2. Schwitter J, et al. Assessment of myocardial perfusion in coronary artery disease by magnetic resonance: a comparison with positron emission tomography and coronary angiography. Circulation. 2001;103(18):2230–2235.
3. Nagel E, et al. Magnetic resonance perfusion measurements for the noninvasive detection of coronary artery disease. Circulation. 2003;108(4):432–437.
4. Klem I, et al. Improved detection of coronary artery disease by stress perfusion cardiovascular magnetic resonance with the use of delayed-enhancement infarction imaging. J Am Coll Cardiol. 2006;47(8):1630–1638.

Teaching File Case 65

60-year-old female with a history of prior myocardial infarction

Category: Viability

Findings

The cine images demonstrate a well-defined aneurysm originating along the inferior wall from the basal to the mid-ventricular level. Undermining of the posterior papillary muscle is apparent, and moderate mitral regurgitation is noted. Although the aneurysm appears to have a narrow neck, as is often associated with a false aneurysm, it can be seen that a thin layer of residual myocardium is present. Significant reduction in the left ventricular ejection fraction is noted, as the basal level usually provides a disproportionate share of the stroke volume.

Delayed-enhancement images with a short inversion time demonstrate extensive infarction of the inferior wall, extending to involve the inferoseptum at the basal and mid-ventricular levels. In addition, laminar thrombus is noted, which appears minimally dark on the short inversion time images, but becomes quite evident on the 2-chamber view of the delayed-enhancement images obtained with a long inversion time (fifth image of the fourth row).

A moderately large pericardial effusion is also noted. Note the diastolic collapse of the right atrial free wall.

Diagnosis

This represents a large true aneurysm of the basal to mid-ventricular inferior wall of the left ventricle, associated with abundant mural thrombus.

Review of the cine images indicates the difficulty with visualization of thrombi on non-contrast enhanced cine MR images, or for that matter, echocardiographic images. Contrast enhanced MR images demonstrate a twofold improvement over echo in the detection of ventricular thrombi.[1,2]

This case also illustrates the distinction between true and false aneurysms. A true aneurysm is one in which layers of residual myocardium persist. A false aneurysm can be best thought of as a contained ventricular rupture, which is bound only by the epicardial adventitia and the pericardium. Therefore, it represents a pseudoaneurysm of the left ventricle, and often involves the inferolateral wall at the base. True aneurysms, in contrast, often involve the anterior wall. Another distinction is that false aneurysms often have a neck that is narrower than the widest part of the aneurysm. This again relates to its nature as a focal area of contained rupture.[3]

This case is somewhat atypical in that this is a true aneurysm that originated in the location often associated with development of false aneurysm. Nonetheless, the demonstration by contrast-enhanced imaging of residual myocardium that makes up the wall of the aneurysm indicates that this is a true and not a false aneurysm.

For further reading regarding the use of MR to distinguish true from false aneurysms, please see the attached references.

References

1. Heatlie GJ, Mohiaddin R. Left ventricular aneurysm: comprehensive assessment of morphology, structure and thrombus using cardiovascular magnetic resonance. Clin Radiol. 2005;60(6):687–692.
2. Srichai MB, et al. Clinical, imaging, and pathological characteristics of left ventricular thrombus: a compari-

son of contrast-enhanced magnetic resonance imaging, transthoracic echocardiography, and transesophageal echocardiography with surgical or pathological validation. Am Heart J. 2006;152(1):75–84.

3. Konen E, et al. True versus false left ventricular aneurysm: differentiation with MR imaging–initial experience. Radiology. 2005;236(1):65–70.

Teaching File Case 66

53-year-old male with atrial fibrillation; the study is performed as a preprocedural evaluation for possible pulmonary vein ablation procedure

Category: Angiography

Findings

Standard morphologic images are obtained, along with angiographic data sets. These have been post-processed, and volume-rendered images have been created. These are demonstrated on the far right of the top row.

The study demonstrates the presence of anomalous pulmonary veins. Specifically, the right middle lobe pulmonary vein joins the left atrium separately from the right upper lobe pulmonary vein. In addition, the superior segmental branch of the right lower lobe pulmonary vein joins the right middle lobe vein as it inserts into the left atrium.

On the left, the lingular segmental pulmonary vein has a separate entrance just inferior to the main left upper lobe pulmonary vein. The left lower lobe pulmonary vein enters separately as well.

The esophagus is noted to be central in location without significant contact with any of the pulmonary veins.[1]

Diagnosis

Anomalous pulmonary veins insert into the left atrium as described. Six separate orifices are seen.

Pulmonary vein anomalies are quite common, with the standard normal configuration occurring in probably less than one-half of cases. Conjoined entry of the left upper and lower lobe pulmonary veins is quite common. An additional variant is separate entry of the right middle lobe pulmonary vein into the left atrium. However, multiple variations are possible as noted in this case. MR imaging is able to resolve the pulmonary vein structures in great detail, allowing accurate procedural planning.[2–4]

In addition, the 3-D volumetric data set created with MR can be imported into various software packages, which then allow cross registration of fluoroscopic images with the previously obtained MR angiographic data sets. This can significantly decrease the imaging time needed to perform the radiofrequency ablation of the pulmonary veins.

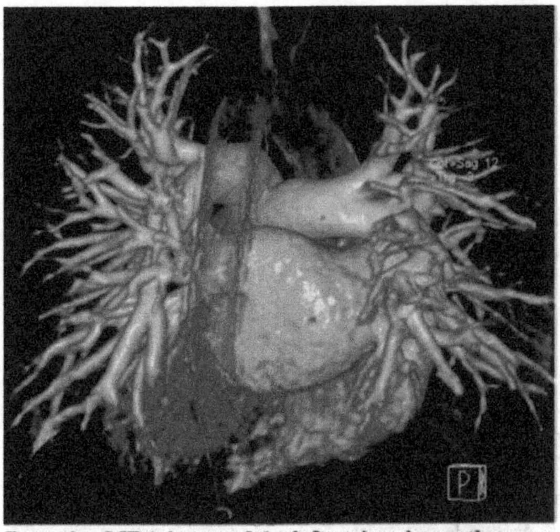

Posterior MRA image of the left atrium in another case

FIGURE 66.1. Posterior view of a 3-D volume rendered MRA image from another case demonstrating the entrance of the pulmonary veins into the left atrium

References

1. Cury RC, et al. Relationship of the esophagus and aorta to the left atrium and pulmonary veins: implications for catheter ablation of atrial fibrillation. Heart Rhythm. 2005;2(12):1317–1323.
2. Vonken EP, et al. Contrast-enhanced MRA and 3D visualization of pulmonary venous anatomy to assist radiofrequency catheter ablation. J Cardiovasc Magn Reson. 2003;5(4):545–551.
3. Pilleul F, Merchant N. MRI of the pulmonary veins: comparison between 3D MR angiography and T1-weighted spin echo. J Comput Assist Tomogr. 2000;24(5):683–687.
4. Mansour M, et al. Three-dimensional anatomy of the left atrium by magnetic resonance angiography: implications for catheter ablation for atrial fibrillation. J Cardiovasc Electrophysiol. 2006;17(7): 719–723.

Teaching File Case 67

14 year-old girl status–post three prior surgical procedures for congenital heart disease

Category: Congenital

Findings

The short-axis views demonstrate normal left ventricular cavity size and function. The ventricular morphology appears normal. The right ventricle is unremarkable in appearance. The 3-chamber view (second row, third image) demonstrates significant turbulence at the level of the aortic valve. Subsequent small field-of-view imaging demonstrates that a bicuspid aortic valve is present. Velocity-encoded images demonstrate a minimal gradient at this level.

Subsequently obtained aortic outflow tract views demonstrate the patient has undergone a prior extra-anatomic bypass graft originating from the proximal ascending aorta and extending posterior and inferior to the heart to anastomose to the descending aorta.

The MR angiographic views with volume rendering demonstrate nicely the postsurgical changes. The extra-anatomic bypass graft is well seen originating from the right lateral margin of the ascending aorta, and connecting to the descending aorta. A second graft is seen originating from the proximal aorta and extending to the proximal descending aorta. However, this is quite tiny in size. There is hypoplasia of the aortic arch between a normal appearing innominate artery and the left common carotid artery. The left subclavian artery is not visualized as a discrete structure, having been incorporated into a patch graft that is anastomosed to the descending aorta.

Diagnosis

This patient has coarctation of the aorta, and is status–post multiple surgeries as described above.

Initially, a graft was attempted from the proximal ascending aorta to the descending aorta in order to bypass the area of constriction. This was unsuccessful. A left subclavian aortoplasty was then performed, with incorporation of the left subclavian artery to enlarge the aortic caliber at this level. However, this was also deemed inadequate, and ultimately the extra-anatomic bypass graft was performed. This results in adequate flow to the descending aorta.

An associated bicuspid aortic valve is noted. A minimal gradient is evident on velocity-encoded imaging, measuring approximately 16 mmHg.

Bicuspid aortic valve is commonly associated with aortic coarctation, being seen in approximately 50–75% of cases.

Patients who are status–post endovascular or surgical correction of coarctation of the aorta should be followed with surveillance MR imaging in order to screen the patient for the development of recurrent coarctation, or post dilatation aneurysm development. Aneurysm may also involve the ascending aorta, particularly in patients with bicuspid aortic valve. For these reasons, yearly or every other yearly follow-up is suggested.[1–5]

References

1. Webb G, Treatment of coarctation and late complications in the adult. Semin Thorac Cardiovasc Surg. 2005;17(2):139–142.
2. Warnes CA, The adult with congenital heart disease: born to be bad? J Am Coll Cardiol. 2005;46(1):1–8.
3. Vriend JW, Mulder BJ. Late complications in patients after repair of aortic coarctation: implications for management. Int J Cardiol. 2005;101(3):399–406.
4. Quenot JP, et al. Usefulness of MRI in the follow-up of patients with repaired aortic coarctation and bicuspid aortic valve. Int J Cardiol. 2005;103(3):312–316.
5. Toro-Salazar OH, et al. Long-term follow-up of patients after coarctation of the aorta repair. Am J Cardiol. 2002;89(5):541–547.

Teaching File Case 68

79-year-old male with evidence of restrictive cardiomyopathy

Category: Cardiomyopathy

History

The study is requested to determine etiology.

Findings

The left ventricular cavity is within normal limits in size. The wall thickness is mildly increased to 1.4 cm.

This is concentric in nature. Evaluation of the wall motion demonstrates normal systolic function. The degree of diastolic impairment is difficult to estimate visually, but the bi-atrial enlargement noted indicates diastolic dysfunction. Other pertinent findings include the thickening in the right ventricular free wall, and on the small field-of-view image of the aortic valve, thrombus is noted in the left atrial appendage.

Delayed-enhancement images demonstrate difficulty in adequately nulling the myocardium. Images obtained with a long inversion time again demonstrate the left atrial appendage thrombus, and in addition clearly demonstrate right atrial appendage thrombus that is difficult to visualize on the cine images.

Subendocardial enhancement is suspected in a diffuse fashion on images where the nulling has been attempted.

Note is also made of the presence of a moderately large pericardial effusion. Bilateral pleural effusions are also evident.

Diagnosis

Amyloidosis.

This patient demonstrates a constellation of findings that when seen in aggregate are highly suspicious for the diagnosis of amyloidosis. Specifically, this disorder produces hypertrophy of the left ventricle, and often of the right ventricle as well.[1] The ejection fraction is often relatively preserved early in the course of the disorder, but diastolic filling impairment is prominent at the time of diagnosis in the majority cases.

Difficulty in nulling the myocardium as distinct from the blood pool is best appreciated on inversion scout images, as these images will demonstrate the abnormal contrast kinetics. Specifically, the gadolinium uptake by the myocardium is abnormally increased, likely due to profound expansion of the extracellular space, and the washout from the blood pool is more rapid in patients with amyloidosis.[2] Diffuse subendocardial enhancement is often reported in addition to the difficulty in adequately nulling the myocardium.[3] For further reading regarding differential diagnosis of cardiomyopathies, please refer to Chapter 3.

It is the most common identified form of restrictive cardiomyopathy in United States.

There are four types of amyloidosis: primary, secondary, senile, and familial. The primary form is the most common, and cardiac involvement is the most common cause of death.

The bi-atrial thrombi noted in this case likely are manifestations of the extensive atrial stasis induced by the restrictive cardiomyopathy present.

References

1. Fattori R, et al. Contribution of magnetic resonance imaging in the differential diagnosis of cardiac amyloidosis and symmetric hypertrophic cardiomyopathy. Am Heart J. 1998;136(5):824–830.
2. Maceira AM, et al. Cardiovascular magnetic resonance in cardiac amyloidosis. Circulation. 2005;111(2):186–193.
3. Sueyoshi E, et al. Cardiac Amyloidosis: Typical Imaging Findings and Diffuse Myocardial Damage Demonstrated by Delayed Contrast-Enhanced MRI. Cardiovasc Intervent Radiol. 2006.

Teaching File Case 69

18-year-old female with the recent development of ascites and leg swelling

Category: Pericardium

Findings

The left ventricle is normal in size and function. The right ventricle has an unusual configuration, and its diastolic excursion appears diminished. The far right short axis image in the top row demonstrates deformity of the apex of the right ventricle, which appears tethered to the inferior pericardial surface. This is noted on the first image of the second row as well.

The first short axis view demonstrates marked dilatation of the inferior vena cava, as well as sluggish flow.

Evaluation of the valves demonstrates minimal aortic insufficiency. Trace mitral insufficiency is seen as well.

Morphologic images seen in the third and fourth rows demonstrate thickening of the pericardium, and review of the cine images demonstrates fusion of the visceral and parietal layers of the pericardium.

Real time images are noted as the fifth and sixth images of the second row. A real-time image is also seen as the first image of the second row. These images demonstrate that inversion of the septum is noted when the patient takes a deep inspiration.

Delayed-enhancement imaging shows no evidence of infarction.

Diagnosis

Constrictive pericarditis.

The static morphologic images strongly suggest this diagnosis based on the abnormal appearance of the pericardium. Although the absolute thickness does not exceed 3 mm, the adherence of the visceral and parietal pericardial layers is distinctly abnormal. In addition, the altered ventricular morphology is consistent with this diagnosis. Marked distention of the inferior vena cava is apparent.[1]

However, it is desirable to have functional and physiologic demonstration of the altered hemodynamics found in constriction. Real-time cine MR imaging can provide confirmation of the hemodynamic abnormalities present in constriction.[2] In this instance, real-time imaging during a deep inspiration demonstrates that the increased right ventricular filling induced by this provocative maneuver results in displacement of the interventricular septum from right-to-left, indicating impaired distensibility of the right ventricle produced by the pericardial abnormality. Therefore, this provides confirmation of the altered physiology present, confirming the abnormality suspected on purely anatomic imaging.

In the former era, pericardial constriction was most often due to tuberculosis. However, constrictive pericarditis is now most often idiopathic or post viral in origin. Prior surgery and prior radiation represent identifiable causes of constriction in the appropriate population.[3]

Surgical pericardiectomy is the procedure of choice in the appropriate patient, and in the present example the patient responded dramatically to this intervention. However, in instances where the constriction has been present for a prolonged period of time, the response may be less dramatic, due to the development of extensive atrophy and fibrosis. Therefore, a high index of suspicion is necessary for a prompt diagnosis and early intervention.[4]

MR imaging provides a comprehensive assessment of the pericardium, with tissue characterization superior to echocardiography or CT. It is not limited by acoustic windows. As seen in the present example, it can provide excellent morphologic and physiologic information.[5] For further reading regarding pericardial disease, see also Chapter 5.

References

1. Breen JF. Imaging of the pericardium. J Thorac Imaging. 2001;16(1):47–54.
2. FranconeM, et al. Real-time cine MRI of ventricular septal motion: a novel approach to assess ventricular coupling. J Magn Reson Imaging. 2005;21(3):305–309.
3. Cameron J, et al. The etiologic spectrum of constrictive pericarditis. Am Heart J. 1987;113(2 Pt 1): 354–360.
4. Nishimura RA. Constrictive pericarditis in the modern era: a diagnostic dilemma. Heart. 2001;86(6):619–623.
5. Grizzard JD, Ang GB. Magnetic resonance imaging of pericardial disease and cardiac masses. Cardiol Clin. 2007;25(1):111–140.

Teaching File Case 70

49-year-old female with a recent myocardial infarction in for a myocardial stress test

Category: Viability

History

Studies at an outside hospital suggested the patient was not a candidate for revascularization.

Findings

The left ventricular cavity size is normal, but the anterior wall thickness is diminished, and the anterior wall from the basal level to the apex is akinetic. Thinning is also noted to involve the anterior septum. The left ventricular systolic function is diminished, with an overall left ventricular ejection fraction of approximately 38%.

The right ventricle is normal in size and function.

Stress imaging demonstrates an extensive perfusion deficit signifying inducible ischemia involving the anterior wall, and the anterior portions of the septum and lateral wall from the basal to the apical levels.

Delayed-enhancement images demonstrate a subendocardial anterior wall infarction at the midventricular level, which becomes focally transmural at the apex. However, significant viability remains in the anterior wall, the antero- septum, and the anterolateral walls.

Diagnosis

Ischemia is noted in the LAD territory, with a small region of infarction. The anterior wall myocardium is predominantly viable, however, even though thinned.

The patient subsequently underwent revascularization, with improvement in wall motion of the anteroseptum and anterior walls at the midventricular and apical levels.

This case illustrates the utility of MR in depicting not only what is viable, but also what is infarcted, as well as the relative percentages.[1] Although the anterior wall is thinned, it is predominantly viable, and not scarred. Therefore, it was expected that revascularization would improve the contractility of the anterior wall. This information was not available with nuclear SPECT imaging, which only demonstrated hypokinetic poorly perfused myocardium in the anterior wall suggestive of scar. Thus, hibernating myocardium that might benefit from surgery was missed.

MR should be strongly considered in circumstances where other imaging suggests the presence of extensive scar not amenable to revascularization, as it can more reliably determine which areas are truly scarred and which are simply hibernating myocardium.[2]

References

1. Kim RJ, Shah DJ. Fundamental concepts in myocardial viability assessment revisited: when knowing how much is "alive" is not enough. Heart. 2004;90(2):137–140.
2. Kuhl HP, et al. Assessment of reversible myocardial dysfunction in chronic ischaemic heart disease: comparison of contrast-enhanced cardiovascular magnetic resonance and a combined positron emission tomography-single photon emission computed tomography imaging protocol. Eur Heart J. 2006;27(7):846–853.

Teaching File Case 71

50-year-old female sent from the emergency department for evaluation of chest pain

Category: Stress test

Findings

The short-axis cine views demonstrate normal regional and global left ventricular function. The wall thickness is normal, measuring 11 mm in diameter.

The right ventricle size and function are normal as well.

Evaluation of the valvular structures demonstrates minimal flow turbulence through a trileaflet aortic valve without evidence of stenosis. No mitral and tricuspid insufficiency is seen.

The stress and rest perfusion images seen in the second and third rows respectively demonstrate that a vertically oriented dark linear band is seen to traverse the lateral portion of the myocardium from top to bottom. No perfusion defect is noted.

Delayed-enhancement images subsequently obtained demonstrate no focus of prior infarction. No thrombus is seen.

Diagnosis

Normal adenosine stress imaging study demonstrating an artifact related to the use parallel imaging technology.

The proper interpretation of MR images requires the appropriate recognition of artifact. In this instance, the vertically oriented linear dark band is recognized as an artifact as it does not correspond with any anatomic structures, and persists on stress and rest images. This form of artifact can often be displaced from the central portion of the image by changing the phase encoding direction, and also by increasing the field-of-view. Rotating the field-of-view may also serve a similar purpose.[1]

This study was negative for inducible ischemia. It has been shown in one study that a negative adenosine stress MR perfusion study is associated with an extremely low risk for major adverse cardiac events in the year following the study.[2] Therefore, even though this study is "negative," it nonetheless provides valuable prognostic information.

References

1. Glockner JF, et al. Parallel MR imaging: a user's guide. Radiographics. 2005;25(5):1279–97.
2. Ingkanisorn WP, et al. Prognosis of negative adenosine stress magnetic resonance in patients presenting to an emergency department with chest pain. J Am Coll Cardiol. 2006;47(7):1427–1432.

Teaching File Case 72

57-year-old woman with hypertension

Category: Angiography

Findings

MR angiography demonstrates an irregular long segment narrowing of the midportion of the abdominal aorta just below the renal arteries. Narrowing of both renal arteries is also apparent. Review of the source images indicated that the vessel wall did not appear to be diffusely thickened, although mild thickening at the site of constriction was apparent.

Additional history subsequently obtained indicating that the patient had had a prior imaging study demonstrating similar findings 10 years previously.

Diagnosis

Mid-aortic syndrome.

This disorder, also known as abdominal coarctation, is usually idiopathic in nature. Associated conditions include thoracic coarctation, Williams syndrome, as well as neurofibromatosis.

Patients with this disorder frequently come to medical attention for evaluation of hypertension, or less commonly, diminished femoral pulses.

Imaging findings demonstrate a diffuse narrowing of the abdominal aorta, sometimes associated with long segment narrowing of the thoracic aorta. Renal artery stenosis is frequently associated, and is often bilateral, as in this case. Surface shaded and volume-rendered images aid in the visualization of these findings.[1–3]

The disorder is distinguished from the more common atherosclerotic disease by its frequent occurrence in young individuals and its stability over time. Often, little progression is seen over a number of years, as was the case in the present example.

References

1. Lewis VD 3rd, et al. The midaortic syndrome: diagnosis and treatment. Radiology. 1988;167(1):111–113.
2. Messina LM, et al. Middle aortic syndrome. Effectiveness and durability of complex arterial revascularization techniques. Ann Surg. 1986;204(3):331–339.
3. Brzezinska-Rajszys G, et al. Middle aortic syndrome treated by stent implantation. Heart. 1999;81(2):166–170.

Teaching File Case 73

72-year-old female with hypertrophic cardiomyopathy presents with chest pain and negative enzymes

Category: Stress test

History

The study is requested to evaluate for possible ischemia.

Findings

The short-axis views confirm the diagnosis of hypertrophic cardiomyopathy, with concentric hypertrophy apparent. In addition, outflow tract obstruction is evident on the 3-chamber view, with turbulence seen along with systolic anterior motion of the mitral valve. Mild mitral regurgitation is noted.

Abnormality of the aortic valve is also seen, with restriction of its movement. Mild aortic stenosis is evident on velocity-encoded images (not shown). In addition, mild aortic insufficiency is noted.

The right ventricular size and function appears normal.

Perfusion images demonstrate a subtle area of diminished contrast uptake in the anterior septum at the basal and mid-ventricular levels. This area appears normal on the rest images.

Delayed-enhancement images demonstrate no evidence of infarction in the anterior septum.

Diagnosis

Anteroseptal ischemia. This is superimposed upon underlying hypertrophic cardiomyopathy.[1]

The perfusion deficit is not accompanied by any significant abnormality on the delayed-enhancement images, indicating that it is due to ischemia and not prior infarction.

Patients with hypertrophic cardiomyopathy are known to be at risk for ischemic disease as well, likely owing to increased metabolic demands as well as diminished perfusion reserve.[2, 3] Impaired diastolic coronary filling is also likely contributory.

References

1. Rickers C, et al. Utility of cardiac magnetic resonance imaging in the diagnosis of hypertrophic cardiomyopathy. Circulation. 2005;12(6):855–861.
2. Matsunaka T, et al. First-pass myocardial perfusion defect and delayed contrast enhancement in hypertrophic cardiomyopathy assessed with MRI. Magn Reson Med Sci. 2003;2(2):61–69.
3. Sipola P, et al. First-pass MR imaging in the assessment of perfusion impairment in patients with hypertrophic cardiomyopathy and the Asp175Asn mutation of the alpha-tropomyosin gene. Radiology. 2003; 226(1):129–137.

Teaching File Case 74

59-year-old male with a history of ventricular septal defect (VSD) and possible pulmonic stenosis

Category: Congenital

Findings

The left ventricle is mildly dilated, and demonstrates mild concentric hypertrophy. The systolic function is mildly reduced, with an ejection fraction of 45%.

The right ventricle is not significantly dilated, but demonstrates hypertrophy and prominent trabeculation. The appearance is consistent with significant right ventricular hypertrophy.

The 3-chamber view (first image in the third row) demonstrates immobility of the right coronary cusp, with both aortic stenosis and aortic insufficiency apparent. In addition, a small jet of flow is seen to extend under the right coronary cusp and into the right ventricular outflow tract. The right coronary cusp is observed to be prolapsed into the right ventricular outflow tract, producing significant obstruction.

The first image of the fourth row demonstrates a jet of contrast extending through the VSD into the right ventricular outflow tract from the left ventricular outflow tract. The third and fourth images of the fifth row are phase contrast in-plane flow studies demonstrating the jet of flow extending from the left ventricular outflow tract into the right ventricular outflow tract underneath the prolapsed right coronary cusp.

The small field-of-view images of the aortic valve (second row, fourth and fifth images) demonstrates the abnormal valvular morphology with immobility of the right coronary cusp which is observed to have prolapsed into the right ventricular outflow tract. Velocity-encoded images demonstrated a mild degree of aortic stenosis with a gradient of 12 mmHg, and volumetric measurements demonstrated a mild degree of aortic insufficiency with a regurgitant fraction of 10%.

Images in the plane of the right ventricular outflow tract (top row, fourth and fifth images, as well as the sixth row, first three images) demonstrate the extensive right ventricular outflow tract obstruction with a high velocity jet seen to extend from the prolapsed coronary cusp into the main pulmonary artery segment. Axial images (observed in the sixth row) across the right ventricular outflow tract demonstrate the high degree of obstruction produced. Velocity-encoded images demonstrated a gradient of 25 mmHg.

Dark-blood HASTE images seen in the seventh row demonstrate that the pulmonary arterial anatomy is reminiscent of that seen with valvular pulmonic stenosis, with dilatation of the main and left pulmonary artery, with less dilatation of the right pulmonary artery.

MR angiographic images demonstrate that the aorta is minimally tortuous. The main pulmonary artery is dilated, as is the left pulmonary artery. The right pulmonary artery is relatively normal in size.

Delayed-enhancement images demonstrate a focus of hyper enhancement seen in the inferior portion of the septum at the septal insertion site; a pattern associated with right ventricular hypertrophy and right ventricular pressure overload states.

Diagnosis

The patient's primary abnormality is a VSD, which affected the outflow septum. This resulted in undermining of the aortic valve, with resultant prolapse of the right coronary cusp through the defect, producing right ventricular outflow tract obstruction.[1,2] This is a known complication of ventricular septal defect. It is usually associated with aortic insufficiency, which can be significant.

The patient likely had a preexistent pulmonic valve abnormality that resulted in abnormal remodeling of the pulmonary artery as described, but this cannot be stated with certainty given the extensive turbulence produced at the present time by the subvalvular outflow tract obstruction. Preexisting pulmonic stenosis would have protected the patient's pulmonary vascular bed from developing pulmonary vascular disease as might have been expected from the left-to-right shunt induced by the VSD.

References

1. Layangool T, Kirawittaya T, Sangtawesin C. Aortic valve prolapse in subpulmonic ventricular septal defect. J Med Assoc Thai. 2003;86(Suppl 3): S549–S555.
2. Eroglu AG, et al. Aortic valve prolapse and aortic regurgitation in patients with ventricular septal defect. Pediatr Cardiol. 2003;24(1):36–39.

Teaching File Case 75

80-year-old female with abnormality noted on recent chest radiography

Category: Mass

Findings

The images in the top row are static morphologic images obtained through the chest. The first and third images are HASTE images, while the second and fourth images are steady-state free precession (SSFP) images. The fifth image (next to the last right image) is a T2 spin-echo sequence, while the far right image is a T1-weighted spin-echo image sequence.

Cine images are noted in the second row.

The HASTE images demonstrate a large rounded structure of medium to low signal intensity bordering the left side of the heart and mediastinum. This same area is noted to be quite high in signal intensity on steady-state free precession images, consistent with a fluid filled structure such as a cyst. The T2-weighted images confirm the high signal intensity consistent with simple fluid. The T1-weighted images demonstrate low signal intensity, also consistent with fluid.

The cine images in the second row demonstrate little impression upon the heart, and no impairment of cardiac function produced by this large cystic structure. Note is made of normal left ventricular size and systolic function. Mild mitral regurgitation is apparent.

The first three images of the third row are perfusion images which are obtained during the first pass of contrast, which are heavily T1-weighted images. These demonstrate that the lesion in question is purely cystic, and does not demonstrate enhancement.

The last three right-sided images of the third row are delayed-enhancement images obtained with a long inversion time. These also demonstrate low signal intensity of the lesion consistent with fluid.

The first image of the fourth row is a VIBE sequence (volumetric interpolated breath-hold exam), an excellent morphologic imaging technique for evaluating abdominal and chest structures. This is a fat-saturated heavily T1-weighted sequence, again demonstrating the cystic nature of the lesion in question.

Additional sequences obtained for tissue characterization are demonstrated in the last two rows. They include static T1 sequences, as well as STIR sequences which allow fat suppression and T2-weighting.

Diagnosis

This represents a large pericardial cyst.

Pericardial cysts are felt to originate from portions of the pericardium pinched off from the remainder of the pericardium during embryologic development. They most commonly occur along the right cardiophrenic angle, and are less commonly left-sided. However, they can occur anywhere along the margin of the pericardium. The differential diagnosis would include other cystic structures including bronchogenic or foregut cysts.

Cystic neoplasm would be significantly less likely, although thymomas may occasionally demonstrate cystic degeneration.

The differential diagnosis for an anterior mediastinal mass would include teratomas as well as thymomas. Lymphoma also can result in an anterior mediastinal mass, but these would not be cystic in nature.

This exam demonstrates the capacity of MR to characterize a variety of lesions. Using a combination of standard T1, T2, and delayed-enhancement images, comprehensive evaluation and characterization of cardiac and pericardiac masses is possible. In addition, the impact of such a lesion upon the myocardium can be well demonstrated. Therefore, MR imaging is now the preferred modality for the study of cardiac and paracardiac masses.[1–3]

References

1. Sechtem U, Tscholakoff D, Higgins CB. MRI of the abnormal pericardium. AJR Am J Roentgenol. 1986;147(2):245–252.
2. Vander Salm TJ, Unusual primary tumors of the heart. Semin Thorac Cardiovasc Surg. 2000;12(2):89–100.
3. Nizzero A, Dobranowski J, Tanser P. Biventricular heart failure secondary to a pericardial cystic mass: case report. Can Assoc Radiol J. 2000;51(1):16–19.

Teaching File Case 76

A 49-year-old female with abnormal echocardiogram

Category: Congenital

Findings

The cine images demonstrate the left ventricle is normal in size and function.

The right atrium is markedly enlarged, with a diminutive right ventricle evident. This is due to apical displacement of the posterior and septal leaflets of the tricuspid valve. The anterior leaflet of the tricuspid valve is somewhat enlarged and dysplastic, but is not significantly displaced. Small field-of-view imaging seen as the third image of the second row demonstrates tricuspid insufficiency and the abnormal tricuspid leaflets.

The other valvular structures are unremarkable.

Morphologic imaging and angiographic datasets demonstrate significant enlargement of the right atrium, along with atrialization of the right ventricle. No evidence of prior infarction is seen on delayed-enhancement imaging.

Diagnosis

Ebstein's anomaly.

This disorder results from apical displacement of the septal and posterolateral leaflets of the tricuspid valve into the right ventricle. This results in "atrialization" of the inflow of the right ventricle, with a resulting decrease in size of the functioning right ventricle.[1,2] Tricuspid regurgitation is frequently noted. Enlargement of the right atrium is usually present. Apical displacement of at least 8 mm of the septal leaflet is usually considered diagnostic.

A shunt may be present at the atrial level either due to a patent foramen ovale or due to an associated atrial septal defect in approximately 50% of patients. In addition, given the high pulmonary vascular resistance present normally at birth, right-to-left shunting in the neonatal period may be extensive. Paradoxical emboli may develop in the adult, and represent an indication for surgical repair.[3–6] The patients are also prone to arrhythmias, and there is an association with accessory conduction pathways seen with this disorder. At least 25% of patients will develop associated atrial tachyarrhythmias,

The clinical presentation varies widely, with some instances of severe abnormality presenting in the neonatal period, while others we'll not present to adulthood and only then with minimal symptoms.

Surgical repair is often preferred to valve replacement when feasible.

MR imaging can be helpful in surgical planning, and can demonstrate any associated abnormalities such as an atrial septal defect, as well as quantitate any shunt present.

References

1. Choi YH, et al. MR imaging of Ebstein's anomaly of the tricuspid valve. AJR Am J Roentgenol. 1994;163(3):539–543.
2. Attenhofer Jost CH, et al. Ebstein's anomaly. Circulation. 2007;115(2):277–285.
3. Knott-Craig CJ, et al. Repair of neonates and young infants with Ebstein's anomaly and related disorders. Ann Thorac Surg. 2007;84(2):587–592; discussion 592–593.
4. Dearani JA, Oleary PW, Danielson GK. Surgical treatment of Ebstein's malformation: state of the art in 2006. Cardiol Young. 2006;16(Suppl 3):12–20.
5. Kanter RJ. Ebstein's anomaly of the tricuspid valve: a Wolf(f) in sheep's clothing. J Cardiovasc Electrophysiol. 2006;17(12):1337–1339.
6. Radmehr H, et al. Repair of Ebstein anomaly: early and mid-term results. Arch Iran Med. 2006;9(4):354–358.

Teaching File Case 77

63-year-old male with an abnormal echocardiogram

Category: Viability

Findings

The images are acquired in nonstandard imaging planes. Nonetheless, it can clearly be seen that there is a large focal outpouching arising along the posterolateral left ventricular wall at the basal level, which demonstrates extensive dyskinesia. The left ventricular wall appears incomplete laterally, and only the pericardium is seen to form the lateral border of the lesion. Still frame images confirm this appearance.

Evaluation of the valvular structures and right ventricle is problematic given the lack of standard imaging planes. However, the right ventricle is felt to be within normal limits.

Diagnosis

False aneurysm of the inferolateral left ventricular wall at the basal level.

A false aneurysm or pseudoaneurysm essentially represents a contained rupture of the myocardium. The pericardium forms the margin of the lesion, and there is complete disruption of all myocardial layers. There is a high risk of progression to complete rupture, with sudden death due to cardiac tamponade.[1–5]

Classic imaging distinctions between true and false aneurysms include the predilection of the true aneurysm to involve the anterior wall, with the false aneurysm tending to involve the inferolateral wall at the basal level. True aneurysms have a wide origin from the ventricular cavity, while a false aneurysm will typically have a definable neck that is smaller than the body of the aneurysm. This reflects its nature as an area of contained rupture.

Recently, MR imaging using delayed-enhancement has been reported to aid in this distinction. In addition to clearly defining the margins of the myocardium, this technique has also been reported to reveal hyperenhancement of the pericardium in cases of contained rupture (false aneurysm).

References

1. Konen E, et al. True versus false left ventricular aneurysm: differentiation with MR imaging–initial experience. Radiology. 2005;236(1):65–70.
2. Heatlie GJ, Mohiaddin R. Left ventricular aneurysm: comprehensive assessment of morphology, structure and thrombus using cardiovascular magnetic resonance. Clin Radiol. 2005;60(6):687–692.
3. Varghese A, Pepper J, Pennell DJ. Cardiovascular magnetic resonance of left ventricular pseudoaneurysm. Heart. 2005;91(4):477.
4. Tran T, et al. Gd-enhanced cardiovascular MR imaging to identify left ventricular pseudoaneurysm. J Cardiovasc Magn Reson. 2005;7(4):717–721.
5. Baks T, et al. Chronic pseudoaneurysm of the left ventricle. Int J Cardiovasc Imaging. 2005:1–3.

Teaching File Case 78

73-year-old female with a retroatrial mass noted on recent echocardiography

Category: Mass

Findings

The short-axis cines demonstrate a large mass posterior to the right and left atria, which is heterogenous in signal intensity having regions of both low and high signal intensity. Elevation of the right atrium is apparent, with minimal effacement of both the right and left atria.

The left ventricular size and function appear normal. The right ventricular size and function are normal.

The aortic valve is abnormal. There is partial fusion of the right coronary leaflet and the non-coronary leaflet. Also, there is partial fusion of the left and right coronary leaflets. The aortic root is normal in diameter, measuring 3.8 cm. The mitral valve is normal as is the tricuspid valve.

Phase contrast velocity measurements through the region of the aortic valve demonstrate a peak gradient of 12 mmHg. Mild aortic insufficiency is also seen with a small regurgitant jet.

The pericardium is normal in thickness.

Delayed-enhancement imaging demonstrates that no evidence of myocardial scar is seen. The large retrocardiac mass is again noted to have heterogenous signal intensity on the delayed-enhancement images as well.

Diagnosis

A large hiatal hernia accounts for the retrocardiac mass described. This is quite apparent on the morphologic images as well as on the cine images. Continuity of the mass with the intra-abdominal structures is apparent.

MR is frequently used as a problem solving technique in the evaluation of cardiac and pericardiac masses. Normal structures or ectopically located normal structures can be a source of confusion on echocardiography. In particular, the eustachian valve and the crista terminalis may be mistaken for masses on echocardiography. In addition, given the heterogeneity and the complexity of the signal of a hiatal hernia, it is easy to understand how it could present a confusing appearance on echocardiography. The multiplanar, multisequence capabilities of MR imaging make it a useful technique for evaluation of cardiac and paracardiac masses.[1–3]

References

1. Link KM, Lesko NM. MR evaluation of cardiac/juxtacardiac masses. Top Magn Reson Imaging. 1995;7(4):232–245.
2. Hoffmann U, et al. Usefulness of magnetic resonance imaging of cardiac and paracardiac masses. Am J Cardiol. 2003;92(7):890–895.
3. Sechtem U, Jungehulsing M. Noninvasive imaging of cardiac masses. Curr Opin Radiol. 1990;2(4):575–580.

Teaching File Case 79

70-year-old male with a history of right nephrectomy for renal cell carcinoma

Category: Viability

History

He also has a history of myocardial infarction. Assess for viability.

Findings

The left ventricle is enlarged, with a diastolic diameter of 8 cm. There is thinning of the anterior wall from the mid-ventricular level to the apex. Evaluation of the regional wall motion demonstrates severe global hypokinesia, with akinesia of the anteroseptal, anterior, and anterolateral walls from the mid-ventricular level to the apex. The true apex is dyskinetic. The left ventricular ejection fraction is 16%.

Evaluation of the valvular structures demonstrates that mild mitral regurgitation is noted, along with moderately severe tricuspid regurgitation. The aortic valve appears to be competent without evidence of insufficiency or stenosis.

Delayed-enhancement images demonstrate extensive, essentially transmural infarction of the anterior wall, the antero-septum, and the antero-lateral walls from the mid-ventricular level to the apex. Involvement of the inferior septum and portions of the inferior wall are apparent at the more apical levels. Extensive infarction of the lateral wall is also seen in the apical segments.

Images with a long inversion time did not demonstrate thrombus.

Note is also made of the presence of MR angiographic images, demonstrating the solitary left kidney, with no evidence of renal artery stenosis. Also noted is the prior performance of aortobifemoral grafting.

Diagnosis

This represents a case of dilated ischemic cardiomyopathy, with little residual preserved viability.

The delayed-enhancement images convincingly demonstrate extensive scarring throughout much of the left ventricle, with significant transmural extent indicating the patient would likely not regain significant myocardial contractile function from revascularization.[1–3]

Cardiac MR using the delayed-enhancement technique is helpful in the evaluation of patients presenting with dilated cardiomyopathy. Studies have demonstrated that virtually all patients with ischemic dilated cardiomyopathy (such as the present patient) demonstrate hyperenhancement in a pattern consistent with coronary artery disease (CAD). Patients with non-ischemic cardiomyopathy either demonstrate no enhancement (approximately 60%), or they demonstrate a mid-wall "stripe" pattern (28–30%) that is clearly different from a CAD pattern. A small percentage (10–12%) will have a subendocardial CAD pattern.[4]

Therefore, an algorithmic approach to interpretation of CMR studies of cardiomyopathies can be developed as follows: Step 1– evaluate for the presence of hyperenhancement. Step 2–If hyperenhancement is noted, classify into CAD or non-CAD pattern. Step 3–If non-CAD hyperenhancement is noted, attempt further classification (e.g. midwall stripe pattern in non-ischemic dilated cardiomyopathy, RV insertion site hyperenhancement in hypertrophic cardiomyopathy, epicardial enhancement along the lateral wall in myocarditis).[5]

References

1. Elliott MD, Kim RJ. Late gadolinium cardiovascular magnetic resonance in the assessment of myocardial viability. Coron Artery Dis. 2005;16(6):365–372.
2. Kuhl HP, et al. Relation of end-diastolic wall thickness and the residual rim of viable myocardium by magnetic resonance imaging to myocardial viability assessed by fluorine-18 deoxyglucose positron emission tomography. Am J Cardiol. 2006;97(4):452–457.
3. Bello D, et al. Gadolinium cardiovascular magnetic resonance predicts reversible myocardial dysfunction and remodeling in patients with heart failure undergoing beta-blocker therapy. Circulation. 2003;108(16): 1945–1953.
4. McCrohon JA, et al. Differentiation of heart failure related to dilated cardiomyopathy and coronary artery disease using gadolinium-enhanced cardiovascular magnetic resonance. Circulation. 2003;108(1): 54–59.
5. Mahrholdt H, et al. Delayed enhancement cardiovascular magnetic resonance assessment of non-ischaemic cardiomyopathies. Eur Heart J. 2005;26(15): 1461–1474.

Teaching File Case 80

38-year-old female with low ejection fraction

Category: Cardiomyopathy

History

She is three months post-partum.

Findings

The short-axis views seen in the top row demonstrate that the left ventricular cavity size is markedly enlarged, with normal wall thickness evident. Diffuse, severe global hypokinesia is evident, with marked reduction of left ventricular ejection fraction. The LVEF measured approximately 18%.

Perfusion images with adenosine stress and also the resting images show no focal perfusion defect. The perfusion images (and the cine images) show a vertically oriented artifact that is due to the parallel imaging technique used.

Evaluation of the valvular structures demonstrates that no significant mitral regurgitation is noted. Trace tricuspid regurgitation is evident. Minimal flow turbulence is seen in the aortic valve, but no evidence of stenosis was seen.

Delayed-enhancement images show no evidence of infarction. No abnormal enhancement is evident.

Diagnosis

Dilated non-ischemic cardiomyopathy, thought secondary to postpartum cardiomyopathy.

The study demonstrates that no evidence of ischemic injury or prior infarction is seen. The perfusion sequence demonstrates no abnormality, and the delayed-enhancement sequences exclude prior infarction. The findings are most consistent with a dilated non-ischemic cardiomyopathy.[1, 2]

Postpartum cardiomyopathy is an uncommon post-pregnancy complication, occurring in less than 0.1% of pregnancies. It is more common in women who become pregnant after the age of 30. A significant percentage of patients will spontaneously improve, but at least half will progress to either death or transplantation.

This case demonstrates the utility of delayed-enhancement imaging to differentiate between ischemic and non-ischemic causes of dilated cardiomyopathy. The lack of subendocardial enhancement is indicative of a non-ischemic etiology in this patient. Using the delayed-enhancement sequence as part of a diagnostic algorithm as outlined in the previous case will usually provide significant insight into the likely etiology in a variety of cardiomyopathies.[3,4]

The vertically oriented artifact seen traversing the myocardium is characteristic of an IPAT or parallel imaging artifact. It could be dealt with by increasing the field of view, but with a resulting decrease in spatial resolution. Alternatively, it could be eliminated by increasing the phase resolution, or by phase oversampling, but with an increase in imaging time.

References

1. Soler R, et al. Magnetic resonance imaging of primary cardiomyopathies. J Comput Assist Tomogr. 2003;27(5):724–734.
2. Young AA, et al. Regional heterogeneity of function in non-ischemic dilated cardiomyopathy. Cardiovasc Res. 2001;49(2):308–318.
3. McCrohon JA, et al. Differentiation of heart failure related to dilated cardiomyopathy and coronary artery disease using gadolinium-enhanced cardiovascular magnetic resonance. Circulation. 2003;108(1):54–59.
4. Mahrholdt H, et al. Delayed enhancement cardiovascular magnetic resonance assessment of non-ischaemic cardiomyopathies. Eur Heart J. 2005;26(15):1461–1474.

Teaching File Case 81

38-year-old female with discrepancy in arm blood pressures

Category: Angiography

Findings

MR angiography was performed in both the thoracic and abdominal regions. The thoracic images are displayed first and demonstrate concentric narrowing of the left subclavian artery just distal to its origin. Narrowing of the right subclavian artery with post-stenotic aneurysmal dilatation is also apparent. The left carotid artery is noted to be significantly smaller in caliber than the right carotid artery.

Review of the axial HASTE images demonstrates concentric soft tissue thickening involving the transverse portion of the aorta, as well as the proximal right and left subclavian arteries. This is confirmed on standard spin-echo images with T1 and T2-weighting seen as the first 2 images of the second row.

Phase contrast images are also seen in the second row and demonstrate retrograde flow in the left vertebral artery as seen in the axial and coronal planes.

Delayed-enhancement imaging was performed as noted in the third row, and demonstrates that no abnormal myocardial enhancement is seen. However, the concentrically hypertrophied proximal aorta is observed to demonstrate apparent wall enhancement. This is easily seen on the sagittal view as seen in the second image of the third row.

Other images demonstrate that the patient has undergone a prior aortic valve replacement, and severe stenosis of the prosthetic valve is apparent. The gradient was measured at 100 mm Hg.

Images in the last row demonstrate that the abdominal aortogram shows no evidence of abnormality in the abdominal aorta. The renal arteries are widely patent as are the celiac axis and superior mesenteric artery. Both iliacs are normal in appearance.

Diagnosis

Focal high-grade stenosis of the left subclavian artery, with milder stenoses of the right subclavian and left common carotid arteries likely due to Takayasu arteritis.[1]

Takaysu arteritis is an inflammatory and obliterative arteritis classically affecting young women who present with pulseless upper extremities. It typically involves the ascending aorta and the proximal great vessels.

The differential diagnosis would include atherosclerotic disease, although the patient's young age and the absence of more widespread involvement argue against this diagnosis. Takayasu arteritis classically involves the aortic branch vessels, usually at their origins. Therefore, this was thought the most likely diagnosis.[2]

Treatment with infliximab has been reported to be helpful in two patients.[3]

Endovascular treatment with stent placement has also been reported, with generally good results.[4]

References

1. Gowda AR, et al. Takayasu arteritis of subclavian artery in a Caucasian. Int J Cardiol. 2004;95(2–3): 351–354.
2. Johnston, S.L., R.J. Lock, and M.M. Gompels, Takayasu arteritis: a review. J Clin Pathol. 2002;55(7): 481–486.
3. Della Rossa, A., et al. Two Takayasu arteritis patients successfully treated with infliximab: a potential disease-modifying agent? Rheumatology (Oxford). 2005; 44(8):1074–1075.
4. Sakaida H, et al. [Stenting for the occlusive carotid and subclavian arteries in Takayasu arteritis]. No Shinkei Geka. 2001;29(11):1033–1041.

Teaching File Case 82

48-year-old male status–post prior patch aortoplasty for supravalvular aortic stenosis

Category: Congenital

Findings

The left ventricular cavity is normal in size, and normal left ventricular systolic function is demonstrated. No evidence of concentric hypertrophy is seen. The right ventricle is normal in size and function.

The mitral valve is unremarkable in appearance.

The aortic valve is noted to be normal in appearance, but there is focal irregularity of the supravalvular aorta at the site of prior repair. Flow turbulence is noted, but no significant gradient is observed at this location.

Above this level, however, there is an area of tubular hypoplasia of the ascending aorta, seen best on the fourth and fifth images of the second row. Velocity-encoded images are seen as the first three images of the third row and demonstrate aliasing at 200 cm/sec but not at 250 cm/ sec, indicative of a gradient between 16 and 25 mm Hg. (The peak velocity measured 220 cm/sec, consistent with a gradient of 19 mm Hg.)

MR angiographic images confirm the narrowing of the ascending aorta.

Delayed-enhancement imaging demonstrates no area of abnormal enhancement to suggest the presence of significant scarring.

Diagnosis

Status-post repair of supravalvular aortic stenosis, with residual tubular hypoplasia of the ascending aorta resulting in a gradient of 19mm Hg at rest.

The patch annuloplasty of the ascending aorta has resulted in a minimal area of irregularity in the supravalvular aorta, but no stenosis in this segment. Tubular hypoplasia of the more distal aorta remains.

The patient's supravalvular aortic stenosis is an uncommon obstructive lesion of the left ventricular outflow tract, and accounts for approximately 8% of congenital left ventricular outflow tract obstructing lesions in children. The characteristic abnormality in this condition is narrowing at the level of the sinotubular junction, which typically results in an hourglass appearance of the supravalvular aorta.[1–3]

Approximately 60% of patients with supravalvular aortic stenosis will demonstrate Williams syndrome, an uncommon disorder characterized by the presence of mild mental retardation, short stature, elfin facies, and supravalvular aortic stenosis. There may also have peripheral pulmonary arterial stenosis and renal artery stenosis along with coarctation of the aorta. This disorder results from mutations involving the elastin gene on chromosome 7q11.23.[4]

References

1. Minakata K, et al. Surgical repair for supravalvular aortic stenosis: intermediate to long-term follow-up. J Card Surg. 1997;12(6):398–402.
2. Uechi Y, Kaneshiro R. Supravalvular aortic stenosis and peripheral pulmonary stenosis coexisting with a straight thoracic spine. Circ J. 2002;66(5): 516–518.
3. Ozergin U, et al. Supravalvular aortic stenosis without Williams syndrome. Thorac Cardiovasc Surg. 1996;44(4):219–221.
4. Keating, M.T., Genetic approaches to cardiovascular disease. Supravalvular aortic stenosis, Williams syndrome, and long-QT syndrome. Circulation. 1995; 92(1):142–147.

Teaching File Case 83

55-year-old female with exercise-induced weakness of the left forearm and hand

Category: Angiography

Findings

The maximum intensity projection images seen in the top row demonstrate occlusion of the left subclavian artery at its origin. The innominate, right subclavian, right carotid and left carotid arteries are all patent. The left vertebral artery is observed to fill as is the more distal portion of the left subclavian artery.

In the second row of images, velocity-encoded images are seen in the transverse and coronal plane. These demonstrate that flow toward the head is displayed as white on the velocity-encoded images, and flow toward the feet is encoded as dark on these images. Therefore, antegrade flow toward the head is observed in both carotid arteries and the right vertebral artery, and retrograde flow is seen in the left vertebral artery with flow directed toward the feet. This is readily appreciated on the coronal in-plane flow study where antegrade flow in the right vertebral is visualized, and retrograde flow is visualized in the left vertebral artery.

Diagnosis

Left subclavian artery occlusion leading to subclavian steal physiology.

Subclavian steal results from a high-grade stenosis or occlusion of the left subclavian artery proximal to the origin of the left vertebral artery. In this disorder, flow to the more distal portion of the left subclavian artery occurs via collateral flow from the right vertebral artery via the basilar artery and then retrograde flow in the left vertebral artery. Therefore, the velocity-encoded images are quite helpful, in that they clearly demonstrate the retrograde nature of the flow in the left vertebral artery confirming the subclavian steal physiology.[1,2]

The classic surgical treatment of this disorder usually consists of left carotid to left subclavian artery bypass grafting. However, endovascular therapy with angioplasty of the stenosis, and subsequent stent placement in the left subclavian artery is currently an area of active investigation.[3,4]

References

1. Sheehy N, et al. Contrast-enhanced MR angiography of subclavian steal syndrome: value of the 2D time-of-flight "localizer" sign. AJR Am J Roentgenol. 2005;185(4):1069–1073.
2. Van Grimberge F, et al. Role of magnetic resonance in the diagnosis of subclavian steal syndrome. J Magn Reson Imaging. 2000;12(2):339–342.
3. Gosselin C, Walker PM. Subclavian steal syndrome: existence, clinical features, diagnosis and management. Semin Vasc Surg. 1996;9(2):93–97.
4. Kerr AJ, Williams MJ, Wilkins GT> Primary stenting as treatment for coronary-subclavian steal syndrome. Aust N Z J Med. 1997;27(1):80–81.

Teaching File Case 84

55-year-old male from the ED with a history of chest pain and negative ECG

Category: Stress test

Findings

The left ventricular cavity size is within normal limits. The wall thickness is increased in a concentric fashion, and measured over 1.4 cm. The systolic function appears normal.

The right ventricular size and function appear normal.

Perfusion images seen in the second and third rows demonstrate that no focal perfusion deficit is noted. Increased myocardial mass is apparent.

Evaluation of valvular structures demonstrates mild mitral regurgitation. Minimal turbulence is seen in the region of the aortic valve, but no true aortic stenosis is present.

Delayed-enhancement imaging shows no area of focal scar formation.

Diagnosis

Hypertrophic cardiomyopathy. No evidence of ischemia.

Although patients with hypertrophic cardiomyopathy are at increased risk for ischemic disease, this patient's study is negative.

The use of MR imaging in the risk assessment of ED patients was studied by Kwong et al who used resting perfusion, delayed-enhancement, and cine imaging in the evaluation of acute coronary syndrome patients. They demonstrated an excellent sensitivity (84%) and specificity (85%) for the detection of acute coronary syndrome (ACS). In addition, 100% of patients with non-ST segment elevation MIs were detected.[1]

A recent study evaluated the predictive power of a negative perfusion MR scan and found a negative adenosine perfusion MR scan to be highly predictive of event free survival for one year following the study. This will need to be validated with larger multicenter studies, but appears consistent with the sensitivity for ischemic disease previously reported.[2]

References

1. Kwong RY, et al. Detecting acute coronary syndrome in the emergency department with cardiac magnetic resonance imaging. Circulation. 2003;107(4):531–537.
2. Ingkanisorn WP, et al. Prognosis of negative adenosine stress magnetic resonance in patients presenting to an emergency department with chest pain. J Am Coll Cardiol. 2006;47(7):1427–1432.

Teaching File Case 85

49-year-old female with chronic pulmonary disease

Category: Cardiomyopathy

Findings

The left ventricular cavity size is normal, as is the overall wall thickness. Minimal increased wall thickness is noted along the right ventricular side of the septum in the apical region.

The right ventricle is normal in size and function.

The 4-chamber views evident as the far right images of the second row demonstrate adenopathy in the right hilum associated with right middle lobe volume loss.

Delayed-enhancement images demonstrate abnormal enhancement along the right ventricular side of the basal and mid ventricular septum. The anteroseptal wall is noted to be involved at the apical level.

Diagnosis

Sarcoidosis.

Clinically, cardiac involvement is diagnosed in only approximately 5% of patients with sarcoidosis. However, at autopsy, up to 25% of patients with sarcoidosis demonstrate cardiac involvement. The Japanese Ministry of Health criteria are commonly used for the diagnosis of cardiac sarcoidosis, but are insensitive, as only approximately 10 to 14% of patients will fulfill the criteria. Endocardial biopsy is also widely used as the gold standard for diagnosis, but sampling error makes this a less than ideal technique. This is particularly true given the patchy nature of involvement.[1, 2]

Two studies comparing delayed-enhancement cardiac MR imaging with SPECT and PET scanning have demonstrated the clear superiority of delayed-enhancement cardiac MR imaging for the detection of cardiac sarcoidosis. In studies evaluating contrast-enhanced MR, basal involvement predominated, with a slight predominance of septal and anterior septal involvement.[3, 4]

Steroid therapy may result in regression of the lesions, with decrease in the enhancement noted, with significant resolution apparent on posttreatment imaging.[5]

The differential diagnosis would be that of any patchy myocarditis. Chagas disease or viral myocarditis could conceivably present with this pattern. However, the coexisting mediastinal adenopathy and lung disease makes sarcoidosis the most likely diagnosis.

References

1. Vignaux O. Cardiac sarcoidosis: spectrum of MRI features. AJR Am J Roentgenol. 2005;184(1): 249–254.
2. Smedema JP, et al. Cardiac involvement in patients with pulmonary sarcoidosis assessed at two university medical centers in the Netherlands. Chest. 2005;128(1):30–35.
3. Smedema JP, et al. Evaluation of the accuracy of gadolinium-enhanced cardiovascular magnetic resonance in the diagnosis of cardiac sarcoidosis. J Am Coll Cardiol. 2005;45(10):1683–1690.
4. Tadamura E, et al. Effectiveness of delayed-enhancement MRI for identification of cardiac sarcoidosis: comparison with radionuclide imaging. AJR Am J Roentgenol. 2005;185(1):110–115.
5. Shimada T, et al. Diagnosis of cardiac sarcoidosis and evaluation of the effects of steroid therapy by gadolinium-DTPA-enhanced magnetic resonance imaging. Am J Med. 2001;110(7):520–527.

Teaching File Case 86

Known congenital heart disease

Category: Congenital

History

The patient is status–post two prior corrective surgeries.

Findings

Standard morphologic images are noted in the upper row, and demonstrate that the heart is midline in position. The apex is noted to point to the right, indicating this represents true dextrocardia. The morphologic right ventricle lies to the left of the morphologic left ventricle, and is the systemic ventricle. These findings are most apparent on the short-axis views seen in the second and first part of the third row. The morphologic right ventricle fills from the left atrium through a deformed tricuspid valve, with findings suggestive of an Ebstein's like malformation of the transposed tricuspid valve. The systemic right ventricle fills a large anteriorly placed aortic through an infundibulum, indicating its right ventricular morphology. The aortic root is significantly dilated, and insufficiency of the aortic valve is noted. The aortic valve is noted to be trileaflet however.

The systemic right ventricle is thick-walled and demonstrates mildly decreased systolic function. A moderately large ventricular septal defect provides communication to the smooth-walled more posteriorly located left ventricle which otherwise has no outlet. No communication between either ventricle and a pulmonary artery segment is seen.

The venous flow is as follows: The left innominate vein joins the superior vena cava, which has been anastomosed to the right pulmonary artery. The inferior vena cava appears to be in continuity with the dilated right atrium, which empties into the left ventricle and subsequently fills the ventricular septal defect and extends into the systemic ventricle. There is no vessel extending from the heart to the left pulmonary artery. Collaterals produce delayed filling of the left pulmonary artery. The right pulmonary artery is filled from the superior vena cava as described.

The pulmonary veins fill in a normal fashion, and the left atrium does not show significant dilatation.

MR angiography is also performed, and demonstrates that the aorta originates anteriorly from the systemic right ventricle as previously described. It is moderately dilated. The branching pattern is normal, with a normally placed innominate artery seen. However, the right subclavian artery is occluded in its proximal portion, having been sacrificed for a prior Blalock-Taussig shunt.

Very large bronchial collaterals and dilated unnamed aortopulmonary collaterals are seen originating from the proximal descending aorta and peripheral anastomoses are seen between dilated intercostal branches and the peripheral pulmonary arteries on the right. The left pulmonary artery appears to fill at the level of left hilum via small collaterals, which are poorly visualized.

Imaging including the upper abdominal aorta demonstrates that abnormal collateralization also occurs from the upper abdominal aortic branches, with a large collateral originating from the upper aspect of the right renal artery extending into the right lung base, and another large collateral originating from the celiac axis and extending into the left lung base.

Diagnosis

This represents a complex cyanotic congenital heart defect. The predominant abnormality is the presence of an L loop transposition associated with absence of the main pulmonary artery segment, consistent with pulmonary atresia. A large ventricular septal defect is also noted. The large anteriorly placed aorta originates from the systemic right ventricle. The left ventricle has no outlet except for the VSD, but does receive inflow from the systemic veins, resulting in admixture at the ventricular level.

Pulmonary blood flow is marginal as described, with a Glenn procedure having been previously performed resulting in flow from the SVC to the right pulmonary artery. The left pulmonary artery fills in a delayed fashion from abundant collaterals, but no large single confluent collateral is noted.

Cardiac MR is extremely helpful in assessing ventricular morphology in complex heart defects. It is also quite useful in assessing patency of shunts and collateral vessels.

Abdominal situs is easily determined, and in this case the abdominal situs is normal (solitus).

The cardiac situs and looping is determined by evaluating the morphology of the ventricles. In this case, the systemic ventricle is the right ventricle as seen by the presence of septal papillary muscles, a trileaflet atrioventricular valve, and the presence of an infundibulum leading to its outflow great vessel. Other findings indicative of right ventricular morphology including heavier trabeculation than the left ventricle, and the presence of a moderator band when detectable.[1,2]

Findings associated with a morphologic left ventricle include a smooth appearing septum, less extensive trabeculation, and fibrous continuity between the mitral and aortic valves. No infundibulum is present in a left-sided ventricle. The left-sided atrioventricular valve should demonstrate a mitral configuration with only 2 leaflets evident.

MR has been shown to be superior to conventional angiography in the detection and characterization of aorto-pulmonary collaterals (which are frequently seen in patients with pulmonary atresia/severe Tetralogy). MR imaging will often allow better treatment planning when unifocalization of these vessels is being considered.[2, 3]

References

1. Choe YH, et al. MR imaging in the morphologic diagnosis of congenital heart disease. Radiographics. 1997;17(2):403–422.
2. Roche KJ, et al. Assessment of vasculature using combined MRI and MR angiography. AJR Am J Roentgenol. 2004;182(4):861–866.
3. Powell AJ, et al. Accuracy of MRI evaluation of pulmonary blood supply in patients with complex pulmonary stenosis or atresia. Int J Card Imaging. 2000;16(3):169–174.

Teaching File Case 87

21-year-old female with suspected pulmonary hypertension

Category: Pulm HTN

Findings

Short-axis cine images seen in the top row demonstrate that the left ventricular cavity and wall thickness are normal. Abnormal leftward motion of the septum is noted, and there is abnormal curvature of the septum with inversion noted on many of the images.

The right ventricle is noted to be enlarged, and demonstrates thickening of its wall consistent with concentric hypertrophy.

Evaluation of the valvular structures demonstrates that the mitral valve is unremarkable, but severe tricuspid regurgitation is noted. The pulmonic valve is somewhat dilated, and demonstrates mild insufficiency as best seen on the fifth and sixth images of the second row.

Pulmonary angiographic images noted in the fourth row demonstrate dilatation of the main and hilar pulmonary arteries, but do not show abrupt termination to suggest the presence of embolic disease. Review of the axial data set also shows no filling defects.

Delayed-enhancement images subsequently obtained demonstrate a small focus of hyperenhancement in the inferior portion of the septum at the septal insertion site.

Real-time imaging performed as noted in the fourth row demonstrates that the septal inversion present does not show respiratory variation.

Diagnosis

Primary pulmonary hypertension.

The differential diagnosis would include reversal of a preexisting left-to-right shunt (Eisenmenger syndrome), but there is no evidence of any septal defect or patent ductus arteriosus in this case.

Chronic thromboembolic pulmonary vascular disease can also result in pulmonary hypertension, but no evidence of pulmonary arterial thrombus or remodeling is seen.[1]

The patient demonstrated normal pulmonary parenchyma on standard chest radiography and CT imaging of the lungs, indicating that underlying parenchymal lung disease was not responsible for the pulmonary hypertension.

Primary pulmonary hypertension is an uncommon disorder that disproportionately affects women, usually in their 30s to 50s. It is of uncertain etiology, although it is often seen in patients with autoimmune symptoms and findings such as Raynaud syndrome. Although vasospasm is felt to be a primary component at onset, over time plexogenic arteriopathy develops with the obliteration of the pulmonary vascular bed, with resultant fixed increased pulmonary vascular resistance and increased pulmonary arterial pressures.

MR imaging has been recently reported to demonstrate findings that correlate with elevated pulmonary arterial pressures. Specifically, the radius of septal curvature compared to the free wall curvature has been shown to correlate with the degree of pulmonary arterial hypertension.[2, 3]

Also, phase contrast velocity-encoded imaging has been demonstrated to correlate with mean pulmonary arterial pressure, as well as the systolic pulmonary arterial pressure and the pulmonary vascular resistance index.[4]

Lastly, hyperenhancement at the RV insertion sites upon the septum has also been described with pulmonary hypertension.

Therefore, MR imaging may prove to be a helpful adjunct in the evaluation of patients presenting with pulmonary arterial hypertension. It can provide evaluation of the pulmonary arterial bed to exclude major vascular embolic disease, and can evaluate left heart structures that may result in secondary causes of pulmonary arterial hypertension. The radius of septal curvature can be assessed, as can the velocity through the main pulmonary artery, and these parameters appear to demonstrate good correlation with invasive measurements of pulmonary arterial pressure.

References

1. Kreitner KF, et al. Chronic thromboembolic pulmonary hypertension - assessment by magnetic resonance imaging. Eur Radiol. 2006.
2. Roeleveld RJ, et al. Interventricular septal configuration at mr imaging and pulmonary arterial pressure in pulmonary hypertension. Radiology. 2005;234(3): 710–717.
3. Dellegrottaglie S, et al. Pulmonary hypertension: accuracy of detection with left ventricular septal-to-free wall curvature ratio measured at cardiac MR. Radiology. 2007;243(1):63–69.
4. Sanz J, et al. Pulmonary arterial hypertension: noninvasive detection with phase-contrast MR imaging. Radiology. 2007;243(1):70–79.

Teaching File Case 88

48-year-old female with end-stage renal disease and a known vascular abnormality, followup evaluation

Category: Aorta

Findings

The study demonstrates that the volume rendered and maximum intensity projection images demonstrate a type B aortic dissection beginning distal to the left subclavian artery, and extending into the abdomen.

The axial images are reconstructed from the coronal data set, and are displayed in the far right image of the top row. These allow visualization of the true and false lumens. Sequential opacification demonstrates that the true lumen is observed to be the smaller and more anteriorly placed of the two lumens.

Evaluation of the filling pattern demonstrates that the true lumen fills the superior mesenteric artery, the left renal artery, and both of the two right renal arteries noted. The false channel actually fills in a retrograde fashion, from the descending aorta near the diaphragm, which is apparent on review of the dynamic images obtained during contrast administration.

The left ventricle is noted to demonstrate mild concentric hypertrophy. The left ventricular cavity size is within normal limits.

The right ventricle is unremarkable in appearance.

The aortic valve is trileaflet and normal in appearance. The mitral valve is likewise normal in appearance. Mild tricuspid insufficiency is noted.

Delayed-enhancement images demonstrate an unusual pattern, simulating that seen with amyloidosis, with diffuse subendocardial enhancement noted.

Diagnosis

Type B aortic dissection, with filling as described above.

Aortic dissections are most readily classified using the Stanford system, in which dissections involving the ascending aorta are termed Type A dissections regardless of the length of propagation, and dissections involving only the descending aorta are termed Type B dissection. Type A dissections require surgery for definitive treatment, while Type B dissections are most commonly treated medically. Endovascular covered stent graft placement is emerging as an alternative therapy for treatment of type B dissection.[1–3]

MR imaging is helpful in evaluating the anatomy of the dissections, and demonstrates the relationships of the true lumen, the false lumen, and the branch vessels. In addition, dissections involving the ascending aorta often involve the aortic root and may involve the aortic valve, an area where gated MR has significantly advantages over CT. It also has advantages over CT for followup in these patients who frequently require multiple examinations, in that no radiation is required.[4]

However, this study was performed prior to the reports of a possible association of the administration of gadolinium containing contrast agents to patients with renal failure and the subsequent development of a rare, potentially fatal disorder known as Nephrogenic Systemic Fibrosis. Although the exact relationship is uncertain, gadolinium-based contrast agents should not be administered to patients with renal insufficiency, particularly those requiring dialysis, unless the study is deemed absolutely necessary and there are no alternatives. In such cases, post-procedural dialysis is advised, although there is no definitive data to indicate that this will be effective in preventing this rare complication. For more information regarding MR safety and NSF, please refer to Chapter 1.

The enhancement pattern noted in this case is very reminiscent of that seen with amyloid. Although the patient had no history of amyloid, she did have a history of long-standing renal insufficiency, and the relationship between the enhancement pattern described, and the long-standing renal insufficiency is uncertain.

References

1. Destrieux-Garnier L, et al. Midterm results of endoluminal stent grafting of the thoracic aorta. Vascular. 2004;12(3):179–185.
2. Eggebrecht H, et al. Interventional management of aortic dissection. Herz. 2002;27(6):539–547.
3. Strotzer M, et al. Morphology and hemodynamics in dissection of the descending aorta. Assessment with MR imaging. Acta Radiol. 2000;41(6):594–600.
4. Krinsky GA, et al. Thoracic aorta: comparison of gadolinium-enhanced three-dimensional MR angiography with conventional MR imaging. Radiology. 1997;202(1):183–193.

Teaching File Case 89

23-year-old black male with a progressive neuromuscular disorder and an abnormal ECG

Category: Cardiomyopathy

Findings

Cine images demonstrate dilatation of the left ventricular cavity, associated with globally impaired systolic function. In addition, focal thinning of the lateral and inferolateral wall at the basal and mid-ventricular levels is apparent. The posterior papillary muscle is noted to be significantly smaller in size than the anterior papillary muscle.

The right ventricular function and size appear normal.

The valvular structures are unremarkable in appearance.

Delayed-enhancement images demonstrate extensive transmural enhancement of the lateral, inferolateral, and inferior walls from the basal to the mid-ventricular levels.

A coronary CTA examination was also performed and demonstrated that the epicardial coronary arteries were normal in appearance.

Diagnosis

Cardiac involvement by Duchenne muscular dystrophy.

This patient has Duchenne muscular dystrophy, accounting for the diffuse cardiomyopathy apparent.[1, 2] In addition, this disorder has been reported to demonstrate focal transmural scar in the lateral and inferolateral walls, particularly at the basal levels. Becker muscular dystrophy has been reported to demonstrate a similar pattern. The predilection of scar involvement of the lateral and inferolateral walls accounts for the ECG abnormality noted in this disorder, and should suggest this diagnosis.[3, 4]

On the basis of the delayed-enhancement images alone, other differential diagnostic considerations would include myocarditis, sarcoidosis, as well as Fabry disease, although the latter disorder would usually be accompanied by significant hypertrophy and not thinning. Chagas disease could also conceivably have this appearance. However, the depressed global LV function is a clue to the correct diagnosis. Obviously, in the real-world clinical setting, the patient's underlying illness would be well known to the examiner.

References

1. Hoogerwaard EM, et al. Signs and symptoms of Duchenne muscular dystrophy and Becker muscular dystrophy among carriers in The Netherlands: a cohort study. Lancet. 1999;53(9170):2116–2119.
2. Muntoni F, Cardiomyopathy in muscular dystrophies. Curr Opin Neurol. 2003;16(5):577–583.
3. Vogel-Claussen J, et al. Delayed-enhancement MR imaging: utility in myocardial assessment. Radiographics. 2006;26(3):795–810.
4. Petrie CJ, Mark PB, Dargie HJ. Cardiomyopathy in Becker muscular dystrophy–does regional fibrosis mimic infarction? J Cardiovasc Magn Reson. 2005;7(5):823–825.

Teaching File Case 90

35-year-old female with a history of non-Hodgkin's lymphoma

Category: Mass

History

Echocardiography suggested the presence of a right atrial mass. MR is requested for further evaluation.

Findings

The short-axis views demonstrate that the left ventricular size and function are within normal limits. The regional wall motion is normal as well. The right ventricular size and function also appear normal.

The morphologic images obtained in the second row demonstrate that no definite mass is appreciated.

The third row is largely comprised of images obtained in the 4-chamber projection, demonstrating a prominent crista terminalis projecting minimally into the right atrium. No other masses are seen.

Images obtained with delayed-enhancement show no evidence of scar, and no additional masses are detected.

Diagnosis

Right atrial pseudomass due to a prominent crista terminalis.

Right atrial pseudomasses are fairly common sources of confusion on echocardiography. A prominent crista terminalis can clearly mimic a mass or have a masslike appearance as is evident in this case. Other causes of right atrial pseudomasses include a prominent eustachian valve.[1–3] Intra-atrial catheters can also present a confusing appearance, and may also coexist with thrombus. Thrombus is the most common cause of a true right atrial mass.

The crista terminalis is an embryologic remnant that marks the site of fusion of the embryologic right atrium (which later becomes the right atrial appendage) with the sinus venosus derived portion of the right atrium. It has a fairly prominent appearance in this case, but is a normal structure. It can be seen on the right ventricular 2-chamber view (the fifth image of the fourth row) as a vertically oriented curvilinear structure that moves in and out of the image plane.

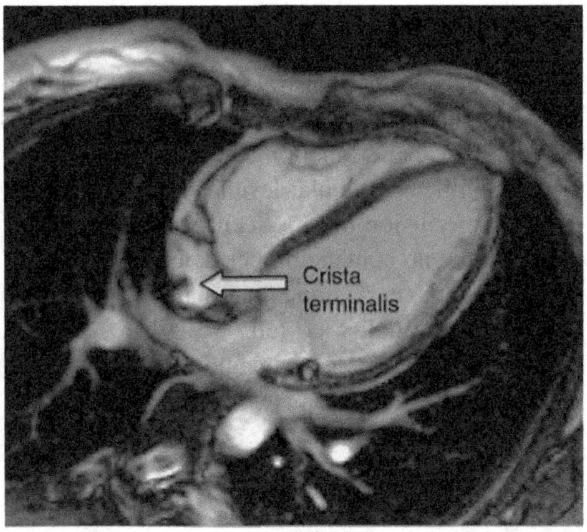

FIGURE 90.1. The arrow points to a prominent crista terminalis seen on this 4-chamber still frame cine image

References

1. Mirowitz SA, Gutierrez FR. Fibromuscular elements of the right atrium: pseudomass at MR imaging. Radiology. 1992;182(1):231–233.
2. Gaudio C, et al. Prominent crista terminalis mimicking a right atrial myxoma: cardiac magnetic resonance aspects. Eur Rev Med Pharmacol Sci. 2004;8(4):165–168.
3. Meier RA, Hartnell GG. MRI of right atrial pseudomass: is it really a diagnostic problem? J Comput Assist Tomogr. 1994;18(3):398–401.

Teaching File Case 91

67-year-old female, status–post coronary artery bypass grafting, now with recurrent chest pain

Category: Stress test

Findings

The cine images demonstrate normal left ventricular size and wall motion. The right ventricle is normal in size and function as well.

No significant valvular lesions are apparent.

Stress perfusion images seen in the second row demonstrate no convincing perfusion defect.

The resting perfusion images in the third row show no abnormality as well.

Delayed-enhancement imaging shows no evidence of prior infarction.

Diagnosis

Normal adenosine stress and rest perfusion imaging.

Perfusion imaging is one of the more challenging aspects of cardiac MR imaging. A few normal cases are included to ensure that the reader has an opportunity to visualize normal studies, and does not presume that all the studies in this Teaching File are abnormal.

Stress testing can be performed with adenosine stress as in this Teaching File, or with the use of dobutamine, similar to the technique of dobutamine stress echo. Although dobutamine has a higher rate of significant side-effects than does adenosine stress, both have excellent diagnostic accuracy and safety profiles.[1,2]

References

1. Wahl A, et al. Safety and feasibility of high-dose dobutamine-atropine stress cardiovascular magnetic resonance for diagnosis of myocardial ischaemia: experience in 1000 consecutive cases. Eur Heart J. 2004;25(14):1230–1236.
2. Klem I, et al. Improved detection of coronary artery disease by stress perfusion cardiovascular magnetic resonance with the use of delayed-enhancement infarction imaging. J Am Coll Cardiol. 2006;47(8):1630–1638.

Teaching File Case 92

75-year-old male with chest pain

Category: Aorta

Findings

The dark-blood images in the top row demonstrate eccentric wall thickening involving the ascending aorta just above the sinotubular junction. The anterior and anteromedial portion of the aortic wall demonstrates focal thickening, particularly on frame 18 of the first image series. In addition, the single frame T2-weighted spin-echo image noted in the still frame images (the second image of the fourth row) demonstrate eccentric high signal along the medial aspect of the ascending aorta interposed between the aortic root and the pulmonary artery. Eccentric thickening of the lateral wall of the descending aorta is noted. The angiographic data set does not show any evidence of an intimal flap.

Imaging of the aortic valve demonstrates that no evidence of insufficiency is seen. No flap or dissection is apparent.

Diagnosis

Intramural hematoma.

Intramural hematoma is recognized as one of the three causes of the acute aortic syndrome, the other two being aortic dissection, and penetrating atherosclerotic ulcer.

Intramural hematoma is recognized as a distinct entity wherein hemorrhage is noted within the wall of the aorta, without continuity with the vessel lumen, and without ulceration or preexisting plaque. Its etiology is not known with certainty, but rupture of the vasa vasorum is suspected as an underlying etiology.[1]

The natural history is variable, with approximately one-third resolving, one-third remaining relatively stable, and one-third progressing to the formation of aortic pseudoaneurysm, classic dissection, and/or rupture.[2, 3] For followup regarding the outcome of this patient, please refer to the next case, performed 6 months after this imaging study.

References

1. Schappert T, et al. Diagnosis and therapeutic consequences of intramural aortic hematoma. J Card Surg. 1994;9(5):508–512; discussion 512–515.
2. Evangelista A, et al. Prognostic value of clinical and morphologic findings in short-term evolution of aortic intramural haematoma. Therapeutic implications. Eur Heart J. 2004;25(1):81–87.
3. Evangelista A, et al. Long-term follow-up of aortic intramural hematoma: predictors of outcome. Circulation. 2003;108(5):583–589.

Teaching File Case 93

75-year-old male, (same patient as in Teaching File Case 92) 6 months after the initial imaging study

Category: Aorta

Findings

The cine short-axis images demonstrate normal left ventricular size and function.

The right ventricle is unremarkable as well. The 3-chamber view demonstrates that the aortic valve remains competent.

The volume-rendered image of the aorta is seen as the far right image in the third row and demonstrates clearly an eccentric outpouching arising from the anteromedial aspect of the ascending aorta, representing a localized pseudoaneurysm. This represents a definite change from the prior study performed 6 months earlier. Persistent wall thickening involving the aorta is apparent as well, consistent with continued intramural hematoma.

Diagnosis

Pseudoaneurysm of the ascending aorta, secondary to prior intramural hematoma.

As stated in the previous example, intramural hematoma is known to carry a risk for progression to either frank aortic dissection, or localized pseudoaneurysm formation.

A study of the long-term followup of aortic intramural hematoma with a focus on the predictors of outcome indicated that the best predictor of regression without complications was a normal aortic diameter in the acute phase.[1, 2]

MR imaging is a superior modality for the surveillance of such aortic syndromes in that an MR imaging study allows multi-planar examination not only of the aorta itself, but of the aortic valve as well. In addition, repeated examinations can be performed without radiation exposure or exposure to potentially nephrotoxic iodinated contrast.

References

1. Evangelista A, et al. Prognostic value of clinical and morphologic findings in short-term evolution of aortic intramural haematoma. Therapeutic implications. Eur Heart J. 2004;25(1):81–87.
2. Evangelista A, et al. Long-term follow-up of aortic intramural hematoma: predictors of outcome. Circulation. 2003;108(5):583–589.

Teaching File Case 94

49-year-old female with a history of hemolytic anemia treated with transfusions

Category: Cardiomyopathy

Findings

The left ventricle is dilated and demonstrates diffuse, global hypokinesia. The right ventricle also demonstrates impaired function and dilatation.

Moderate tricuspid and mitral regurgitation are apparent.

A small pericardial effusion is noted.

The signal intensity of the entire myocardium is abnormally low. In addition, abnormal low signal intensity is seen diffusely in the subcutaneous tissues and the liver is noted to be markedly low in signal intensity.

Diagnosis

Secondary hemochromatosis (erythropoietic hemochromatosis).

Primary hemochromatosis is an autosomal recessive condition characterized by abnormal excessive intestinal absorption of iron, which leads to deposition of iron in the liver, heart, pancreas, and other organs. Treatment with phlebotomy can markedly diminish the degree of organ damage. Females tend to present later than males secondary to menstrual blood loss.

Secondary hemochromatosis most often results from disorders such as thalassemia. In this disorder, ineffective erythropoiesis combined with multiple transfusions results in a state of iron overload. This can often be distinguished from primary hemochromatosis in that the spleen is frequently abnormal in signal intensity in secondary hemochromatosis but is relatively normal in signal intensity in primary hemochromatosis.

Hemochromatosis most often results in a dilated cardiomyopathy with impairment of systolic and diastolic function. The degree of dysfunction can be determined by alternative modalities such as echocardiography, but MR imaging can facilitate a specific diagnosis when the above-described findings are seen. Gradient echo T2* imaging can help quantitate the myocardial iron, and has advantages over endomyocardial biopsy which is prone to sampling error.[1–4]

References

1. Ptaszek LM, et al. Early diagnosis of hemochromatosis-related cardiomyopathy with magnetic resonance imaging. J Cardiovasc Magn Reson. 2005;7(4):689–692.
2. Blankenberg F, et al. Use of cine gradient echo (GRE) MR in the imaging of cardiac hemochromatosis. J Comput Assist Tomogr. 1994;18(1):136–138.
3. Liu P, Olivieri N, Iron overload cardiomyopathies: new insights into an old disease. Cardiovasc Drugs Ther. 1994;8(1):101–110.
4. Cheong B, et al. Evaluation of myocardial iron overload by T2* cardiovascular magnetic resonance imaging. Tex Heart Inst J. 2005;32(3):448–449.

Teaching File Case 95

19-year-old with a history of recent onset of chest pain

Category: Cardiomyopathy

History

The patient is also taking stimulant drugs for treatment of attention deficit disorder, and admits to ingestion of greater than the prescribed amount.

Findings

The left ventricular cavity size is normal. There is subtle hypokinesia of the anterolateral and inferolateral segments at the basal and mid-ventricular levels, with less extensive involvement of the apical lateral wall. These walls also appear minimally thicker than the adjacent segments. The left ventricular ejection fraction is reduced, measured to be 45%. The top row images are obtained prior to contrast administration while those in the first four images of the second row are post-contrast images. Note the differential enhancement of the epicardial portion of the lateral wall, as well as its reduced function.

The right ventricle is unremarkable in appearance. The valvular structures are within normal limits.

Delayed-enhancement imaging demonstrates abnormal epicardial hyperenhancement of the anterolateral and inferolateral wall at the basal and mid-ventricular levels, with involvement of the lateral wall at the apical level.

T2-weighted images seen in the bottom row demonstrate mildly increased signal and edema in the anterolateral and inferior lateral walls similar to the distribution of abnormal enhancement.

Diagnosis

The appearance is consistent with viral myocarditis. Of note, the patient underwent coronary angiography, which was entirely within normal limits.

Viral myocarditis has been reported to result in predominantly epicardial enhancement of the lateral walls involving the basal and mid-ventricular levels. In a study reported from Germany, parvovirus B19 was the most common etiologic agent, and demonstrated a tendency to involve the epicardial portion of the lateral wall. Herpes simplex 6 was also a common etiologic agent, particularly when the disorder involved the interventricular septum.[1] Not infrequently, the clinical presentation may mimic an acute myocardial infarction.[2, 3]

In general, the prognosis is quite favorable, particularly when the etiologic agent is parvovirus. Markers for a greater risk of disease progression include septal involvement and involvement with herpes simplex 6.[4]

The differential diagnosis of this epicardial pattern of enhancement includes viral myocarditis, as well as nonviral myocarditis as may be seen with sarcoidosis and Chagas disease. Although Anderson-Fabry disease can also involve the lateral wall, particularly at the basal levels, that disorder is usually accompanied by significant hypertrophy, which is not seen in this case. In addition, the enhancement in that disorder is most often mid-myocardial and not epicardial.

References

1. Mahrholdt H, et al. Cardiovascular magnetic resonance assessment of human myocarditis: a comparison to histology and molecular pathology. Circulation. 2004;109(10):1250–1258.
2. Desai A, Patel S, Book S. "Myocardial infarction" in adolescents: do we have the correct diagnosis? Pediatr Cardiol. 2005;26(5):627–631.
3. Laissy JP, et al. Differentiating acute myocardial infarction from myocarditis: diagnostic value of early- and delayed-perfusion cardiac MR imaging. Radiology. 2005;237(1):75–82.
4. Mahrholdt H, et al. Presentation, patterns of myocardial damage, and clinical course of viral myocarditis. Circulation. 2006;114(15):1581–1590.

Teaching File Case 96

56-year-old male with chest pain

Category: Stress test

History

He presented to the emergency room, and had a stress echocardiogram that was negative for coronary artery disease.

Findings

The short-axis views demonstrate that the left ventricular wall thickness and function appear normal. The left ventricular cavity size is normal as well.

The right ventricular size and function appear normal.

The valvular structures are unremarkable, without evidence of significant mitral or aortic disease.

Adenosine stress perfusion images in the second row demonstrate a well-defined area of diminished perfusion in the inferior wall at the mid-ventricular and apical levels. This region appears normal on the resting images in the third row.

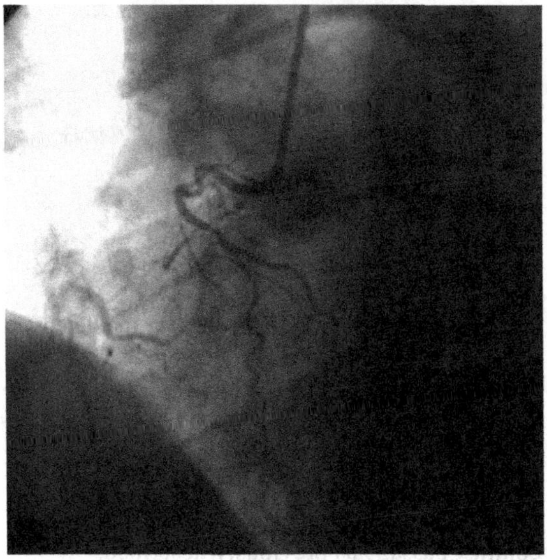

FIGURE 96.1. Still frame image from the patient's right coronary artery catheterization demonstrating occlusion of the proximal right coronary with reconstitution distally via collateral vessels

Delayed-enhancement images show no evidence of prior infarction involving the inferior wall. The left ventricular myocardium is viable throughout.

Diagnosis

Inferior wall ischemia.

The patient subsequently underwent coronary catheterization, which demonstrated complete occlusion of the right coronary artery just distal to the acute marginal branch.

Adenosine stress perfusion is the predominant technique used for provocative testing in most clinical cardiac MR laboratories. It has a favorable safety profile. In addition, image interpretation is straightforward.

Contraindications to the use of adenosine include heart block, as well as a history of asthma or significant obstructive lung disease. Resting hypotension and significant bradycardia would also represent relative contraindications.

The adenosine is administered at a rate of 140 ug/kg/min, usually for approximately 3 minutes. (Adenosine usually produces maximum vasodilatation within 2 minutes following initiation). It has a very rapid onset and offset of action, with a short half-life, contributing to its favorable safety profile.

Recent reports indicate that MR perfusion imaging may prove very helpful in the triage of patients presenting to the ED with chest pain.[1,2] MR demonstrated excellent sensitivity and specificity in the detection of CAD. This was particularly true in the study by Plein, which also evaluated the utility of the various components (perfusion, delayed-enhancement, etc) of the comprehensive CMR exam.

In addition, a negative scan has been reported to have excellent negative predictive value, with no patient with a negative scan demonstrating an adverse outcome at one year follow-up.[3]

References

1. Kwong RY, et al. Detecting acute coronary syndrome in the emergency department with cardiac magnetic resonance imaging. Circulation. 2003;107(4):531–537.
2. Plein S, et al. Assessment of non-ST-segment elevation acute coronary syndromes with cardiac magnetic resonance imaging. J Am Coll Cardiol. 2004;44(11):2173–2181.
3. Ingkanisorn WP, et al. Prognosis of negative adenosine stress magnetic resonance in patients presenting to an emergency department with chest pain. J Am Coll Cardiol. 2006;47(7):1427–1432.

Teaching File Case 97

61-year-old male with increasing creatinine level

Category: Angiography

Findings

MR angiographic data sets demonstrate a focal short segment stenosis of the proximal right renal artery, which on thin section image review approximated 75% narrowing. The left renal artery is single and widely patent.

The celiac axis and SMA are widely patent. A tight stenosis of the origin of the inferior mesenteric artery is apparent. The iliac arteries are widely patent.

Renal cysts are apparent as well.

Diagnosis

Focal high-grade right renal artery stenosis.

MR angiography has been shown in multiple series to have a diagnostic accuracy of approximately 95% in the detection of significant renal artery stenosis when compared with conventional catheter angiography. In fact, the three-dimensional nature of MR angiography provides some advantages over catheter angiography, in that eccentric narrowing can often be better appreciated on the multi-planar image review possible with the 3-D data set obtained with MR imaging as opposed to the two-dimensional projectional images available from conventional catheter angiography.[1] It also has significant advantages relative to captopril renography or Doppler ultrasound for the detection of renal artery stenosis.[2]

High-resolution imaging is necessary, and slice thickness of approximately 1mm is desirable. The images are acquired with breath-holding in order to eliminate respiratory motion artifact. Image acquisition is synchronized to the arterial phase of contrast passage as previously described.

In this age group, atherosclerotic disease is by far the most common etiology of focal renal artery narrowing.[3, 4] It may be accompanied by elevation of the patient's blood pressure, and elevated creatinine values may be seen as well as noted in this instance.

References

1. Gilfeather M, et al. Renal artery stenosis: evaluation with conventional angiography versus gadolinium-enhanced MR angiography. Radiology. 1999;210(2): 367–372.
2. Qanadli SD, et al. Detection of renal artery stenosis: prospective comparison of captopril-enhanced Doppler sonography, captopril-enhanced scintigraphy, and MR angiography. AJR Am J Roentgenol. 2001;177(5):1123–1129.
3. Uzu T, et al. Prevalence and outcome of renal artery stenosis in atherosclerotic patients with renal dysfunction. Hypertens Res. 2002;25(4):537–542.
4. Ozsarlak O, Parizel PM. Role of mr angiography in the evaluation of renovascular hypertension. Jbr-Btr. 2004;87(1):36–42.

Teaching File Case 98

9-month-old with congestive heart failure

Category: Congenital

History

Echocardiography noted excessive trabeculation. The study is requested to evaluate for possible noncompaction.

Findings

The left ventricle is dilated and demonstrates diminished systolic function. In particular, the anterior wall demonstrates diminished thickening, beginning at the basal level, and is noted to demonstrate severe hypokinesia progressing to akinesia and then dyskinesia as one proceeds from the basal and mid-ventricular levels to the apex. This is most apparent on the 2-chamber views (third and fifth images of the second row). The contractility of the inferior wall is relatively preserved.

The trabeculation of the left ventricle does appear to be mildly increased, becoming more highly trabeculated in a circumferential pattern as one proceeds to the apex. However, the degree of trabeculation is not consistent with a diagnosis of noncompaction.

The right ventricular function appears relatively preserved. It is within normal limits in size.

Moderate mitral regurgitation is noted. The aortic valve appears normal.

Perfusion images are difficult to interpret given the patient's small size. However, there is a suggestion that the patient has significant disparity in perfusion with normal perfusion of the right ventricular myocardium as well as the myocardium in the inferoseptum and inferior wall, with reduced perfusion of the entire anterior one-half of the left ventricle as well as the lateral wall of the left ventricle. These findings are quite subtle, however.

Delayed-enhancement images demonstrate diffuse, nearly circumferential subendocardial enhancement with minimal sparing of the inferoseptal and inferior wall, affecting the majority of the left ventricle.

Diagnosis

Anomalous left coronary artery originating from the pulmonary artery. This has resulted in extensive ischemic injury of the left ventricle, with resultant dilated cardiomyopathy, and evidence of infarction in a diffuse fashion on the delayed-enhancement images. The patient subsequently underwent reimplantation of the anomalous left coronary, and a repeat scan demonstrated improvement in the patient's systolic function.[1]

Anomalous left coronary artery has a variable presentation, depending on the degree of collateralization and the degree of shunting from the right coronary artery with resultant steal through the left ventricular myocardium.[2] As in this case, it can present in early infancy, usually at a point in time after the pulmonary vascular resistance falls, and the resultant steal phenomena begins.[3] The affected infants typically present with a history of feeding intolerance, and may manifest findings of diaphoresis, and pallor, similar to findings seen in adults who are suffering a myocardial infarction. This diagnosis should be strongly considered in an infant presenting with heart failure, particularly in the absence of a preexisting or underlying shunt lesion.

Echocardiography is usually diagnostic, but as in this case, there are occasionally false negatives.[4] MR imaging can be quite helpful in that it clearly demonstrates the abnormal enhancement induced by the ischemic injury. The perfusion sequence findings are subtle, but appear to demonstrate regional heterogeneity of enhancement.

References

1. Ikeda U, Murakami Y, Shimada K. Left ventricular wall thickening after surgical correction of anomalous origin of left coronary artery from pulmonary artery. Heart. 1999;81(2):205.
2. Schwerzmann M, et al. Images in cardiovascular medicine. Anomalous origin of the left coronary artery from the main pulmonary artery in adults: coronary collateralization at its best. Circulation. 2004;110(21):e511–e513.
3. Schwartz ML, Jonas RA, Colan SD. Anomalous origin of left coronary artery from pulmonary artery: recovery of left ventricular function after dual coronary repair. J Am Coll Cardiol. 1997;30(2):547–553.
4. Kaku B, et al. Detection of anomalous origin of the left coronary artery by transesophageal echocardiography and magnetic resonance imaging. Jpn Heart J. 1994;35(3):383–388.

Teaching File Case 99

64-year-old male with ischemic cardiomyopathy

Category: Viability

History

Evaluate for possible ventricular reconstructive surgery.

Findings

Marked left ventricular dilatation is noted, with diffusely impaired function. Relatively better preservation of function is noted in the basilar segments, but severe global hypokinesia is noted. Extensive adverse remodeling is noted. Dyskinesia of the anterior wall and apex is apparent.

Note the extensive thinning in the anterior wall beginning at the mid-ventricular level and extending to the apex. This measures less than 6 mm in thickness.

The right ventricle is mildly dilated and demonstrates a mild to moderate decrease in function as well.

Evaluation of the valvular structures demonstrates a minimal amount of mitral regurgitation. Very mild aortic insufficiency is noted.

Perfusion imaging demonstrates no significant perfusion deficit at rest.

Delayed-enhancement imaging demonstrates that subendocardial hyperenhancement of the anterior wall is noted beginning at the mid-ventricular level. The hyperenhancement is less than 25% transmural at the mid-ventricular level, but becomes nearly 100% transmural at the apical level. The inferior wall at the apical level is also transmurally infarcted, with subendocardial infarction noted in the more basal segments.

Subendocardial hyperenhancement is also noted in the septal and lateral walls at the mid-ventricular level, but is less than 50% in transmural extent. In the apical region, the infarction becomes more extensively transmural.

Diagnosis

Ischemic cardiomyopathy is apparent. Despite the anterior wall thinning, significant residual viability is noted in the anterior wall, as well as in portions of the lateral wall and septum.[1,2] In addition, given the extensive adverse remodeling noted and the significant loss of viability in the apex, the patient was felt to be a candidate for ventricular reconstruction as well as revascularization.[3]

Please see the following image series for the followup study after surgery.

References

1. Kim RJ, et al. The use of contrast-enhanced magnetic resonance imaging to identify reversible myocardial dysfunction. N Engl J Med. 2000;343(20):1445–1453
2. Choi KM, et al. Transmural extent of acute myocardial infarction predicts long-term improvement in contractile function. Circulation. 2001;104(10):1101–1107
3. Kramer CM, et al. Reverse remodeling and improved regional function after repair of left ventricular aneurysm. J Thorac Cardiovasc Surg. 2002;123(4):700–706.

Teaching File Case 100

64-year-old male (the same patient as Teaching File Case 99) after revascularization and ventricular reconstructive surgery

Category: Viability

Findings

Since the prior study, there has been improvement in the wall thickness and global and regional systolic function of the left ventricle. The apex remains akinetic, with a suggestion of focal dyskinesia, but overall there is significant improvement in left ventricular function in comparison to the prior study. The left ventricular ejection fraction has improved from approximately 17% to approximately 35%. The left ventricular cavity size has significantly decreased.

The anterior wall, which was previously thinned and poorly functioning now demonstrates significant improvement in thickness as well as thickening. These changes are quite marked at the basal and mid-ventricular levels.

The right ventricle also appears smaller in size, with improved function.

Evaluation of the valvular structures demonstrates no significant change in the mild aortic insufficiency. No definite mitral regurgitation is now seen.

The delayed-enhancement images demonstrate changes consistent with the ventricular reconstructive surgery. Areas of residual infarction in the apical region are again apparent, with subendocardial infarction noted in the lateral and septal walls in the mid-ventricular level and apex as well.

Diagnosis

Significant improvement in left ventricular function after revascularization and ventricular reconstruction guided by magnetic resonance viability imaging.

The viability assessment provided by magnetic resonance imaging proved invaluable in guiding the surgical reconstruction and revascularization. Although the left ventricular wall was thin and poorly functioning, and demonstrated extensive adverse remodeling, appropriate surgical intervention based upon the magnetic resonance imaging findings resulted in improvement.

The viability imaging in the preceding Teaching File case demonstrated that residual viability was noted in the thin and poorly functioning anterior wall. Other areas of subendocardial infarction of less than 50% transmural extent were also noted. The apex, which was transmurally infarcted, was resected, and the ventricle reconstructed. The resulting improvement is significant.[1]

One can easily imagine that other viability imaging in such a patient might result in a diagnosis of extensive nonviability and scar involving virtually the entire anterior left ventricular wall. For example, echocardiography would note the extensive thinning of the myocardium particularly in the anterior wall where the thickness measured less than 6 mm, and might diagnose scar without significant viability.

From such an example, one can understand the utility of performing viability imaging with MR, particularly in patients deemed not revascularizable by other modalities. The viability information provided by cardiac MR imaging was invaluable in this patient.[2]

References

1. Kramer CM, et al. Reverse remodeling and improved regional function after repair of left ventricular aneurysm. J Thorac Cardiovasc Surg. 2002;123(4):700–706.
2. Kim RJ, Shah DJ. Fundamental concepts in myocardial viability assessment revisited: when knowing how much is "alive" is not enough. Heart. 2004;90(2): 137–140.

Teaching File Case 101

69-year-old female with abnormal echocardiogram

Category: Mass

Findings

The left ventricle is normal in size and function.

The right ventricle is noted to contain a large mass. The mass originates within the right ventricular free wall, and has both intramural and intracavitary components. In addition, several septations are noted within the lesion. The most superior portion of the lesion appears to have slightly different signal intensity than the remainder of the lesion.

The lesion is noted to nearly obstruct the right ventricular outflow tract, and extends almost up to the level of the pulmonary valve.

Morphologic HASTE images noted in the third row obtained without (fourth image) and with fat saturation (fifth image) demonstrate that the lesion does not change significantly on fat saturation imaging, and is high in signal on these relatively T2-weighted images, indicating that the majority of the lesion is fluid filled.

Perfusion images (which are heavily T1 weighted) are seen in the fourth row, and demonstrate that the lesion is quite low in signal, with slightly greater signal intensity of its most superior component.

Inversion recovery images with a long inversion time demonstrate a near-total absence of signal within the lesion, with only a few septations noted. The most superior component of the lesion is slightly higher in signal intensity on long inversion recovery images.

Diagnosis

Probable lymphangioma.

The exact diagnosis is not known with certainty. However, extensive review of the patient's records indicates that the patient had a cardiac catheterization that demonstrated a large filling defect in the right ventricle approximately 30 years prior to the

MR imaging study. She has had serial echocardiograms demonstrating stability of a septated predominantly fluid filled mass in the right ventricular free wall for the last 15 years. Therefore, the lesion has certainly behaved in a benign fashion.

The differential diagnosis of benign lesions of the heart is quite extensive.[1,2] The most common benign lesion is atrial myxoma, which makes up more than 50% of all primary benign cardiac tumors. These are usually attached to the fossa ovalis, and are rarely present within the ventricle. In addition, they do not originate in an intramural location as noted in the present case. Their consistency can be quite gelatinous, but would not be expected to be fluid filled as is the present example.

Other benign lesions that are solid in nature including rhabdomyomas and fibromas are unlikely in this case of a septated, cystic mass. Paragangliomas would also be solid in consistency, and usually demonstrate intense enhancement as opposed to the present example.

The fat saturation pulse sequence excludes lipoma, as the lesion does not diminish in signal intensity.

Hemangioma is not favored given the relatively low signal on T1-weighted images. In addition, these should demonstrate delayed-enhancement, which is absent in this case. Therefore, lymphangioma is favored.

Cardiac lymphangiomas are uncommon tumors characterized by the presence of septated fluid filled spaces. As differentiated from hemangiomas, these endothelial-lined spaces are filled with lymphatic fluid rather than blood.[3, 4] They may be intramural or epicardial in location, and frequently extend to involve the pericardium is well. Although a tissue diagnosis was not obtained, this is the presumptive diagnosis made in this case. Other diagnoses are certainly possible, but are thought less likely as described above. For a tabular display of differentiating characteristics of cardiac masses, please refer to Chapter 5, Table 5.1.

References

1. Araoz PA, et al. CT and MR imaging of benign primary cardiac neoplasms with echocardiographic correlation. Radiographics. 2000;20(5):1303–1319.
2. Schvartzman PR, White RD. Imaging of cardiac and paracardiac masses. J Thorac Imaging. 2000;15(4): 265–273.
3. Kaji T, et al. Cardiac lymphangioma: case report and review of the literature. J Pediatr Surg. 2002; 37(10):E32.
4. Jougon J, et al. Cystic lymphangioma of the heart mimicking a mediastinal tumor. Eur J Cardiothorac Surg. 2002;22(3):476–478.

Teaching File Case 102

69-year-old male with abnormality suspected on recent cardiac catheterization

Category: Coronary MRA

History

MR confirmation was desired.

Findings

The left ventricular size and global function appeared normal. The wall thickness is at the upper limits of normal.

The right ventricular size and function appears normal. No significant mitral or aortic abnormality is seen. Trace tricuspid regurgitation is suspected.

Perfusion images demonstrate no abnormality in these resting images.

High-resolution SSFP thin section angiographic images are seen in the far right images of the second row. These images demonstrate that the right coronary artery is seen to originate from the medial margin of the left coronary cusp, and is observed to pass between the right ventricular outflow tract and the aorta.

Delayed-enhancement images show a small focal area of hyperenhancement in the anterior wall of the mid-ventricular level.

Diagnosis

Anomalous origin of the right coronary artery from the left coronary cusp.

This is a potentially dangerous variant in that it passes between the great vessels. An inter-arterial passage of an anomalous coronary artery is considered a malignant anomaly, and often will prompt surgical bypass, as it is associated with a risk of sudden cardiac death. However, given the patient's age, intervention was not immediately elected in this patient.

Coronary artery anomalies are fairly common, occurring in approximate 1 to 2% of the population.[1] The most common anomaly is an origin of the left circumflex coronary artery from the right coronary artery cusp or from the right coronary artery itself, with retroaortic passage of the anomalous circumflex. This requires no specific therapy. However, malignant varieties characterized by inter-arterial passage of the vessel often mandate surgical therapy.[2] Specifically, anomalous origin of the right coronary from the left cusp or anomalous origin of the left coronary from the right cusp with passage of the anomalous vessel between the aorta and pulmonary artery are considered potentially dangerous variants.

A small focus of scarring noted in the anterior wall may be related to prior placement of a stent in the diagonal branch of the left anterior descending coronary artery.

A variety of MR sequences are used for coronary artery imaging including FLASH, T2 prepared steady-state free-precession imaging (as in the present example), as well as contrast enhanced imaging using agents with prolonged intravascular retention; many of these can be performed using navigator-gated free-breathing techniques. A variety of reports indicate that for proximal coronary artery imaging, CMR can achieve sensitivity and specificity of approximately 90+%. Although the rapid progress made by coronary CT angiography along with its superior spatial resolution will likely result in preferential adoption of CT for non-invasive coronary artery imaging, significant coronary anomalies are usually well depicted by MR imaging.[3, 4]

References

1. Cademartiri F, et al. Coronary artery anomalies: incidence, pathophysiology, clinical relevance and role of diagnostic imaging. Radiol Med (Torino). 2006;111(3):376–391.
2. Varghese A, Keegan J, Pennell DJ. Cardiovascular magnetic resonance of anomalous coronary arteries. Coron Artery Dis. 2005;16(6):355–364.
3. Manning WJ, et al. Coronary magnetic resonance imaging: current status. Curr Probl Cardiol. 2002;27(7):275–333.
4. McConnell MV, Stuber M, Manning WJ. Clinical role of coronary magnetic resonance angiography in the diagnosis of anomalous coronary arteries. J Cardiovasc Magn Reson. 2000;2(3):217–224.

Teaching File Case 103

68-year-old male with lower limb ischemia

Category: Angiography

Findings

MR angiographic images demonstrate that the abdominal aorta is normal in contour and caliber. No aneurysm is seen. The renal arteries appear widely patent. The iliac arteries are patent. The common femoral arteries and proximal superficial femoral arteries appear normal.

The second set of images demonstrates normal appearance of the superficial femoral arteries throughout the upper legs.

Images obtained in the region of the lower leg demonstrate that on the right, narrowing of the tibioperoneal trunk is apparent. Occlusion of the anterior tibial artery is seen at its origin. The posterior tibial artery demonstrates multiple focal areas of moderately severe narrowing in its proximal and mid portions. The distal posterior tibial artery appears to be occluded. The peroneal artery is patent to a level just above the ankle.

On the left, the anterior tibial artery is occluded proximally, and focal narrowing is seen within the tibioperoneal trunk, with irregularity throughout the posterior tibial and peroneal arteries. The left peroneal artery is patent. The left posterior tibial is patent as it crosses the ankle.

Diagnosis

Extensive distal peripheral vascular disease, with poor distal runoff.

This pattern of relatively well-preserved inflow, with poor distal runoff is commonly seen in patients with diabetes. In these patients, small vessel disease frequently predominates, often with relative preservation of the inflow vessels. This patient was diabetic.[1]

Given the peripheral nature of the disease, bypass surgery is often problematic.[2] This patient underwent percutaneous intervention on the distal right posterior tibial artery, with restoration of flow across the ankle.

The images were obtained with time-resolved imaging performed initially at the lower leg level. These sequences provide visualization of the distal arteries free of venous contamination even in circumstances where the patient has rapid arterial flow, and/or rapid arteriovenous shunting as may be seen in cases of cellulitis.

References

1. Lapeyre M, et al. Assessment of critical limb ischemia in patients with diabetes: comparison of MR angiography and digital subtraction angiography. AJR Am J Roentgenol. 2005;185(6):1641–1650.
2. Conte MS, et al. Impact of increasing comorbidity on infrainguinal reconstruction: a 20-year perspective. Ann Surg. 2001;233(3):445–452.

Teaching File Case 104

57-year-old male with recent ST segment elevation MI

Category: Viability

History

Status-post stent placement.

Findings

The left ventricular cavity size is normal and the overall wall thickness is normal as well. Focal thickening of the anterior septum at the basal and mid-ventricular levels is apparent. This segment also demonstrates mild decrease in thickening.

The right ventricle is normal in size and function.

Evaluation of the valvular structures demonstrates minimal turbulence in the region of the aortic valve. The mitral valve demonstrates trace mitral regurgitation. No significant tricuspid regurgitation is noted.

Delayed enhanced images demonstrate an area of infarction involving the anterior septum at the basal and mid-ventricular levels. T2-weighted images are seen in the second row of static images, and demonstrate subtle increased signal in the anterior septum at the baseline mid-ventricular levels.

A small focus of low signal intensity seen within the hyperintense region in the last row of delayed enhanced images likely represents a small no-reflow zone.

Diagnosis

Acute myocardial infarction.

Recent reports have indicated that T2-weighted images obtained up to 2 days post infarction represent a reliable and reproducible measure of the area of ischemic risk. The area of hyperenhancement demarcates the area of infarction, while the area of T2 signal hyperintensity represents both the irreversibly injured as well as reversibly injured regions of myocardium.[1]

T2 imaging can distinguish acute from chronic myocardial infarctions as well, as chronic infarctions will not be hyperintense on T2-weighted images, while acute infarctions will.[2] However, as seen above, using T2 images to demonstrate infarction does not allow accurate distinction between areas of reversible and irreversible ischemic injury, and thus must be used with caution.

This patient subsequently underwent repeat scanning at 30 days post the initial event, which demonstrated decreased but persistent T2 signal abnormality (see the following case). The delayed enhancement imaging showed less significant change in size as one would expect.

References

1. Aletras AH, et al. Retrospective determination of the area at risk for reperfused acute myocardial infarction with T2-weighted cardiac magnetic resonance imaging: histopathological and displacement encoding with stimulated echoes (DENSE) functional validations. Circulation. 2006;113(15):1865–1870.
2. Abdel-Aty H, et al. Delayed enhancement and T2-weighted cardiovascular magnetic resonance imaging differentiate acute from chronic myocardial infarction. Circulation. 2004;109(20):2411–2416.

Teaching File Case 105

57-year-old male (same patient as in Teaching File Case 104) one month after the initial post infarction study

Category: Viability

Findings

The left ventricular cavity size and function remained within normal limits. The overall wall thickness and thickening is normal as well.

Evaluation of valvular structures shows no focal abnormality.

Delayed enhancement images again demonstrate the presence of an anteroseptal infarction beginning at the basal level, and extending nearly to the apex. When compared to the prior study performed one month earlier, the area of hyperenhancement appears more clearly defined and slightly smaller in size.

The T2-weighted images also demonstrate decrease in size of the area of abnormal high signal.

Diagnosis

Followup imaging study, 30 days post acute myocardial infarction and revascularization.

The present examination demonstrates the slight decrease in size of the region of hyperenhancement when followup imaging is performed.

The area of delayed enhancement represents the area of prior infarction, while the area of high signal on T2-weighted images reflects a mix of infarction and edema. It is well known that infarctions appear to shrink over time, as the nonviable myocytes are replaced by collagenous scar.[1]

Both acute and chronic myocardial infarctions will demonstrate hyperenhancement, as has been well demonstrated in a series of articles studying the gross anatomic-pathologic correlations of delayed enhancement imaging as performed above.[2] These studies have clearly demonstrated that the apparent change in infarct size mirrors the actual remodeling that occurs in vivo. It is not a function of artifactual mis-estimation of the infarct volume.[3]

Other studies that have evaluated the apparent variability of infarct sizing by MR imaging have found excellent correlation between the size of the infarction visualized on MR imaging, and that found on histologic evaluation when the appropriate inversion time has been chosen.[4] Use of a constant, fixed inversion time that has not been adjusted to appropriately null the myocardium has resulted in mis-estimation of infarct size, and is inappropriate for clinical use.[5,6]

References

1. Fieno DS, et al. Contrast-enhanced magnetic resonance imaging of myocardium at risk: distinction between reversible and irreversible injury throughout infarct healing. J Am Coll Cardiol. 2000;36(6):1985–1991.
2. Kim RJ, et al. Relationship of MRI delayed contrast enhancement to irreversible injury, infarct age, and contractile function. Circulation. 1999;100(19):1992–2002.
3. Mahrholdt H, et al. Reproducibility of chronic infarct size measurement by contrast-enhanced magnetic resonance imaging. Circulation. 2002;106(18):2322–2327.
4. Wagner A, et al. Effects of time, dose, and inversion time for acute myocardial infarct size measurements based on magnetic resonance imaging-delayed contrast enhancement. J Am Coll Cardiol. 2006;47(10):2027–2033.
5. Oshinski JN, et al. Imaging time after Gd-DTPA injection is critical in using delayed enhancement to determine infarct size accurately with magnetic resonance imaging. Circulation. 2001;104(23):2838–2842.
6. Judd RM, Kim RJ. Imaging time after Gd-DTPA injection is critical in using delayed enhancement to determine infarct size accurately with magnetic resonance imaging. Circulation. 2002;106(2):e6; author reply e6.

Teaching File Case 106

78-year-old male in for followup of a known aortic dissection

Category: Aorta

Findings

Morphologic images seen in the top row demonstrate an aortic dissection beginning in the descending thoracic aorta distal to the left subclavian artery. A cine image seen in the first row confirms flow in the upper portion of the dissection. A similar view obtained in the fourth row on the far right image demonstrates opacified and thrombosed portions of the dissection.

Incidental note is made of marked thyroid enlargement.

The thin section multi-planar reformations from the contrast-enhanced angiogram demonstrate communication between the true and false lumens at the level of the proximal descending thoracic aorta (third and fourth images of the bottom row).

The postcontrast volumetric 3-D image noted in the far left of the fourth row demonstrates well the thrombosed (dark) and opacified portions of the dissection.

Cine images demonstrate normal left ventricular function. The right ventricle is also normal in appearance.

Diagnosis

Partially thrombosed dissection of the aorta.

Aortic dissections will occasionally undergo spontaneous thrombosis of the false lumen. In this instance, the dissection may decrease in size. However, decrease in flow through the false lumen may have a deleterious effect on organs supplied by it.

Complications of aortic dissection include rupture, as well as diminished perfusion of the false lumen as well as the vessels supplied by the false lumen, resulting in the impairment of flow to visceral organs. Compromise of the true lumen may also result from enlargement of the false lumen.[1,2]

Timing of the image acquisition in dissection cases can be difficult, as the two lumens may have significantly different rates of filling. This can be easily assessed if the timing bolus technique is used to trigger the study. In this instance, sequential filling of the true and false lumens can be directly observed, and adjustment made to insure appropriate triggering.

In the case where fluoroscopic triggering is used, a slight delay in starting the acquisition may be helpful. Also, the flow rate of the contrast can be slightly reduced so as to prolong the injection duration. In addition, the ordering of K-space acquisition, which is usually performed with centric ordering when using bolus-triggering, can be switched to a linear acquisition scheme. Finally, rapidly repeating the acquisition is often helpful in cases of marked flow discrepancy.

References

1. Strotzer M, et al. Morphology and hemodynamics in dissection of the descending aorta. Assessment with MR imaging. Acta Radiol. 2000;41(6):594–600.
2. Srichai MB, et al. Acute dissection of the descending aorta: noncommunicating versus communicating forms. Ann Thorac Surg. 2004;77(6):2012–20; discussion 2020.

Teaching File Case 107

62-year-old male with persistent bacteremia, status–post aortic graft placement and repair of prior dissection

Category: Mass

History

Evaluate the prosthetic valve.

Findings

The patient had difficulty suspending respiration. Thus, the standard segmented image acquisitions are degraded in image quality. Real time imaging was also performed as can be seen in the second and third images of the upper row.

Review of the short-axis images indicates that there is normal left ventricular cavity size, with focal thinning of the inferolateral wall at the basal and mid-ventricular levels. This region is also hypocontractile.

Note is made of a focal rounded outpouching from the left ventricular apex, which on perfusion images (last 3 right-sided images of the top row) is seen to be in continuity with the blood pool.

Imaging of the prosthetic aortic valve demonstrates minimal turbulence, but velocity-encoded measurements indicate that no significant gradient is present. Insignificant insufficiency is seen.

Single-shot delayed-enhancement images were obtained due to patient difficulty with suspending respiration. These are demonstrated in the far right-sided images of the third row. These confirm the small inferolateral infarction at the mid-ventricular level. No enhancement is seen in the left ventricular apex at the site of the outpouching.

Rotating volume-rendered images of the aorta are demonstrated in the fourth row. Redundancy of the graft is noted, resulting in buckling of the ascending aorta. However, no significant turbulence is produced.

Diagnosis

Focal pseudoaneurysm of the left ventricular apex.

The patient is status–post aortic valve replacement, with graft placement in the ascending aorta. Redundancy of the graft is noted, resulting in buckling. Note that the prosthetic valve is not a contraindication to MR scanning, and does not produce image degradation.

Note the small prior infarction in the left circumflex artery territory. Only single-shot imaging was performed due to the patient's inability to hold his breath. Nonetheless, a small, subendocardial infarction is evident. As previously discussed, the single-shot technique is an excellent substitute for the standard segmented inversion recovery delayed-enhancement images in such a situation, with only a slight decrease in sensitivity when compared with the standard technique.

The rounded outpouching is shown to be in continuity with the blood pool. Definite myocardial tissue surrounding this lesion is not seen, which would make it a pseudoaneurysm rather than a true aneurysm or diverticulum.[1, 2] A diverticulum should demonstrate contractility, rather than the paradoxical motion noted on this exam.[3, 4] This pseudoaneurysm was likely postsurgical in nature, possibly relating to trauma to the left ventricular apex at the time of surgery. No adjacent infarction is noted to suggest that it represents a post-infarction contained rupture.

Perfusion imaging was helpful in this case by demonstrating conclusively the presence of continuity between the rounded outpouching and the left ventricular blood pool.

References

1. Tran T, et al. Gd-enhanced cardiovascular MR imaging to identify left ventricular pseudoaneurysm. J Cardiovasc Magn Reson. 2005;7(4):717–721.
2. Baks T, et al. Chronic pseudoaneurysm of the left ventricle. Int J Cardiovasc Imaging. 2005;1–3.
3. Marijon E, et al. Diagnosis and outcome in congenital ventricular diverticulum and aneurysm. J Thorac Cardiovasc Surg. 2006;131(2):433–437.
4. Yamashita C, et al. Left ventricular diverticulum with hypertrophy of the left ventricular apex. Ann Thorac Surg. 1992;54(4):761–763.

Teaching File Case 108

51-year-old male with known cardiac abnormality

Category: Cardiomyopathy

Findings

Concentric left ventricular hypertrophy is evident. Normal systolic function is demonstrated. The left ventricular cavity size is at the lower limits of normal.

The right ventricle size and function are normal.

Evaluation of valvular structures demonstrates mild mitral regurgitation. The aortic valve is normal in appearance. Mild tricuspid regurgitation is also seen. No significant systolic anterior motion of the mitral valve is apparent. No asymmetric septal thickening is seen.

Delayed-enhancement images demonstrate focal areas of abnormal enhancement in the midportion of the anterior septal and inferior walls at the RV insertion sites.

Diagnosis

Hypertrophic cardiomyopathy (HCM).

The differential diagnosis would include disorders that produce concentric ventricular hypertrophy. The sparing of the right ventricle is a finding that favors HCM rather than amyloid, which often involves the right ventricle as well.[1] Fabry disease can mimic hypertrophic cardiomyopathy, particularly when the pattern is that of a concentric hypertrophy as in the present case.[2]

Hypertrophic cardiomyopathy is the most common genetically transmitted cardiac disorder, with an incidence of 1 in 500. Typically it has one of 3 patterns: asymmetric septal hypertrophy often resulting in some degree of ventricular outflow tract obstruction is the most common pattern, accounting for approximately 60% of cases. Approximately 25 to 30% of cases are concentric in configuration, while apical hypertrophic cardiomyopathy makes up approximately 10% of cases. In the Far East, hypertrophic cardiomyopathy of the apical form is more common.

Delayed-enhancement imaging has been reported to be positive in approximately 80% of patients with HCM. The most common pattern is that of enhancement of the mid-myocardium at the septal insertion sites. Areas that demonstrate the greatest thickening at rest and the poorest systolic function also tend to demonstrate the greatest enhancement.[3] The degree of enhancement correlates with the impairment of function, and with the risk of progression.[4]

Patient with hypertrophic cardiomyopathy are at risk for sudden death. In addition to standard risk stratification using measurements of ventricular outflow tract obstruction and wall thickness, as well as historical factors, MR imaging with delayed enhancement has been reported to add incremental information. Specifically, the degree of left ventricular hyperenhancement as a percentage of total cardiac mass has been shown to correlate with the risk of sudden death and progressive disease. These preliminary observations will need to be extended in larger studies, but the technique demonstrates promise.[4]

References

1. Fattori R, et al. Contribution of magnetic resonance imaging in the differential diagnosis of cardiac amyloidosis and symmetric hypertrophic cardiomyopathy. Am Heart J. 1998;136(5):824–830.
2. Beer G, et al. Fabry disease in patients with hypertrophic cardiomyopathy (HCM). Z Kardiol. 2002;91(12): 992–1002.
3. Choudhury L, et al. Myocardial scarring in asymptomatic or mildly symptomatic patients with hypertrophic cardiomyopathy. J Am Coll Cardiol. 2002;40(12):2156–2164.
4. Moon JC, et al. Toward clinical risk assessment in hypertrophic cardiomyopathy with gadolinium cardiovascular magnetic resonance. J Am Coll Cardiol. 2003;41(9):1561–1567.

Teaching File Case 109

77-year-old female with known end-stage renal disease and pericardial effusion

Category: Pericardium

History

The patient has had recurrent episodes of right heart failure. The study is requested to assess the possible hemodynamic significance of the effusion.

Findings

Dark-blood and bright-blood images confirm the presence of a large pericardial effusion. Cine imaging was attempted, as can be seen in the upper row, but only a few images could be adequately obtained using standard retrospective gating techniques. Apparent diastolic collapse of the atria is apparent. For further evaluation, real-time imaging was performed as seen in the last four images of the second row.

The first three images obtained with real-time technique demonstrate minimal septal flattening as the patient takes an inspiration. The last image on the far right of the second row was obtained with real-time imaging while the patient was asked to take a deep inspiration. Note the more extensive septal flattening observed.

Other findings include left ventricular hypertrophy, and turbulent flow noted through the aortic valve on the 3-chamber view. The delayed-enhancement images did not show any definite focal scar.

Diagnosis

Hemodynamically significant pericardial effusion.

The pericardium normally has some degree of distensibility and usually only limits right ventricular filling in the extreme case of marked increase in right ventricular volume. Pericardial effusions that accumulate slowly over time result in gradual distention of the pericardium, and hemodynamic effects can be minimal. The acute development of a similar amount of pericardial fluid would result in cardiac compromise and would not be tolerated in the acute setting.

Techniques for assessing the significance of the effusion include the use of real-time imaging. This has two benefits: First, it can be used even in the absence of gating which is problematic in this patient with a low amplitude ECG signal.[1] Secondly, it allows assessment of real-time hemodynamics, including provocative maneuvers such as having the patient take a deep inspiration.

In this case, the use of provocative maneuvers during real-time imaging provided assessment of the hemodynamic significance of the effusion noted.[2] Specifically, the augmentation of right ventricular filling resulting from a deep inspiration results in displacement of the septum from right-to-left, indicating that the pericardium has reached its maximum capacity. Therefore, any further increase in right ventricular filling will result in decrease of the filling of the left ventricle.

Similar provocative maneuvers can be used to study patients with constrictive pericarditis. A study by Francone et al found that real-time MR during deep inspiration could reliably distinguish between restrictive cardiomyopathy (no septal displacement), constrictive pericarditis (septal displacement produced by augmented RV filling during deep inspiration), and cor pulmonale (septal displacement independent of the phase of respiration).[2]

References

1. Kuhl HP, et al. Assessment of myocardial function with interactive non-breath-hold real-time MR imaging: comparison with echocardiography and breath-hold Cine MR imaging. Radiology. 2004;231(1):198–207.
2. Francone M, et al. Real-time cine MRI of ventricular septal motion: a novel approach to assess ventricular coupling. J Magn Reson Imaging. 2005;21(3): 305–309.

Teaching File Case 110

24-year-old male status–post repair of congenital heart disease in childhood

Category: Congenital

Findings

The left ventricle is mildly dilated, and normal in wall thickness. The global systolic function is markedly reduced, in a diffuse fashion.

The right ventricle is markedly dilated, and demonstrates mild wall thickening, and globally reduced systolic function. Paradoxical septal motion is apparent.

Evaluation of the valvular structures demonstrates that no significant mitral regurgitation is noted. The aortic valve is trileaflet and otherwise normal in appearance. Moderately severe tricuspid regurgitation is noted, with an eccentric jet noted

The most striking abnormality is absence of the pulmonary valve, with free pulmonic insufficiency.

Diagnosis

Tetralogy of Fallot, status–post patch annuloplasty, and resection of the pulmonary valve.

The patient now has severe biventricular failure, and will likely require transplantation.

The four components of the Tetralogy are all related to the embryologic malformation of the cono-truncal septum and hypoplasia of the infundibulum, with resultant overriding of the aorta, and a malalignment VSD. In addition, the abnormal rotation of the cono-truncal septum results in narrowing of the right ventricular outflow tract, and often an associated dysplasia of the pulmonary valve as well. Right ventricular hypertrophy results from the right ventricular outflow tract obstruction.

Surgery was formerly directed toward relieving the right ventricular outflow tract obstruction, and patch annuloplasty was frequently performed. The resultant pulmonic insufficiency was thought likely to be well tolerated. However, over time, the pulmonic insufficiency is not well tolerated, and right ventricular failure may ensue. Therefore, timely placement of a pulmonary valve prosthesis is of critical importance in these individuals.[1, 2]

Discernment of the optimal time for valve replacement can be a complex undertaking, and the reader is referred to the attached articles.[3, 4]

Note that the finding of paradoxical septal motion characteristically seen with constrictive pericarditis may be seen in other disorders; specifically, those that result in RV pressure or volume overload as in the present example.

References

1. Davlouros, P.A., et al. Timing and type of surgery for severe pulmonary regurgitation after repair of tetralogy of Fallot. Int J Cardiol. 2004;97 Suppl 1:91–101.
2. Davlouros, P.A., et al. Right ventricular function in adults with repaired tetralogy of Fallot assessed with cardiovascular magnetic resonance imaging: detrimental role of right ventricular outflow aneurysms or akinesia and adverse right-to-left ventricular interaction. J Am Coll Cardiol. 2002;40(11):2044–52.
3. Geva, T., Indications and timing of pulmonary valve replacement after tetralogy of Fallot repair. Semin Thorac Cardiovasc Surg Pediatr Card Surg Annu. 2006: 11–22.
4. Cheung, M.M., I.E. Konstantinov, and A.N. Redington, Late complications of repair of tetralogy of Fallot and indications for pulmonary valve replacement. Semin Thorac Cardiovasc Surg. 2005;17(2):155–9.

Teaching File Case 111

53-year-old male with a history of prior episode of deep venous thrombosis involving the subclavian vein on the left

Category: Angiography

History

The study is performed in followup post thrombolytic treatment.

Findings

Initial morphologic images demonstrate that no mass is seen encasing the subclavian vein.

Subsequently, MR venography was performed by direct injection of dilute gadolinium into the left arm venous system at the level of the forearm. The initial image with contrast displayed as the fifth image of the top row was obtained prior to placing a tourniquet at the level of the elbow. The far right image was obtained after placing a tourniquet at the level of the elbow and repeating the injection. The first image of the second row is a volume rendered image of the same study.

The images demonstrate patency of the axillary and subclavian veins on the left, with free flow of contrast into the superior vena cava. No evidence of collateralization is seen.

Diagnosis

Patency of the left subclavian venous system is demonstrated.

MR venography can be performed in two ways.[1–3] First, injection can be performed into the contralateral venous system using standard gadolinium with saline flush, with imaging first in the arterial phase, followed by delayed imaging to capture the venous phase. This is termed indirect MR venography.

Alternatively, if one can obtain venous access in the affected limb, direct injection of gadolinium diluted 1 to 10 with saline can be performed, with scan initiation beginning after approximately two-thirds of the contrast has been injected. The patient should be told not to perform a Valsalva maneuver as this will compromise venous return by raising intrathoracic pressure, and result in a pseudostenosis appearance as the left subclavian vein transits underneath the first rib and becomes truly intrathoracic. Direct injection was used in the present example. As noted in this study, placement of a tourniquet above the injection site in order to diminish superficial venous filling and force contrast into the deep venous system is often helpful.

References

1. Tanju S, et al. Direct contrast-enhanced 3D MR venography evaluation of upper extremity deep venous system. Diagn Interv Radiol. 2006;12(2):74–79.
2. Lin J, et al. Vena cava 3D contrast-enhanced MR venography: a pictorial review. Cardiovasc Intervent Radiol. 2005;28(6):795–805.
3. Vogt FM, Herborn CU, Goyen M. MR venography. Magn Reson Imaging Clin N Am. 2005;13(1): 113–129, vi.

Teaching File Case 112

28-year-old male with a history of prior abnormal echocardiogram

Category: Cardiomyopathy

Findings

The left ventricle is mildly dilated, and heavily trabeculated, in a nearly concentric fashion involving the apical one-half of the myocardium. The abnormal trabeculation begins at the mid-ventricular level and extends to the apex with relatively greater involvement of the lateral wall. The left ventricular systolic function is mildly reduced, with an LVEF of 41%.

The right ventricle is also mildly dilated, and also demonstrates excessive trabeculation and reduced systolic function.

Incidentally noted is a small tag of abnormal tissue in the right ventricular outflow tract evident on the 3-chamber view. Cine images subsequently obtained directly in the plane of this lesion demonstrate that it appears to be excess conal tissue attached along the anterior margin of the undersurface of the aortic valve.

Perfusion images show no abnormality.

Delayed-enhancement images show the excessive trabeculation, but no abnormal enhancement is seen. Breathing artifact minimally degrades the high-resolution segmented images, but the single-shot inversion recovery images are normal in appearance other than the heavy trabeculation.

Diagnosis

This patient has noncompaction of the left ventricular myocardium.

This is felt to represent a distinct cardiomyopathy of unknown origin,[1] although a familial predilection has been reported. It is characterized by abnormal heavy trabeculation, often preferentially involving the lateral and apical walls. It is speculated that this order is due to an embryologic defect, with arrest of the normal compaction of the myocardium.[2, 3]

The diagnosis is based on the finding of a trabecular meshwork that is two times thicker than the adjacent compacted myocardium as measured in systole. In addition, it is noted that the trabecular meshwork fills from the endocardial blood pool. Lastly, the disorder should not accompany any other structural heart disease such as a congenital valvular lesion.

The prognosis demonstrates variability, but the disorder often progresses to impaired systolic function, and heart failure. Some reports indicate an increased incidence of embolic events as well.[4–6]

References

1. Petersen SE, et al. Left ventricular non-compaction: insights from cardiovascular magnetic resonance imaging. J Am Coll Cardiol. 2005;46(1):101–105.
2. Varnava AM, Isolated left ventricular non-compaction: a distinct cardiomyopathy? Heart. 2001;86(6):599–600.
3. Oechslin E, Jenni R. Isolated left ventricular non-compaction: increasing recognition of this distinct, yet 'unclassified' cardiomyopathy. Eur J Echocardiogr. 2002;3(4):250–251.
4. Murphy RT, et al. Natural history and familial characteristics of isolated left ventricular non-compaction. Eur Heart J. 2005;26(2):187–192.
5. Lilje C, et al. Complications of non-compaction of the left ventricular myocardium in a paediatric population: a prospective study. Eur Heart J. 2006;27(15): 1855–1860.
6. Ker J, Van Der Merwe C. Isolated left ventricular non-compaction as a cause of thrombo-embolic stroke: a case report and review. Cardiovasc J S Afr. 2006;17(3):146–147.

Teaching File Case 113

61-year-old male with a recent equivocal nuclear medicine study, which suggested a possible inferior wall defect versus artifact

Category: Viability

Findings

Cine images in the short-axis plane demonstrate thinning and impaired wall motion of the inferior wall from the base to the mid-ventricular level. The more distal inferior wall appears normal in appearance. The cavity size is normal. The wall thickness is mildly increased in regions other than the thinned inferior wall, suggesting concentric hypertrophy.

The right ventricle is normal in appearance. The valvular structures are unremarkable.

Resting perfusion images demonstrate abnormal perfusion of the inferior wall.

Delayed-enhancement images demonstrate extensive transmural infarction of the inferior wall from the base to the mid-ventricular level. Corresponding T2-weighted images demonstrate no increased signal in the inferior wall at the site of the abnormal enhancement.

Diagnosis

Chronic infarction of the inferior wall.

The delayed-enhancement images are consistent in appearance with an area of transmural infarction involving the inferior wall from the base to the mid-ventricular level, consistent with infarction in the territory of the right coronary artery. These images, however, do not distinguish between acute and chronic infarcts.

The perfusion images demonstrate that abnormal perfusion persists in the region of scar. This indicates residual microvascular impairment in the area of prior infarction.

The T2-weighted images demonstrate no significant edema, indicating that this represents an area of old, chronic infarction. An acute infarction would be expected to demonstrate high signal on the T2-weighted images.[1] In addition, the thinning implies some degree of chronicity as well.

Contrast-enhanced MR imaging has been shown to be helpful in the evaluation of equivocal nuclear SPECT abnormalities. In particular, inferior wall attenuation by diaphragmatic structures is a frequent source of difficulty on SPECT images, which can be readily resolved with MR imaging.[2] In a study by Lee et al, 20 patients with equivocal SPECT studies underwent CE-MRI. The study demonstrated that 50% of the equivocal findings involved the inferior wall, and that 24% were due to infarction, with the remaining 76% the result of artifact. Interestingly, 29 segments in 8 patients were noted to demonstrate infarct at MR that had not been suspected at SPECT imaging, including 3 patients not known clinically to have had an MI.

References

1. Abdel-Aty H, et al. Delayed-enhancement and T2-weighted cardiovascular magnetic resonance imaging differentiate acute from chronic myocardial infarction. Circulation. 2004;109(20):2411–2416.
2. Lee VS, et al. MR imaging evaluation of myocardial viability in the setting of equivocal SPECT results with (99m)Tc sestamibi. Radiology. 2004;230(1): 191–197.

Teaching File Case 114

51-year-old female with reduced blood pressure in the left arm

Category: Angiography

Findings

Volume-rendered and maximum intensity projection images demonstrate a 99% stenosis of the proximal left subclavian artery, with patency of the more distal subclavian artery and the left vertebral artery apparent. In addition, there is an apparent stenosis in the right subclavian artery, at the point where the subclavian vein crosses the artery. Repeat imaging in the venous phase (last image of the top row) demonstrates no evidence of right subclavian stenosis.

Diagnosis

Left subclavian stenosis, with the anatomic substrate for subclavian steal present.[1, 2] In this syndrome, a stenosis or occlusion of the subclavian artery proximal to the vertebral artery results in reversed flow in the vertebral artery in order to supply the affected arm.

Pseudostenosis of the right subclavian artery is evident, related to inflow artifact from undiluted gadolinium entering from the right subclavian venous injection.[3]

The pseudostenosis appearance produced by injection of the veins of the affected arm is a well-recognized pitfall, and its nature can be clarified by repeat imaging in the venous phase. This pitfall results from susceptibility effects induced by the passage of undiluted gadolinium through the subclavian vein closely adjacent to the imaged artery. Images obtained in the venous phase demonstrate that the dense contrast has washed out of the vein, leaving only dilute contrast, and the susceptibility effects are no longer present.

References

1. Van Grimberge F, et al. Role of magnetic resonance in the diagnosis of subclavian steal syndrome. J Magn Reson Imaging. 2000;12(2):339–342.
2. Gosselin C, Walker PM. Subclavian steal syndrome: existence, clinical features, diagnosis and management. Semin Vasc Surg. 1996;9(2):93–97.
3. Bitar R, et al. MR angiography of subclavian steal syndrome: pitfalls and solutions. AJR Am J Roentgenol. 2004;183(6):1840–1841.

Teaching File Case 115

62-year-old female with mitral regurgitation

Category: Cardiomyopathy

Findings

The left ventricular cavity size is normal. The posterior wall thickness is normal, but focal asymmetric thickening of the septum is noted, to a diameter approaching 2 cm. The septum demonstrates minimally diminished thickening.

The right ventricular size and function are normal.

Evaluation of the valvular structures demonstrates mild to moderate mitral regurgitation. Mild tricuspid regurgitation is evident.

There is partial fusion of the left and the noncoronary cusps of the aortic valve, which results in mild aortic stenosis, with an estimated pressure gradient of 12 mmHg based on a peak velocity of 160 cm/sec. The aortic valve area by planimetry measures 2.1 sq cm.

Delayed-enhancement images demonstrate irregular midwall enhancement in the region of abnormal antero-septal thickening at the basal level. In addition, a small area of subendocardial infarction is noted in the anterior and inferior septum from the mid-ventricular level to the apex.

Diagnosis

The asymmetric septal hypertrophy is consistent with hypertrophic cardiomyopathy. The abnormal enhancement seen in the septal insertion site and in the area of abnormal thickening is commonly seen in this disorder.[1]

Superimposed on this pattern is a pattern of subendocardial infarction, from the mid-ventricular level to the apex involving the septum.

Hypertrophic cardiomyopathy is the most common genetically transmitted cardiac disorder. It may result in concentric left ventricular hypertrophy, but asymmetric septal hypertrophy is actually more common. The septal hypertrophy, when extensive, can result in outflow tract obstruction.[2] In addition, systolic anterior motion of the mitral valve is often associated, and may contribute to the dynamic left ventricular outflow tract obstruction.

The apical variant of hypertrophic cardiomyopathy is uncommon in the United States, but is commonly seen in the Far East. It accounts for approximately 10% of cases in the United States.[3]

Patients with hypertrophic cardiomyopathy are noted to be at increased risk for ischemic events, given their abnormal perfusion parameters, and increased myocardial mass.[4] Thus, this patient demonstrates a mixture of non-ischemic and ischemic patterns.

Although the patient has significant asymmetric septal hypertrophy, no systolic anterior motion of the mitral valve is seen. The mitral regurgitation noted was mild to moderate by visual assessment. If precise quantification is needed, through-plane flow studies with velocity-encoded sequences can be obtained. Alternatively, flow through the aortic valve can be measured and compared with the stroke volume as determined from tracing the endocardial contours in diastole and systole. The regurgitant volume is the difference between the LV stroke volume and the flow through the aortic valve. An alternative method to calculate the regurgitant volume would be to compare the antegrade flow through the mitral valve with the flow through the aortic valve; the difference represents the mitral regurgitant volume.

References

1. Soler R, et al. Magnetic resonance imaging of delayed-enhancement in hypertrophic cardiomyopathy: relationship with left ventricular perfusion and contractile function. J Comput Assist Tomogr. 2006;30(3):412–420.

2. Amano Y, et al. Delayed hyper-enhancement of myocardium in hypertrophic cardiomyopathy with asymmetrical septal hypertrophy: comparison with global and regional cardiac MR imaging appearances. J Magn Reson Imaging. 2004;20(4):595–600.
3. Moon, J.C., et al. Detection of apical hypertrophic cardiomyopathy by cardiovascular magnetic resonance in patients with non-diagnostic echocardiography. Heart. 2004;90(6):645–649.
4. Matsunaka T, et al. First-pass myocardial perfusion defect and delayed contrast enhancement in hypertrophic cardiomyopathy assessed with MRI. Magn Reson Med Sci. 2003;2(2):61–69.

Teaching File Case 116

25-year-old male with recent chest pain

Category: Cardiomyopathy

Findings

The left ventricular size is normal. The wall thickness is normal at the basal level, but increased thickness of the anterior wall at the mid and apical levels is noted. Impaired contractility of these same segments is apparent as well.

T2-weighted images are demonstrated in the second row, with the far left and far right images representing T2-weighted 2-chamber views. Short-axis views are noted in the remainder of this row of images. These demonstrate that beginning at the mid-ventricular level and extending to the apex, abnormal high signal is noted that is almost completely transmural in most regions. A small focal area of relative sparing of the apex is evident.

The 2-chamber cine views confirm abnormal contractility of the anterior wall with focal dyskinesia noted at the apex. A small focus of involvement of the inferior wall in the apical region is noted. The second through fourth images of the third row are post-contrast cines and demonstrate contrast enhancement of the affected regions.

The right ventricular size and function appear normal. No definite involvement of the right ventricle is seen.

Delayed-enhancement images obtained after the administration of contrast demonstrate abnormal enhancement of the anterior wall in the same segments that demonstrate abnormal thickness at rest. The involvement is predominantly epicardial, although nearly transmural in the apical region. Some sparing of subendocardial portions of the myocardium is noted. The overall pattern is not consistent with coronary artery disease.

Diagnosis

Myocarditis.

The patient initially underwent cardiac catheterization which demonstrated normal coronary arteries. Subsequently MRI was performed, and demonstrated the findings described. The pattern noted is not consistent with coronary artery disease, and is far more consistent with a focal myocarditis, likely viral in origin.[1]

Although inferolateral left ventricular epicardial involvement is most common, any area of the heart may be involved.[2]

A wide variety of viral agents have been implicated in the development of myocarditis. In particular, parvovirus B 19 and herpes simplex 6 viruses are frequently seen. Enterovirus and Coxsackie virus also can produce myocarditis.

Other etiologies are more common in other portions of the world, with Chagas disease being the most common cause in Central and South America.

MR imaging is probably the best noninvasive means of making the diagnosis of myocarditis. Labeled anti-myosin antibodies are fairly sensitive, but not sufficiently specific, with specificity less than 45%. Endomyocardial biopsy is problematic in that that sampling errors are known to occur. MR can direct the performance of biopsy with high accuracy, however.

When performing MR imaging, a combination of T2 and delayed-enhancement imaging is most helpful, as the combined sensitivity in the detection of myocarditis exceeds the sensitivity of either type of sequence alone.[3, 4]

References

1. Laissy JP, et al. Differentiating acute myocardial infarction from myocarditis: diagnostic value of early- and delayed-perfusion cardiac MR imaging. Radiology. 2005;237(1):75–82.
2. Mahrholdt H, et al. Cardiovascular magnetic resonance assessment of human myocarditis: a comparison to histology and molecular pathology. Circulation. 2004;109(10):1250–1258.
3. Abdel-Aty H, et al. Diagnostic performance of cardiovascular magnetic resonance in patients with suspected acute myocarditis: comparison of different approaches. J Am Coll Cardiol. 2005;45(11): 1815–1822.
4. Laissy JP, et al. MRI of acute myocarditis: a comprehensive approach based on various imaging sequences. Chest. 2002;122(5):1638–1648.

Teaching File Case 117

17-year-old male status–post stab wound to the heart

Category: Pericardium

History

Abundant hemopericardium was noted at surgery. The study is requested to evaluate for residual pericardial abnormality.

Findings

Evaluation of the wall motion demonstrates that the left ventricular cavity size is normal, as is the right ventricular cavity size. No regional wall motion abnormality is seen. However, abnormal anterior movement of the entire heart toward the chest wall is noted during systol.

The second row of images demonstrates abnormal diastolic movement of the septum from right-to-left in early diastole. This is most apparent on the second through the fifth images of the second row.

The short-axis views also demonstrate abnormal signal material within the pericardium, and the visceral and parietal layers of the pericardium appear fused over the anterior cardiac margin.

The images seen in the third row are real-time cine images. The first set is obtained with the patient initially breathing with quiet respiration. The second image of the third row demonstrates the patient coughing, and then taking in a deep inspiration, resulting in marked displacement of the septum from right-to-left. This finding is confirmed on multiple subsequent images obtained with deep inspiration as well.

Delayed-enhancement images demonstrate no significant myocardial injury. However, abnormal signal is noted within the pericardial sac, consistent with thrombus. This can be seen in the second image of the second row as a small area of diminished signal superior to the right ventricle within the pericardium.

Diagnosis

This represents a case of pericardial constriction, produced by intrapericardial hemorrhage with subsequent fibrosis. Some residual thrombus is noted as described above.

The paradoxical septal motion noted in early diastole is sometimes referred to as a shivering septum, or a septal bounce. This finding is seen in approximately 85% in cases of pericardial constriction. It implies abnormal filling dynamics of the right ventricle.

Real-time imaging with the patient instructed to take a deep inspiration has been reported to be helpful in the differentiation between constrictive pericarditis and restrictive cardiomyopathy. In cases of pericardial constriction, septal displacement from right-to-left is noted, or the septum may be excessively straightened. No septal displacement is noted in restrictive disorders.[1–3]

References

1. Wang ZJ, et al. CT and MR imaging of pericardial disease. Radiographics. 2003;23(Spec No):S167–S80.
2. Francone M, et al. Real-time cine MRI of ventricular septal motion: a novel approach to assess ventricular coupling. J Magn Reson Imaging. 2005;21(3):305–309.
3. Giorgi B, et al. Clinically suspected constrictive pericarditis: MR imaging assessment of ventricular septal motion and configuration in patients and healthy subjects. Radiology. 2003;228(2):417–424.

Teaching File Case 118

62-year-old male with hypertension and a prior echocardiogram showing diminished ejection fraction

Category: Stress test

History

The study is performed to evaluate for possible ischemic disease.

Findings

The anterior wall is thinned from the basal level to the apex. In addition, it demonstrates impaired contraction, and essentially is akinetic or minimally dyskinetic in the mid-ventricular level. The 2-chamber view in the fourth row demonstrates the abnormality of the anterior wall very well. In addition, the inferior wall at the apical level also demonstrates thinning and dyskinesia.

The right ventricle is normal in size and function.

Evaluation of the valvular structures demonstrates mild mitral regurgitation. Trace tricuspid regurgitation is also apparent. Mild turbulent flow is seen through the aortic valve, but no true stenosis is present.

Stress and rest perfusion images are seen in the second and third rows, and demonstrate a large area of inducible ischemia in the anterior wall seen in the second row of images that has a more normal appearance on the resting images in the third row.

Delayed-enhancement images demonstrate a subendocardial infarction involving the anteroseptum and anterior wall at the basal and mid-ventricular levels extending to the apex. It comprises less than 25% of the wall thickness however.

Diagnosis

Extensive anterior wall ischemia, with significant residual viability despite markedly impaired function.[1]

Although a subendocardial infarction is noted, the anterior wall is predominantly viable as demonstrated by delayed-enhancement imaging. It likely has become thinned not from significant infarction, but from chronic low-grade ischemia, resulting in myocardial hibernation. However, given that significant viability is demonstrated, the literature would support revascularization with the expectation of a reasonable likelihood of recovery of function.[2, 3]

References

1. Arai AE, Magnetic resonance first-pass myocardial perfusion imaging. Top Magn Reson Imaging. 2000;11(6):383–398.
2. Beek AM, et al. Delayed contrast-enhanced magnetic resonance imaging for the prediction of regional functional improvement after acute myocardial infarction. J Am Coll Cardiol. 2003;42(5):895–901.
3. Choi KM, et al. Transmural extent of acute myocardial infarction predicts long-term improvement in contractile function. Circulation. 2001;104(10):1101–1107.

Teaching File Case 119

64-year-old male with known MI, assess for viability

Category: Viability

Findings

The left ventricular cavity is mildly dilated. Globally reduced systolic function is noted. Evaluation of the regional wall motion demonstrates akinesia of the lateral wall at the basal level involving both the anterior and inferior lateral walls. The anterior wall is noted to be hypokinetic beginning in the mid-ventricular level, and extending to the apex, where dyskinesia is apparent.

The overall left ventricular ejection fraction is approximately 25%.

The right ventricular size and function appear normal.

Evaluation of the valvular structures demonstrates that no mitral regurgitation is seen. Mild aortic stenosis is apparent, with mild aortic insufficiency noted as well. No significant tricuspid regurgitation is seen.

Delayed-enhancement images show a transmural infarction of the anterior lateral wall at the basal level, with less extensive involvement of the inferolateral basal wall. The infarction becomes less transmural proceeding toward the apex. A dark central area within the region of hyperenhancement is noted, representing a no-reflow zone within this lateral wall infarction at the basal level.

Subendocardial infarction is noted in the anterior wall, beginning at the mid-ventricular level and extending to the apex. The infarction is approximately 50% transmural at the mid-ventricular level, but becomes greater than 75% transmural at the apex. The inferior wall is viable throughout, as is the inferior septum in the basal and mid-ventricular levels.

Diagnosis

Transmural basal lateral wall infarction with no-reflow zone evident.[1–3]

The no-reflow zone is evident on delayed-enhancement images as a dark central focus within the hyperenhanced infarct. It is thought to represent the necrotic, poorly perfused central core of an infarction.

Transmural infarction is noted in the lateral wall of the basal segment, involving both the anterior lateral and inferior lateral segments. The presence of a no-reflow zone implies that this finding is likely acute. Anterior wall infarction is noted, and is approximately 25 to 50% in transmural thickness in the majority of segments, although at the apical level it becomes greater than 75% transmural. Overall, there is likely some preserved viability in the anterior wall in the mid ventricle and portions of the apical segments.

The presence of microvascular obstruction as typified by the presence of a no-reflow zone is strongly associated with adverse outcomes in the setting of myocardial infarction.[4, 5] Specifically, adverse remodeling, impaired systolic function, and an increased incidence of cardiac death are associated with this finding. Serial imaging studies have shown that this finding may be noted in acute myocardial infarctions, but gradually becomes less apparent over time, and usually is no longer seen by 6–8 weeks post-infarction.

The microvascular impairment sometimes evident in areas of prior infarction on first-pass perfusion imaging may persist, however.[6]

References

1. Rezkalla SH, Kloner RA. Coronary No-reflow Phenomenon. Curr Treat Options Cardiovasc Med. 2005;7(1):75–80.
2. Reffelmann T, Kloner RA. The “no-reflow” phenomenon: basic science and clinical correlates. Heart. 2002;87(2):162–168.
3. Reffelmann T, et al. Relationship between no-reflow and infarct size as influenced by the duration of ischemia and reperfusion. Am J Physiol Heart Circ Physiol. 2002;282(2):H766–H772.
4. Wu KC, et al. Prognostic significance of microvascular obstruction by magnetic resonance imaging in patients with acute myocardial infarction. Circulation. 1998;97(8):765–772.
5. Wu KC, et al. Quantification and time course of microvascular obstruction by contrast-enhanced echocardiography and magnetic resonance imaging following acute myocardial infarction and reperfusion. J Am Coll Cardiol. 1998;32(6):1756–1764.
6. Arai AE, Magnetic resonance first-pass myocardial perfusion imaging. Top Magn Reson Imaging. 2000;11(6):383–398.

Teaching File Case 120

25-year-old patient with end-stage renal disease on dialysis, now with Gram-positive bacteremia

Category: Mass

Findings

The left ventricular cavity is mildly dilated, and the left ventricular wall thickness is at the upper limits of normal measuring 1.2 cm. Mild generalized hypokinesia is noted, with reduced systolic ejection fraction. The LVEF was measured at 40%.

The right ventricle demonstrates normal size and function.

Evaluation of valvular structures demonstrates that the mitral valve is normal in appearance. The aortic valve is trileaflet, and normal in appearance as well. Mild tricuspid regurgitation is noted, with no evidence of regurgitation seen. The pulmonic valve is imaged on the short-axis views and appears unremarkable as well.

Images through the superior vena cava (far right image of the second row) demonstrate extensive thrombus that appears to be adherent to a catheter which is noted to extend up into the right internal jugular vein. The thrombus is quite bulky in its inferior portion, measuring over 1.5 cm in diameter.

Delayed-enhancement imaging shows no focal enhancement to suggest the presence of scar.

Diagnosis

A large pericatheter thrombus is noted, extending from the level of the internal jugular vein into the superior vena cava.

Long-term central venous catheters frequently develop adherent thrombus,[1–3] although the volume of thrombus in this case appears to be greater than usual. The presence of bacteremia indicated the likely presence of infection, and this catheter was subsequently removed and proven on cultures to be infected.

Interestingly, no definite evidence of septic pulmonary embolism was seen on this study. No valvular vegetations were seen.

References

1. Negulescu O, et al. Large atrial thrombus formation associated with tunneled cuffed hemodialysis catheters. Clin Nephrol. 2003;59(1):40–46.
2. Kingdon EJ, et al. Atrial thrombus and central venous dialysis catheters. Am J Kidney Dis. 2001;38(3):631–639.
3. Mark PB, Wan RK. Infected right atrial thrombus associated with a tunneled hemodialysis catheter. Kidney Int. 2006;69(9):1489.

Teaching File Case 121

66-year-old male with fatigability and increasing heart failure

Category: Cardiomyopathy

Findings

A dilated cardiomyopathy is noted, with marked enlargement of the left ventricular cavity, and preservation of wall thickness. No focal thinning is seen. The overall left ventricular mass is significantly increased. The left ventricular ejection fraction is less than 15%.

The right ventricle is dilated as well. Its function also appears significantly reduced.

Mild mitral regurgitation is noted. Mild tricuspid regurgitation is seen as well.

Delayed-enhancement images demonstrate extensive midwall enhancement involving the septum from the base to the mid-ventricular level. No subendocardial involvement is seen.

Note the dark-band artifact seen extending across the apex in multiple views in the second row.

Diagnosis

Non-ischemic cardiomyopathy.

The pattern of enhancement noted is characteristic of dilated non-ischemic cardiomyopathy. The midwall enhancement pattern described may also occasionally be seen with myocarditis, but the distinction can usually be made on the basis of history, as patients with myocarditis typically present with chest pain, and may have enzyme abnormalities as well. Chronic myocarditis may in fact represent a precursor event to the development of non-ischemic dilated cardiomyopathy.

Most patients with dilated non-ischemic cardiomyopathy do not demonstrate enhancement on delayed-enhancement imaging.[1, 2] In one series, with cardiac catheterization correlation, approximately 60% of patients with dilated non-ischemic cardiomyopathy showed no evidence of delayed-enhancement. Of the 40% who demonstrated hyperenhancement, 2/3 demonstrated the pattern evident in this case, with midwall enhancement noted, a pattern clearly distinguishable from subendocardial enhancement seen with coronary artery disease. In approximately 13% of patients, a pattern with subendocardial enhancement indistinguishable from that seen with coronary artery disease was noted. The authors of that study speculated that the enhancement observed represented occasions of true coronary artery obstruction resulting in infarction with subsequent recanalization.[1]

In addition to defining the etiology of heart failure, MR imaging is the best modality for serial evaluations of cardiac function. It has superior interobserver and intraobserver variability compared with echo, and studies have shown that this allows significant (up to 10 fold) reduction in sample sizes for studies designed to detect small changes in LVEF.[3–5]

The dark-band artifact noted is characteristic of the SSFP sequence. It can be shifted in position by re-shimming the magnet, and it can be minimized by having a very homogenous magnetic field, and by using a high bandwidth and very low TE/TR.

References

1. McCrohon JA, et al. Differentiation of heart failure related to dilated cardiomyopathy and coronary artery disease using gadolinium-enhanced cardiovascular magnetic resonance. Circulation. 2003;108(1): 54–59.
2. Soriano CJ, et al. Noninvasive diagnosis of coronary artery disease in patients with heart failure and systolic dysfunction of uncertain etiology, using late gadolinium-enhanced cardiovascular magnetic resonance. J Am Coll Cardiol. 2005;45(5):743–748.

3. Bellenger NG, et al. Reduction in sample size for studies of remodeling in heart failure by the use of cardiovascular magnetic resonance. J Cardiovasc Magn Reson. 2000;2(4):271–278.
4. Bellenger NG, et al. Comparison of left ventricular ejection fraction and volumes in heart failure by echocardiography, radionuclide ventriculography and cardiovascular magnetic resonance; are they interchangeable? Eur Heart J. 2000;21(16):1387–1396.
5. Bellenger NG, et al. Quantification of right and left ventricular function by cardiovascular magnetic resonance. Herz. 2000;25(4):392–399.

Teaching File Case 122

65-year-old female status–post repair of a bicuspid aortic valve

Category: Angiography

History

She subsequently underwent surgical repair of a type A dissection, with placement of an "elephant trunk" graft.

Findings

MR angiographic images of the abdomen were obtained first, followed by MR angiographic imaging of the aorta. The sequences were performed in this order so that dense contrast would not be present within the kidneys and renal venous structures from prior thoracic imaging. The thoracic images are obtained after a 10-minute delay, in order to allow washout of the contrast, and subtraction is used to minimize the impact of residual intravascular contrast.

The study demonstrates clearly the presence of a dissection of the thoracic aorta, with communication between the true and false lumen noted just distal to the subclavian artery. This is well depicted on the volume rendered images, the first two images of the top row. Review of the axial source images provides depiction of the filling of branch vessels.

The dissection continues into the abdomen, as can be seen on the abdominal series of images. The first two images of the third row are obtained immediately following the injection contrast, at which time only the true lumen is filled. The third image of the third row is obtained with a short delay, and allows visualization of the false lumen as well. The fourth image of the third row is obtained after that same delay, while the fifth image is obtained in the early arterial phase and demonstrates only the true lumen.

The celiac axis, superior mesenteric artery, and left renal artery are all noted to originate from the true lumen. The right renal artery is noted to originate from the false lumen, and supplies a markedly atrophic right kidney. This is likely on the basis of diminished perfusion via the false lumen. The dissection is noted to continue into the right common iliac artery, and the proximal portion of the right external iliac artery. The left common iliac artery shows no evidence of dissection

Evaluation of the cardiac images demonstrates the presence of a prosthetic aortic valve. Velocity-encoded images demonstrate that no significant gradient is present, and are only minimally degraded by susceptibility artifact induced by the metallic stent annulus. No significant valvular insufficiency is seen.

Diagnosis

Aortic dissection extending from the descending thoracic aorta throughout the abdomen and into the right iliac arterial system.

When visualization of the aorta from the level of the arch down through the bifurcation and into the iliac arteries is desired, and the patient is larger than the field-of-view allowed by the scanner, 2 injections of contrast are required. Although a single bolus might be attempted, with stepping of the table between stations, the complexities of timing and the likelihood of impaired image quality usually mandate that two injections be performed in a sequential fashion.

Imaging of the abdomen was performed first, as the abdominal organs tend to retain contrast for a prolonged period of time, which would likely impair visualization of some of the arterial structures. Imaging of the chest was then performed second, and subtraction techniques used to minimize the effects of residual intravascular contrast.

The prosthetic aortic valve present produces minimal artifact, and does not significantly impair the analysis of its function.

Dissections are most commonly associated with long-standing hypertension, but also occur at an increased rate in patients with Marfan syndrome, Ehlers-Danlos syndrome, and in patients with bicuspid aortic valves.[1–4]

References

1. Braverman AC, et al. The bicuspid aortic valve. Curr Probl Cardiol. 2005;30(9):470–522.
2. Zalzstein E, et al. Aortic dissection in children and young adults: diagnosis, patients at risk, and outcomes. Cardiol Young. 2003;13(4):341–344.
3. Milano AD, et al. Fate of coronary ostial anastomoses after the modified Bentall procedure. Ann Thorac Surg. 2003;75(6):1797–801; discussion 1802.
4. Parai JL, et al. Aortic medial changes associated with bicuspid aortic valve: myth or reality? Can J Cardiol. 1999;15(11):1233–1238.

Teaching File Case 123

22-year-old female with a mildly enlarged right ventricle noted on echocardiography

Category: Congenital

History

Evaluate the first 3 rows before looking further.

Findings

The first row of images is a series of short-axis views obtained from the mid-ventricular level to the apex. The second row of images was also obtained in the short-axis plane, but they proceed from the mid-ventricular level to the base of the heart and into the atria. The third row of images begins with four 4-chamber views obtained sequentially from the bottom of the heart to the level of the aortic valve. The two far right-sided images of the third row are morphologic images through the chest.

The study demonstrates that the left ventricle is normal in overall size and function. The right ventricle appears to be mildly enlarged, with normal function. No abnormal outpouching of the right ventricular free wall to suggest the presence of ARVD is seen. No evidence of severe tricuspid regurgitation is noted to explain the right ventricular dilatation. No atrial septal defect is seen on these images through the interatrial septum in two planes.

Evaluation of the morphologic images through the chest demonstrates that the left upper and lower lobe pulmonary veins are clearly seen entering the left atrium, as is the right lower lobe pulmonary vein. The right upper lobe pulmonary vein appears to enter the posterolateral margin of the superior vena cava as does the right middle lobe vein.

In the fourth row, third image, a slice is then obtained in the coronal plane at the point where the anomalous pulmonary veins join the superior vena cava. The fourth image of this row demonstrates an axial image showing the anomalous vein connecting to the SVC with flow seen to extend from the pulmonary vein into the superior vena cava.

The fifth and sixth images of the fourth row represent perfusion sequences during the dynamic administration of contrast material. These demonstrate abnormal anomalous connection of the right upper lobe (RUL) pulmonary vein to the superior vena cava, as well as absence of a normal appearing RUL pulmonary vein attaching to the left atrium.

Angiographic images in the bottom row clearly demonstrate the absence of the insertion of the right upper lobe pulmonary vein onto the left atrium on images viewed from the posterior aspect of the left atrium. The rotating images obtained with volumetric display demonstrate the anomalous pulmonary venous connection.

Flow studies obtained through the pulmonic and aortic valves indicated a Qp/Qs ratio of 1.4/1.

Diagnosis

Partial anomalous pulmonary venous return of the right middle and right upper lobe pulmonary veins to the superior vena cava.

The differential diagnosis of right ventricular enlargement would include pulmonic insufficiency, tricuspid insufficiency, Ebstein's anomaly, and ARVD as well as a shunt lesion. Of the possible shunt lesions, an ASD or partial anomalous pulmonary venous return would be the prime considerations.

Partial anomalous pulmonary venous return is frequently associated with a sinus venosus type ASD, but such was not found in the present case. Partial anomalous pulmonary venous return most commonly involves the right upper lobe pulmonary vein, as seen in this example.

Note that given the differential diagnoses described above, MR imaging can provide a rapid and unequivocal diagnosis, without requiring additional imaging.[1, 2] Valvular lesions, primary cardiomyopathy of the right ventricle, and anomalous venous return as well as ASD lesions can be well depicted with MR imaging in a single exam. In addition, the Qp/Qs ratio can be obtained noninvasively, in order to quantify any shunt present.[3]

References

1. Prasad SK, et al. Role of magnetic resonance angiography in the diagnosis of major aortopulmonary collateral arteries and partial anomalous pulmonary venous drainage. Circulation. 2004;109(2):207–214.
2. Ferrari VA, et al. Ultrafast three-dimensional contrast-enhanced magnetic resonance angiography and imaging in the diagnosis of partial anomalous pulmonary venous drainage. J Am Coll Cardiol. 2001;37(4):1120–1128.
3. Wang ZJ, et al. Cardiovascular shunts: MR imaging evaluation. Radiographics. 2003;23(Spec No):S181–S194.

Teaching File Case 124

50-year-old male with recurrent arrhythmias

Category: Cardiomyopathy

Findings

The left ventricular size and function are normal. However, the right ventricle is mildly enlarged, and demonstrates areas of focal dyskinesia, with microaneurysm formation noted on the short-axis views involving the right ventricular anterior wall. Abnormal heavy trabeculation is seen involving the apical portion of the right ventricle as well. The right ventricular systolic function is depressed.

The pulmonic valve is noted to be normal in appearance as is the aortic valve. Trace mitral and tricuspid regurgitation is apparent.

Delayed-enhancement images demonstrate extensive enhancement of the right ventricular free wall, from the base to near the apical levels. No abnormal left ventricular enhancement is seen.

Diagnosis

This represents a case of arrhythmogenic right ventricular dysplasia (ARVD).

This is an uncommon cardiomyopathy characterized by thinning of the right ventricle, fibrofatty infiltration of the right ventricle, and depressed right ventricular systolic function. This has a familial basis in many cases, often with an autosomal dominant inheritance pattern.

The diagnosis is based on a combination of clinical, ECG, and imaging criteria developed by a task force on ARVD.[1] Imaging findings included enlargement of the right ventricle with impairment of systolic function as is seen in this case.[2] Abnormal trabeculation is often seen as well. Cine imaging demonstrating systolic dysfunction with microaneurysm formation is very helpful.

Fatty infiltration was formerly often sought as part of the imaging diagnosis of this disorder, but recent studies have indicated that many normal individuals will have a small amount of epicardial fat present along the right ventricular surface, and over-diagnosis of ARVD can occur based on this imaging criterion alone.[3]

Abnormal right ventricular delayed-enhancement may prove to be a more robust diagnostic criterion, as it is infrequently seen with other disorders. In a small series reported previously, approximately two-thirds of patients with this disorder demonstrated abnormalities of delayed-enhancement imaging with abnormal right ventricular enhancement apparent. In addition, the abnormal enhancement correlated with the likelihood of inducible arrhythmia.[4]

References

1. Kayser HW, et al. Diagnosis of arrhythmogenic right ventricular dysplasia: a review. Radiographics. 2002;22(3):639–648; discussion 649–650.
2. Bluemke DA, et al. MR Imaging of arrhythmogenic right ventricular cardiomyopathy: morphologic findings and interobserver reliability. Cardiology. 2003;99(3): 153–162.
3. Bomma C, et al. Misdiagnosis of arrhythmogenic right ventricular dysplasia/cardiomyopathy. J Cardiovasc Electrophysiol. 2004;15(3):300–306.
4. Tandri H, et al. Noninvasive detection of myocardial fibrosis in arrhythmogenic right ventricular cardiomyopathy using delayed-enhancement magnetic resonance imaging. J Am Coll Cardiol. 2005;45(1):98–103.

Teaching File Case 125

67-year-old male referred for evaluation of a right atrial mass noted on echocardiography

Category: Mass

Findings

The overall left ventricular wall thickness is at the upper limits of normal, with focal thinning noted along the inferior wall at the mid-ventricular level. Mild hypokinesia is noted in this region as well.

The right ventricle is normal in size and function. An inter-atrial septal aneurysm is noted on the cine images.

The most remarkable abnormality is the presence of a rounded mass noted along the lateral margin of the right atrium. The lesion has soft tissue signal intensity along its periphery, with a central area of apparent high signal. Perfusion images noted as the third and fourth images of the third row demonstrate apparent enhancement of the central focus, but not of the peripheral rim. The coronal and axial VIBE images seen as the fifth and sixth images of the third row demonstrate a long segment tubular area of enhancement with surrounding low attenuation material. This is consistent with aneurysmal dilatation of a saphenous vein graft originating along the right anterior margin of the aorta and extending along the lateral wall of the right atrium to anastomose with the posterior descending coronary artery at the base of the heart.

Delayed-enhancement images demonstrate an area of prior infarction involving the inferior wall.

Diagnosis

Fusiform aneurysmal dilatation of a saphenous vein bypass graft, with extensive mural thrombus noted in multiple locations. This results in a mass-like appearance, with indentation of the right lateral atrial wall. Extensive mural thrombus is an associated finding, and can serve as a source of embolic material.

In this instance, the diagnosis, which was not apparent on echo, was easily resolved with cardiac MR imaging. The perfusion images demonstrate enhancement in the arterial phase, coincident with aortic opacification, indicating the vascular nature of the finding. Three-dimensional imaging provided by the VIBE sequence provided a definitive diagnosis.

Similar to aneurysms occurring in the native coronary arteries, aneurysms originating in saphenous vein bypass grafts may serve as a source of embolic material, and may become occluded.[1] Occasionally, they may rupture or develop fistulous connections to the cardiac chambers.[2] As in the present case, they also may cause mass-effect upon adjacent structures.[3, 4] Surgical repair is often advised, although a clear-cut benefit is difficult to discern from a review of the literature.[5]

References

1. Almanaseer Y, et al. Severe dilatation of saphenous vein grafts: a late complication of coronary surgery in which the diagnosis is suggested by chest x-ray. Cardiology. 2005;104(3):150–155.
2. Davey P, Gwilt D, Forfar C. Spontaneous rupture of a saphenous vein graft. Postgrad Med J. 1999; 75(884):363–364.
3. Abrishamchian AR, Gowdamarajan A, Michler RE. Saphenous vein graft aneurysm: potential for mistaken identity. J Card Surg. 2002;17(4):295–297.
4. Carasso S, et al. A large saphenous vein graft aneurysm presenting as a right atrial mass: a case report. Echocardiography. 2006;23(6):499–502.
5. Dieter RS, et al. Conservative vs. invasive treatment of aortocoronary saphenous vein graft aneurysms: Treatment algorithm based upon a large series. Cardiovasc Surg. 2003;11(6):507–513.

Teaching File Case 126

Intermittent abdominal pain

Category: Angiography

Findings

MR angiographic images demonstrate occlusion of the celiac axis at its origin, with reconstitution via collaterals through the pancreaticoduodenal arcade from the SMA. The SMA is widely patent as are both renal arteries. The inferior mesenteric artery is widely patent, as best seen on the appropriately windowed images.

Diagnosis

Occlusion of the celiac axis is noted. The SMA and IMA are patent.

However, the patient does not have the anatomic substrate for mesenteric ischemia. In this condition, stenoses or occlusions of two of the three vessels supplying the GI tract (the celiac axis, SMA, and IMA) result in ischemia of the bowel, usually induced by meals. Avoidance of food may result in profound weight loss. Surgical treatment has historically been advised, with bypass grafting performed. However, endovascular approaches are being investigated.[1–3]

MR angiography can clearly display the origins as well as the collateral supply of the main visceral vessels, limiting catheter angiographic approaches to situations requiring intervention.[4]

References

1. Silva JA, et al. Endovascular therapy for chronic mesenteric ischemia. J Am Coll Cardiol. 2006;47(5):944–950.
2. Landis MS, et al. Percutaneous management of chronic mesenteric ischemia: outcomes after intervention. J Vasc Interv Radiol. 2005;16(10):1319–1325.
3. Razavi M, Chung HH. Endovascular management of chronic mesenteric ischemia. Tech Vasc Interv Radiol. 2004;7(3):155–159.
4. Laissy JP, Trillaud H, Douek P. MR angiography: noninvasive vascular imaging of the abdomen. Abdom Imaging. 2002;27(5):488–506.

Teaching File Case 127

58-year-old male with a history of colon cancer and abnormal PET/CT study

Category: Mass

Findings

Short and long axis views demonstrate that the left ventricle is normal in size and function. The mitral and aortic valves are unremarkable.

Evaluation of the right ventricle demonstrates a filling defect near the right ventricular apex, best appreciated on the 4-chamber view (third image, second row), but also evident on the short-axis views (first and second images, second row).

Small field-of-view cine images are obtained, in both the 2-chamber and 4-chamber views, and are seen in the third row. Clicking on these images will enlarge them, and will better demonstrate the intracavitary lesion in the right ventricular apex.

Delayed-enhancement images demonstrate extensive hyperenhancement of the intracavitary lesion, again best appreciated on the 4-chamber view of the delayed-enhancement images.

Diagnosis

Metastatic deposit in the right ventricular apex.

MR imaging has become the preferred means of evaluating cardiac masses for several reasons. It has superior tissue contrast resolution relative to either CT or echocardiography. In addition, it has the capacity for unrestricted imaging, without limitation by acoustic windows or scan plane.[1–3] The multisequence, multiplanar capacity of MR makes it a clearly superior technique. In addition, new techniques involving delayed-enhancement imaging allow improved evaluation and differentiation of masses from thrombi.

The differential diagnosis of an intracavitary lesion would include a myxoma, but these are exceedingly uncommon in the ventricles, accounting for less than 5% of myxoma cases.[4] In addition, the right ventricle would be the least common location for this entity.

Thrombus would be a consideration in the differential diagnosis, but the signal characteristics are not consistent with this diagnosis. Thrombus would be expected to be homogenously dark in signal on delayed-enhancement images obtained with a long inversion time.

Metastatic lesions are usually intramural or epicardial in location, although they may be endocardial. Metastatic lesions are estimated to be 40 times more common than primary cardiac tumors.

In this instance, the patient had a PET/CT scan that demonstrated a suspicious abnormality projected over the right ventricle. The MR was confirmatory of this abnormality, and excluded thrombus.[5]

References

1. Restrepo CS, et al. CT and MR imaging findings of malignant cardiac tumors. Curr Probl Diagn Radiol. 2005;34(1):1–11.
2. Luna A, et al. Evaluation of cardiac tumors with magnetic resonance imaging. Eur Radiol. 2005;15(7):1446–1455.
3. Hoffmann U, et al. Usefulness of magnetic resonance imaging of cardiac and paracardiac masses. Am J Cardiol. 2003;92(7):890–895.
4. Alter P, et al. Right ventricular cardiac myxoma. Diagnostic usefulness of cardiac magnetic resonance imaging. Herz. 2005;30(7):663–667.
5. Plutchok JJ, et al. Differentiation of cardiac tumor from thrombus by combined MRI and F-18 FDG PET imaging. Clin Nucl Med. 1998;23(5):324–325.

Teaching File Case 128

58-year-old male status–post prior myocardial infarction and prior coronary artery bypass grafting

Category: Viability

History

Recent cardiac catheterization suggests significant RCA territory disease. The patient is under consideration for possible intervention.

Findings

Evidence of prior median sternotomy is seen, with sternal wires noted.

The left ventricular cavity is mildly dilated to a diameter of approximately 6 cm. Reduced global systolic function is apparent, with extensive regional wall abnormality noted involving the lateral wall from the base to nearly the apical levels, associated with thinning of the lateral wall at the basal and mid-ventricular levels. The left ventricular ejection fraction is measured at 41%. Mild hypokinesia of the inferior wall at the mid-ventricular level is noted. Otherwise the inferior and septal walls demonstrate normal thickening throughout.

The right ventricle is normal in size and function.

Evaluation of the valvular structures demonstrates mild mitral regurgitation. Mitral valve morphology is unremarkable. Aortic valve is trileaflet and normal in appearance. The tricuspid valve shows no significant regurgitation.

Delayed-enhancement imaging demonstrates extensive scar in the anterolateral and inferolateral walls at the basal and mid-ventricular levels, which is transmural at the mid-ventricular level, and involves 25 to 50% of the lateral wall at the apical level.

The anterolateral wall demonstrates greater than 75% transmural enhancement in the mid-ventricular level, but less extensive transmurality is noted in the basal level.

A tiny focus of hyperenhancement is seen in the inferior wall at the mid-ventricular level. The remainder of the RCA territory is viable.

Diagnosis

Extensive prior infarction in the circumflex artery territory, which is essentially transmural, and therefore unlikely to regain function. However, the inferior wall remains almost completely viable, despite its minimally reduced function as evident on the cine images.[1,2]

There is evidence that indicates that dysfunctional but viable myocardium may benefit from revascularization.[3,4] DE-MR is being increasingly used in the preoperative and preinterventional evaluation of patients with complex reconstructions under consideration, in order to have the most complete preoperative estimate of viability.

References

1. Beek AM, et al. Delayed contrast-enhanced magnetic resonance imaging for the prediction of regional functional improvement after acute myocardial infarction. J Am Coll Cardiol. 2003;42(5):895–901.
2. Kuhl HP, et al. Relation of end-diastolic wall thickness and the residual rim of viable myocardium by magnetic resonance imaging to myocardial viability assessed by fluorine-18 deoxyglucose positron emission tomography. Am J Cardiol. 2006;97(4):452–457.
3. Elliott MD, Kim RJ. Late gadolinium cardiovascular magnetic resonance in the assessment of myocardial viability. Coron Artery Dis. 2005;16(6):365–372.
4. Kim RJ, et al. The use of contrast-enhanced magnetic resonance imaging to identify reversible myocardial dysfunction. N Engl J Med. 2000;343(20):1445–1453.

Teaching File Case 129

71-year-old female in for evaluation of an abnormality noted on echocardiography

Category: Mass

Findings

Short-axis views demonstrate that the left ventricular cavity size and function are normal. The wall thickness is normal as well.

The 4-chamber views seen in the second row demonstrates increased thickness of the interatrial septum, with sparing of the fossa ovalis.

Standard HASTE images are seen in the fifth image of the second row. These confirm the thickening of the interatrial septum.

Perfusion images demonstrate that no hypervascularity is seen. The area of thickening appears high in signal on precontrast heavily T1-weighted images as comprise the perfusion sequence.

Delayed-enhancement images demonstrate no evidence of prior infarction. No thrombus formation is seen.

Diagnosis

Lipomatous hypertrophy of the interatrial septum.

This is not a neoplasm, but rather a hyperplasia of normal fat cells within the interatrial septum. It is most often seen in elderly females, and has increased prevalence among the obese. The disorder is usually asymptomatic, although occasional patients are noted to develop supraventricular tachyarrhythmias.

The lesion is recognized on MR imaging by its characteristic "barbell" appearance, with the thin segment of the barbell representing the fossa ovalis which is spared the lipomatous hypertrophy present throughout the remainder of the interatrial septum.[1]

MR imaging with its capacity for tissue characterization is well-suited for the evaluation of suspected cardiac masses.[2–4] Note that the abnormality is high in signal on the precontrast images of the perfusion sequences (a T1-weighted sequence), consistent with its fatty nature. Fat-suppressed images (not shown) also confirm the fatty nature of the lesion.

References

1. Salanitri JC, Pereles FS. Cardiac lipoma and lipomatous hypertrophy of the interatrial septum: cardiac magnetic resonance imaging findings. J Comput Assist Tomogr. 2004;28(6):852–856.
2. Luna A, et al. Evaluation of cardiac tumors with magnetic resonance imaging. Eur Radiol. 2005;15(7):1446–1455.
3. Restrepo CS, et al. CT and MR imaging findings of benign cardiac tumors. Curr Probl Diagn Radiol. 2005;34(1):12–21.
4. Araoz PA, et al. CT and MR imaging of benign primary cardiac neoplasms with echocardiographic correlation. Radiographics. 2000;20(5):1303–1319.

Teaching File Case 130

72-year-old male with difficult-to-control hypertension

Category: Angiography

Findings

A high-grade stenosis of the proximal left renal artery is noted. There are 2 right renal arteries, with weblike stenosis seen in the proximal portion of the more superior of the 2 right renal arteries. A slightly less severe narrowing is noted at the origin of the more inferior right renal artery.

The celiac axis and superior mesenteric artery are normal in appearance.

Aneurysmal dilatation of the infrarenal abdominal aorta is also noted. Stents are seen in the proximal common iliac arteries bilaterally, resulting in significant artifact.

Morphologic images demonstrate the presence of a large left renal cyst, with smaller cysts noted bilaterally.

Diagnosis

Bilateral renal artery stenoses.

Irregular proximal left renal artery stenosis is noted, and appears to be severe. Duplicated right renal arteries are noted, each demonstrating a moderately severe stenosis.

MR imaging is highly accurate in the detection and characterization of renal artery stenoses. It has significant advantages over nuclear medicine renography,[1] in that bilateral lesions are detected more readily, and any associated vascular pathology such as the aneurysm noted in this case can be easily visualized. In addition, appropriate endovascular approaches can be planned, given that the iliofemoral systems can be imaged at the same setting.[2]

References

1. Qanadli SD, et al. Detection of renal artery stenosis: prospective comparison of captopril-enhanced Doppler sonography, captopril-enhanced scintigraphy, and MR angiography. AJR Am J Roentgenol. 2001;177(5):1123–1129.
2. Hany TF, et al. Evaluation of the aortoiliac and renal arteries: comparison of breath-hold, contrast-enhanced, three-dimensional MR angiography with conventional catheter angiography. Radiology. 1997;204(2):357–362.

Teaching File Case 131

35-year-old female with a history of corrective cardiac surgery in childhood

Category: Congenital

History

In for follow-up evaluation.

Findings

The left ventricle is mildly dilated, and demonstrates thinning of the anterior septum from the basal level to the apex. Dyskinesia of the anterior septum is noted. Thinning of the anterior wall is noted from the basal level to the apex as well. This area is dyskinetic.

The right ventricle is moderately dilated, and demonstrates diminished systolic function. Marked dilatation of the right ventricular outflow tract and proximal pulmonary artery is apparent, with an aneurysmal appearance. No pulmonic valve is evident. To-and-fro motion of the blood pool in the region of the right ventricular outflow tract is seen.

Velocity-encoded images confirm this to-and-fro motion, with free pulmonic regurgitation noted.

Evaluation of the aortic valve demonstrates a thin jet of trace aortic insufficiency on the aortic outflow tract view in the second row. The velocity-encoded images demonstrate that the aortic valve is trileaflet and the degree of insufficiency is minimal.

Delayed-enhancement images are seen in the fourth, fifth, and sixth rows, and demonstrate extensive scar in the anterior septum and anterior wall the left ventricle extending from the basal level to the apex, with ballooning of the apex.

The MR angiographic images are displayed with volume rendering in a variety of projections. These demonstrate marked dilatation of the main pulmonary artery as well as the left pulmonary artery. However, the right pulmonary artery demonstrates a moderately severe stenosis. A right aortic arch is noted, with mirror image branching. A left-sided innominate artery is noted which bifurcates proximally into the left carotid and left subclavian arteries. The next branch is the right carotid artery followed by the right subclavian artery.

Diagnosis

Tetralogy of Fallot, status–post corrective surgery in childhood, with resection of the right ventricular outflow tract obstruction and performance of patch annuloplasty. Aneurysmal dilatation of the right ventricular outflow tract and main pulmonary artery segment are apparent, along with absence of the pulmonic valve with free pulmonic insufficiency.[1, 2]

Marked compromise of the right ventricular function is noted, with moderate decrease in left ventricular function.

Extensive infarction of the anterior septum and anterior wall of the left ventricle is also apparent. This finding suggests possible transection of an anomalous coronary artery at the time of the right ventricular outflow tract reconstruction, with resultant infarction in the left anterior descending coronary artery territory.

A right aortic arch is seen an approximate 25% of patients with Tetralogy of Fallot. It is usually of the mirror image type, as in this case. The other form of right aortic arch is not associated with congenital heart disease, and is characterized by the presence of an aberrant left subclavian artery, which originates as the last branch from the arch.

Coronary artery anomalies are present in approximately 3% of patients with Tetralogy of Fallot, with an aberrant left anterior descending coronary artery originating from the right coronary artery being the most common form. This is a particularly dangerous variant, as the anomalous left anterior descending coronary artery crosses the right ventricular outflow tract in the region of the ventricular reconstruction, and therefore is susceptible to injury.[3–5] It is speculated that such may have occurred in this case.

References

1. Davlouros PA, et al. Right ventricular function in adults with repaired tetralogy of Fallot assessed with cardiovascular magnetic resonance imaging: detrimental role of right ventricular outflow aneurysms or akinesia and adverse right-to-left ventricular interaction. J Am Coll Cardiol. 2002;40(11):2044–2052.
2. Warnes CA, The adult with congenital heart disease: born to be bad? J Am Coll Cardiol. 2005; 46(1):1–8.
3. Ozkara A, et al. Right ventricular outflow tract reconstruction for tetralogy of fallot with abnormal coronary artery: experience with 35 patients. J Card Surg. 2006;21(2):131–136.
4. Backer CL, Tetralogy of fallot with abnormal coronary artery: importance of the "safety zone." J Card Surg. 2006;21(2):137–138.
5. Ruzmetov M, et al. Repair of tetralogy of Fallot with anomalous coronary arteries coursing across the obstructed right ventricular outflow tract. Pediatr Cardiol. 2005;26(5):537–542.

Teaching File Case 132

17-year-old female with known congenital heart disease, with no prior surgery

Category: Congenital

Findings

The short-axis cine views in the top row demonstrate absence of the inferior portion of the atrial septum and the upper portion of the interventricular septum, with a large valve leaflet seen to extend from the left side of the heart to the right side of the heart. The third image of the second row demonstrates this finding quite clearly. A large bridging valvular structure is seen extending from the tricuspid annulus to the mitral annulus. Extensive tricuspid regurgitation is noted.

The ventricles are normally arranged.

The aortic valve appears to be competent. The pulmonary outflow tract appears diminutive. MR angiographic images subsequently obtained are demonstrated in the fifth and sixth images of the third row, and demonstrate extensive right ventricular and main pulmonary artery segment narrowing. Mild branch pulmonary artery stenosis is apparent as well.

Diagnosis

Complete atrioventricular canal.

In this abnormality, there is absence of the central portion of the skeleton of the heart, with absence of the upper portion of the ventricular septum and the inferior portion of the atrial septum. A large bridging atrioventricular valve is seen, and extensive admixture of blood is usually found in this condition.

In the majority of cases, this disorder is found in patients with trisomy 21, and is often accompanied by the rapid development of pulmonary hypertension. In fact, in some trisomy 21 related cases, it appears that the high pulmonary artery pressures present at birth never significantly regress.[1]

However, in this case, the disorder was seen in an otherwise normal individual. Pulmonary hypertension and pulmonary vascular disease were effectively prevented in this case by the coexisting presence of extensive right ventricular outflow tract obstruction and pulmonary stenosis.[2] As a result, the patient had cyanosis, but no evidence of pulmonary vascular disease.

References

1. Calabro R, Limongelli G. Complete atrioventricular canal. Orphanet J Rare Dis. 2006;1:8.
2. Prifti E, et al. Repair of complete atrioventricular septal defect with tetralogy of fallot: our experience and literature review. J Card Surg. 2004;19(2): 175–183.

Teaching File Case 133

68-year-old male with known peripheral vascular disease

Category: Angiography

History

Assess for possible surgical intervention.

Findings

The abdominal aorta shows no evidence of aneurysm. In the right iliac artery, just above the bifurcation, an ulcerated plaque is apparent. Irregularity and mild to moderate narrowing of the left common iliac artery is noted. There is apparent occlusion of the left common femoral artery on imaging of the abdomen and pelvis, but it has a normal appearance on imaging of the upper leg.

Bilateral SFA occlusions are noted, which are strikingly symmetric in appearance. Reconstitution of the popliteal arteries at the level of the adductor canals is apparent bilaterally, occurring via collaterals from the profunda femoris arteries. Excellent distal runoff is noted.

The time-resolved images are degraded by patient movement. Given that these are subtraction images, patient movement of the right leg in particular in between the scans has resulted in significant limitations.

Diagnosis

Bilateral SFA occlusions. Bilateral iliac artery disease is noted.

Spurious apparent occlusion of the left common femoral artery is due to poor slice positioning, resulting in the exclusion of the left common femoral artery from the imaging volume at the abdomen/pelvis level. Fortunately, this segment of the artery was included adequately on the upper leg image level, and is seen to be normal.

It is important when performing peripheral MR angiography to carefully review the source images in multiple planes. This is important for several reasons. First, positioning errors as in the present case can result in artifactual occlusions or stenoses that are not real. Secondly, intraluminal filling defects can be missed on maximum intensity projection images if they are surrounded by high signal material. These can be easily detected on review of source images.[1, 2]

References

1. Lee VS, et al. Gadolinium-enhanced MR angiography: artifacts and pitfalls. AJR Am J Roentgenol. 2000;175(1):197–205.
2. Ersoy H, Zhang H, Prince MR. Peripheral MR angiography. J Cardiovasc Magn Reson. 2006;8(3): 517–528.

Teaching File Case 134

53-year-old male in for cardiac evaluation

Category: Cardiomyopathy

Findings

Concentric hypertrophy of the left ventricle is noted. No asymmetric involvement of the septum is seen. The regional and global wall motion is within normal limits. The left ventricular ejection fraction is within normal limits.

No turbulence is noted in the region of the left ventricular outflow tract.

The valvular structures are unremarkable in appearance. No evidence of aortic stenosis is seen.

Delayed-enhancement images demonstrate patchy midwall enhancement of the inferolateral wall at the basal level. The remainder is normal in appearance.

Diagnosis

Fabry disease.

This is an X linked recessive genetically transmitted disorder characterized by an enzyme deficiency (alpha galactosidase), resulting in the deposition of abnormal metabolite in various body structures, including the heart and kidneys. Impairment of renal function and cardiac function are the usual causes of death. The disorder is also associated with various neurologic abnormalities, as well as chronic skin abnormalities. (angiokeratoma corporosis diffusum). As one would expect, males are predominantly affected, although female carriers show variable involvement.[1]

In literature reports, between 3 and 5% of a population of hypertrophic cardiomyopathy patients were found to actually have Fabry disease based on enzyme testing.[2, 3] The distinction is an important one, as a specific therapy is now available for Fabry's disease, involving enzyme replacement.[4] This has been shown to diminish levels of abnormal metabolite within the heart.

Fabry disease can result in a characteristic MR imaging appearance of concentric left ventricular hypertrophy, often associated with midwall enhancement in the lateral basal wall.[5, 6] The reason for this focal segmental enhancement pattern is not certain, but likely relates to the abnormal metabolite deposition and regional fibrosis. It is more commonly seen in cases of more severe involvement. The degree of concentric hypertrophy and hyperenhancement correlate with increasing severity of metabolite deposition.[7]

Differential diagnosis for this lateral basal midwall enhancement pattern could conceivably include sarcoidosis, or myocarditis.[8] However, the clinical circumstance would usually be significantly different in these disorders, and they would be unlikely to result in diagnostic confusion.

References

1. Kampmann C, et al. Cardiac manifestations of Anderson-Fabry disease in heterozygous females. J Am Coll Cardiol. 2002;40(9):1668–1674.
2. Sachdev B, et al. Prevalence of Anderson-Fabry disease in male patients with late onset hypertrophic cardiomyopathy. Circulation. 2002;105(12):1407–1411.
3. Nakao S, et al. An atypical variant of Fabry's disease in men with left ventricular hypertrophy. N Engl J Med. 1995;333(5):288–293.
4. Mignani R, Cagnoli L. Enzyme replacement therapy in Fabry's disease: recent advances and clinical applications. J Nephrol. 2004;17(3):354–363.
5. Moon JC, et al. Gadolinium enhanced cardiovascular magnetic resonance in Anderson-Fabry disease. Evidence for a disease specific abnormality of the myocardial interstitium. Eur Heart J. 2003;24(23): 2151–2155.
6. Moon JC, et al. The histological basis of late gadolinium enhancement cardiovascular magnetic resonance in a patient with Anderson-Fabry disease. J Cardiovasc Magn Reson. 2006;8(3):479–482.
7. Weidemann F, et al. The variation of morphological and functional cardiac manifestation in Fabry disease: potential implications for the time course of the disease. Eur Heart J. 2005;26(12):1221–1227.
8. Mahrholdt H, et al. Delayed-enhancement cardiovascular magnetic resonance assessment of non-ischaemic cardiomyopathies. Eur Heart J. 2005;26(15):1461–1474.

Teaching File Case 135

67-year-old male with a history of nephrectomy 18 months earlier, with persistent back and chest pain

Category: Mass

Findings

The short-axis views demonstrate a large mass infiltrating the inferior aspect of the basal myocardium, extending toward the inferior septum. A second rounded area of mass-effect is noted in the anterior wall at the basal level. These findings are well demonstrated on the 2-chamber view seen in the second row of images.

The 4-chamber view demonstrates infiltration of the septum. A large pericardial effusion is noted.

The total chest imaging provided by the HASTE images demonstrates multiple pulmonary parenchymal lesions in addition to the extensive cardiac infiltration described.

Perfusion images are demonstrated in the third row, and demonstrate marked hypervascularity of the infiltrative lesions of the inferior and anterior walls of the basal left ventricle.[1] Abnormal enhancement of pulmonary metastases is also apparent.

Delayed-enhancement imaging demonstrates that most of the infiltrative deposits demonstrate extensive abnormal enhancement and are quite high in signal on the delayed-enhancement images.

Diagnosis

Renal cell carcinoma metastases producing extensive infiltration of the heart. Pulmonary parenchymal metastases are evident. Malignant pericardial effusion is noted.

In adults, metastatic lesions far outweigh primary cardiac tumors. An intramural mass in an adult has a high probability of representing a metastatic lesion. The differential diagnosis in an adult is quite minimal, as the lesions in question would represent metastatic deposits until proven otherwise.[2]

Cardiac metastatic deposits most often arise from lung cancer and breast cancer, along with melanoma and lymphoma. Renal cell carcinoma may demonstrate hematogenous spread as in the present case, or may reach the heart by direct extension via the inferior vena cava.[3]

In the pediatric age group, rhabdomyomas and fibromas would be the most likely causes of intramural masses, particularly in the neonatal and infancy periods.

In this instance, the multiple sequences available with MR allow depiction of the infiltration of the myocardium on the cine images, along with the capacity to characterize these findings as hypervascular on the perfusion images.[1]

The delayed-enhancement images allow clear differentiation of the lesions from normal myocardium.

Survey images of the lungs are also readily obtained with a very short imaging time of approximately 1 to 2 minutes.

References

1. Foster E, Gerber IL. Masses of the heart: perfusing the "good" from the bad. J Am Coll Cardiol. 2004;43(8):1420–1422.
2. Hoffmann U, et al. Usefulness of magnetic resonance imaging of cardiac and paracardiac masses. Am J Cardiol. 2003;92(7):890–895.
3. Chiles C, et al. Metastatic involvement of the heart and pericardium: CT and MR imaging. Radiographics. 2001;21(2):439–449.

Teaching File Case 136

51-year-old male with an echo diagnosis of dilated cardiomyopathy

Category: Cardiomyopathy

History

Assess etiology and viability.

Findings

The left ventricle is noted to be markedly dilated and poorly contractile in a global fashion. The hypokinesia is profound throughout, but there is anterior wall akinesia progressing to dyskinesia at the apical level. Minimal thinning of the anterior wall in the apical region is apparent as well.

The right ventricle is normal in size, but demonstrates mildly reduced function.

Evaluation of the valves demonstrates no significant mitral and tricuspid regurgitation. The aortic valve is trileaflet and normal in appearance.

Delayed-enhancement imaging with a short inversion time demonstrates extensive infarction of the anterior wall and anterior portion of the septum from the mid-ventricular level to the apex. The infarction is initially approximately 50% transmural, but progresses to 100% transmurality at the apical levels and the true apex. The inferior wall of the apex also demonstrates transmural infarction, as does the lateral wall in the apical region.

Multiple ventricular thrombi are noted, best appreciated on delayed enhanced images with a long inversion time. These are noted adjacent to sites of hyperenhancement in the apical region.

Diagnosis

This represents a case of dilated ischemic cardiomyopathy, complicated by multiple left ventricular thrombi.

As discussed in previous cases, MR imaging is an excellent means of distinguishing ischemic from non-ischemic dilated cardiomyopathy. The pattern noted in the present case is characteristic of an ischemic etiology. Non-ischemic disease would most often show either no delayed enhancement (~60%), or a mid-wall enhancement pattern (~30%) clearly different from the present pattern.[1, 2]

The intraventricular thrombi present are noted to be adherent to areas of prior infarction. It is likely that the disruption of endothelial/endocardial integrity by an infarction results in the formation of a thrombogenic focus, and may explain the greater prevalence of thrombi in dilated ischemic vs. non-ischemic cardiomyopathy.

In the evaluation of myocardial viability, it is important to think of the left ventricle in a three-dimensional sense. Evaluation of the stack of short axis images is helpful, but review of orthogonal views such as the 2 and 4-chamber views is necessary for full evaluation. Reporting of the imaging findings using the standard 17-segment model is recommended.[3]

References

1. Soriano CJ, et al. Noninvasive diagnosis of coronary artery disease in patients with heart failure and systolic dysfunction of uncertain etiology, using late gadolinium-enhanced cardiovascular magnetic resonance. J Am Coll Cardiol. 2005;45(5):743–748.
2. McCrohon JA, et al. Differentiation of heart failure related to dilated cardiomyopathy and coronary artery disease using gadolinium-enhanced cardiovascular magnetic resonance. Circulation. 2003;108(1):54–59.
3. Cerqueira MD, et al. Standardized myocardial segmentation and nomenclature for tomographic imaging of the heart. A statement for healthcare professionals from the Cardiac Imaging Committee of the Council on Clinical Cardiology of the American Heart Association. Int J Cardiovasc Imaging. 2002;18(1):539–542.

Teaching File Case 137

49-year-old patient with end-stage renal disease

Category: Angiography

History

The study is requested for possible arteriovenous fistula creation.

Findings

Venous injection of the upper extremities results in filling of a collateral vein along the left flank, which is observed to anastomose with the left iliac venous system, with resultant opacification of the inferior vena cava. This results in persistent venous opacification of the IVC even during the arterial phase of imaging. This occurred because the patient has complete occlusion of both subclavian veins, resulting in extensive collateral formation. These subclavian occlusions also necessitate that the AV fistula created for dialysis be placed in the upper leg.

The arterial images are unremarkable in appearance. Review of the source images indicates that a dialysis access catheter is present in the left iliac vein extending into the inferior vena cava.

Diagnosis

Bilateral subclavian vein obstruction, with extensive collateral formation resulting in filling of the inferior vena cava from a left arm injection.

A similar finding may be seen in cases of superior vena cava obstruction. This also will result in aberrant filling of the inferior vena cava as a collateral pathway.[1,2] This can result in mistiming of the image acquisition if opacification of the IVC is mistaken for opacification of the aorta.

References

1. Prince MR, Sostman, HD. MR venography: unsung and underutilized. Radiology. 2003;226(3): 630–632.
2. Pagnan L, et al. Direct contrast enhanced MR in the study of central venous accesses in children receiving total parenteral nutrition. Radiol Med (Torino). 2005;110(3):241–248.

Teaching File Case 138

27-year-old woman who presented with chest pain

Category: Cardiomyopathy

History

She was noted to have a minimal elevation of troponin levels.

Cardiac catheterization was performed and demonstrated normal coronary arteries. The study was requested for further evaluation.

Findings

The left ventricular cavity is normal in size, and the global systolic function is at the lower limits of normal. Diminished contractility of the inferolateral wall from the mid-ventricular level to the apex is noted. This is best appreciated on the 3-chamber views, both before and after contrast, as seen in the far right-sided images of the second row.

The right ventricle size and function appeared normal. The valvular structures are unremarkable. A small pericardial effusion is noted.

Delayed-enhancement images with a short inversion time as well as a long inversion time were obtained and demonstrate hyperenhancement of the inferolateral wall from the mid-ventricular level to the apex. Less extensive involvement of the basilar segments is apparent. No subendocardial scar is noted to suggest the presence of infarction secondary to coronary disease.

Diagnosis

The pattern of hyperenhancement in the inferolateral wall is highly consistent with the diagnosis of viral myocarditis.

In this case, the coexisting pericardial effusion renders the interpretation slightly more difficult, as the delayed-enhancement images with a short inversion time resulted in a bright appearance of the pericardial effusion. Therefore, the hyperenhancement of the inferolateral wall becomes difficult to distinguish from the adjacent effusion.

However, the delayed-enhancement images obtained with a long inversion time demonstrate the abnormal enhancement of the lateral wall, as the pericardial effusion is low in signal on this image sequence. The long inversion time delayed-enhancement images are seen as the first, third, and fifth images of the third row.

The pattern described is fairly characteristic for viral myocarditis, particularly that due to parvovirus B 19.[1] Although there is a differential diagnosis including other entities such as sarcoidosis, it certainly is not consistent with a pattern seen with coronary artery disease.[2]

Laissy etal reported a series in which they found that first-pass perfusion imaging, in addition to standard delayed-enhancement imaging, was helpful in distinguishing patients with acute MI from those with myocarditis. Patients with myocarditis did not have perfusion abnormalities, while the MI patients frequently did.[3]

References

1. Mahrholdt H, et al. Cardiovascular magnetic resonance assessment of human myocarditis: a comparison to histology and molecular pathology. Circulation. 2004;109(10):1250–1258.
2. Laissy JP, et al. MRI of acute myocarditis: a comprehensive approach based on various imaging sequences. Chest. 2002;122(5):1638–1648.
3. Laissy JP, et al. Differentiating acute myocardial infarction from myocarditis: diagnostic value of early- and delayed-perfusion cardiac MR imaging. Radiology. 2005;237(1):75–82.

Teaching File Case 139

66-year-old female with a murmur

Category: Congenital

Findings

The images are displayed as a series of 4-chamber views in the top row and through most of the second row. They begin at the upper margin of the heart at the level of the right ventricular outflow tract, and extend down to the bottom of the heart.

The left ventricular cavity size and function appear normal. The right ventricular cavity appears mildly dilated, but the wall thickness appears normal. The systolic function appears normal as well. These findings provide a clue to the diagnosis.

The mitral valve is unremarkable in appearance in the images given. The tricuspid valve demonstrates mild to moderate regurgitant flow.

Note is made of apparent flow traversing the interatrial septum. Although the region of the fossa ovalis is often somewhat difficult to visualize on gradient echo images, actual flow traversing the interatrial septum appears to be present on these images.

A series of perfusion images are presented in the far right image of the second row. These demonstrate that as the contrast opacifies the right atrium, unopacified blood streaming across the atrial septal defect into the right atrium from the left atrium dilutes the opacified contrast. Subsequently, in the left atrial phase, persistent opacification of the right heart via flow from the left atrium is apparent.

In the third row, velocity-encoded images obtained with the imaging plane placed parallel to the interatrial septum demonstrate flow coming from left-to-right through an atrial septal defect.

The atrial septal defect can be seen is an area of dark signal on the second image of the third row.

Pulmonary vein images are obtained in the third image of the third row, and demonstrate normal pulmonary venous anatomy.

Delayed-enhancement images show no focal area of scar.

Diagnosis

Ostium secundum ASD.

Atrial septal defects are a common form of congenital heart disease, but infrequently come to MR imaging. MR imaging does allow noninvasive assessment of the size of the defect, as well as quantification of the Qp/Qs ratio.[1] In addition, three-dimensional depiction of the defect and also exclusion of anomalous pulmonary veins are additional reasons to consider cardiac MR imaging in such patients.

The most common form of atrial septal defect is the secundum defect involving the region of the fossa ovalis as seen in the present case. Other forms of atrial septal defect include the ostium primum defect involving the inferior septum, which is a mild form of atrioventricular septal defect, and sinus venosus defect, which may involve the superior or inferior portions of the interatrial septum. Uncommon atrial septal defects include the coronary sinus defect and the confluent/common atrium.[2]

Non-operative management now includes the placement of atrial septal occluder devices such as the Amplatzer device. These have a high rate of success in the appropriate setting, and are often considered the first line of therapy for the appropriate defect.

Postprocedural studies can also be performed in those individuals who undergo closure with atrial septal occluding devices. These produce only minimal artifact, and diagnostic studies can usually be obtained.[3]

Atrial septal defects are not infrequently associated with anomalous pulmonary venous drainage, particularly involving the right upper lobe, most often seen with the superior form of sinus venosus defect. Detailed evaluation of the pulmonary venous connections is therefore necessary in suspected cases of atrial septal defect.[4]

References

1. Piaw CS, et al. Use of non-invasive phase contrast magnetic resonance imaging for estimation of atrial septal defect size and morphology: a comparison with transesophageal echo. Cardiovasc Intervent Radiol. 2006;29(2):230–234.
2. Brickner ME, Hillis LD, Lange RA. Congenital heart disease in adults. First of two parts. N Engl J Med. 2000;342(4):256–263.
3. Schoen SP, et al. Transcatheter closure of atrial septal defects improves right ventricular volume, mass, function, pulmonary pressure, and functional class: a magnetic resonance imaging study. Heart. 2006;92(6):821–826.
4. Cragun DT, Lax D, Butman SM. Look before you close: atrial septal defect with undiagnosed partial anomalous pulmonary venous return. Catheter Cardiovasc Interv. 2005;66(3):432–435.

Teaching File Case 140

66-year-old male with recurrent left leg swelling

Category: Angiography

Findings

The initial angiographic images demonstrate that the abdominal aorta is normal in contour and caliber, with mild tortuosity noted. However, faint visualization of the left femoral vein as well as a portion of the left common iliac vein is apparent.

The upper leg level demonstrates extensive opacification of the left superficial femoral vein throughout the upper leg, although the right leg shows no venous filling, and appears to be in the arterial phase. Therefore, inappropriate timing is thought an unlikely explanation for the findings.

The third and fourth images of each row demonstrate images obtained at the lower leg level. The fourth image of the top row is a time-resolved sequence, which demonstrates near simultaneous opacification of the arteries and the vein on the left.

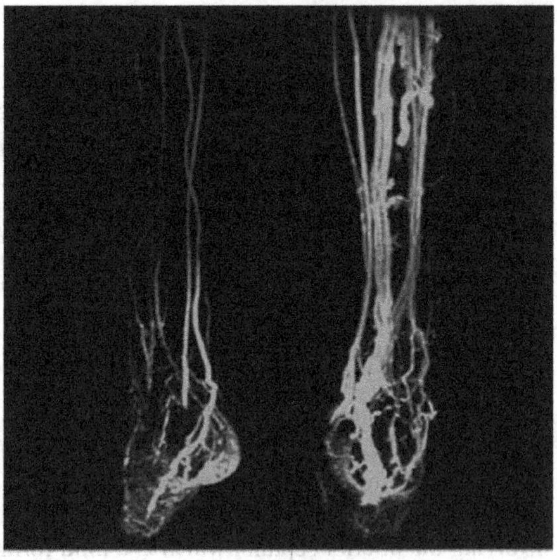

FIGURE 140.1. Magnetic resonance angiogram demonstrating an arteriovenous malformation of the patient's left foot, which resulted in early venous filling

Diagnosis

Left foot arteriovenous malformation.

The differential diagnosis for the above images would include inappropriate triggering of the image acquisition resulting in venous contamination. However, the differential opacification of the right and left lower extremities suggests that this is likely not the case. The presence of venous filling during the arterial phase should always raise the suspicion that an abnormal arteriovenous connection is present.

Arteriovenous malformations may be an isolated abnormality, or may be part of a more extensive vascular syndrome affecting the lower legs. Klippel-Trenaunay-Weber syndrome is a constellation of vascular abnormalities characterized by abnormal venous connections and hypertrophic changes of the lower extremity. Atrophy may also occur as part of this syndrome.[1] Parks-Weber syndrome is a variant of Klippel-Trenaunay-Weber, and usually is accompanied by high flow states, secondary to arteriovenous fistulae. This is usually a more significant and troublesome abnormality.

The present example simply represents an isolated arteriovenous malformation of the foot. Please see the enclosed image.[2]

References

1. Fontana A, Olivetti L. Peripheral MR angiography of Klippel-Trenaunay syndrome. Cardiovasc Intervent Radiol. 2004;27(3):297–299.
2. Herborn CU, et al. Comprehensive time-resolved MRI of peripheral vascular malformations. AJR Am J Roentgenol. 2003;181(3):729–735.

Teaching File Case 141

69-year-old female with chest pain and abnormal enzymes

Category: Cardiomyopathy

Findings

The overall left ventricular cavity size is within normal limits, and the wall thickness is normal as well. Evaluation of the wall motion demonstrates that as one examines from the base to apex, progressive hypokinesia in a circumferential fashion is noted. This is apparent on the 2-chamber and 4-chamber views of the second row as well.

Evaluation of the valvular structures demonstrates that no significant mitral regurgitation is noted. Mild tricuspid regurgitation is evident. The aortic valve is trileaflet and normal in appearance.

Delayed-enhancement images demonstrate no evidence of infarction.

Diagnosis

Apical ballooning syndrome, also known as Takotsubo cardiomyopathy.

This is a disorder that predominantly affects middle-aged and elderly women, usually occurring in the setting of severe emotional or physical stress.[1, 2] The disorder is characterized by profound dysfunction of the apical segments, with relative hypercontractility of the basal segments, resulting in the characteristic appearance, which is likened to the pot used to catch octopi (Takotsubo).[3, 4]

The etiology is unclear, but has been speculated to involve catecholamine excess, with resultant transient myocardial dysfunction. The disorder usually resolves without sequela.

The differential diagnosis would include myocardial stunning from a variety of causes including coronary artery disease, but this would usually be expected in a distribution corresponding to a vascular territory, which is not seen in this case. Regional myocarditis might produce this appearance, but would be expected to produce signal abnormality on postcontrast images.

References

1. Sharkey SW, et al. Acute and reversible cardiomyopathy provoked by stress in women from the United States. Circulation. 2005;111(4):472–479.
2. Dec GW, Recognition of the apical ballooning syndrome in the United States. Circulation. 2005;111(4): 388–390.
3. Teraoka K, et al. Images in cardiovascular medicine. No delayed-enhancement on contrast magnetic resonance imaging with Takotsubo cardiomyopathy. Circulation. 2005;111(16):e261–e262.
4. Haghi D, et al. Delayed hyperenhancement in a case of Takotsubo cardiomyopathy. J Cardiovasc Magn Reson. 2005;7(5):845–847.

Teaching File Case 142

45-year-old male status–post recent electrophysiological procedure

Category: Cardiomyopathy

Findings

Cine images demonstrate that the left ventricular cavity size and function appear normal. The regional wall motion is normal. Evaluation of the right ventricle demonstrates normal size and function as well. A focal area of minimally abnormal signal intensity is noted at the RV insertion site upon the ventricular septum inferiorly.

The series of 4-chamber views noted in the second row did not show any significant right ventricular hypokinesia or abnormalities of the right ventricular free wall as may be seen with ARVD.

Evaluation of the valvular structures demonstrates that no significant mitral or aortic abnormality is seen. Mild tricuspid regurgitation is noted.

Delayed-enhancement images demonstrate a focal area of high signal at the inferior aspect of the septum along the right ventricular surface of the septum. This is nearly transmural in extent. A small focus of hyperenhancement is seen on the left ventricular side of the basilar septum.

Diagnosis

The patient is status–post ablation procedure for an arrhythmogenic focus along the inferior septum at the basal mid-ventricular levels predominantly involving the right ventricular side of the septum. A minimal amount of involvement is also seen in the left ventricular side of the septum. Ablation procedures were performed in both of these locations.

The differential diagnosis for septal insertion site hyperenhancement would include pulmonary hypertension, with right ventricular overload, as well as hypertrophic cardiomyopathy. ARVD can produce right ventricular hyperenhancement, but no wall motion abnormalities are seen to support this diagnosis, and no hyperenhancement is seen in the right ventricular free wall. Focal sarcoidosis could result in a similar appearance, but no clinical or radiographic evidence of sarcoidosis was present in this patient.

Consultation with the referring electrophysiologist indicated that the ablation procedure was performed in the exact locations described above.[1]

Reference

1. Dickfeld T, et al. Characterization of radiofrequency ablation lesions with gadolinium-enhanced cardiovascular magnetic resonance imaging. J Am Coll Cardiol. 2006;47(2):370–378.

Teaching File Case 143

73-year-old male status–post endovascular repair of an abdominal aortic aneurysm

Category: Angiography

History

Evaluate for endograft leak.

Findings

The rotating maximum intensity projection images demonstrate the two limbs of the patient's endograft which extend from just below the renal arteries to the common iliac arteries bilaterally. The endografts are noted to spiral about each other.

The volumetric images obtained with a slight delay are demonstrated in the third and fourth images of the top row, and demonstrate abundant mural thrombus surrounding the endograft within the aneurysmal sac. However, no flow is seen within the aneurysm sac, and therefore, no endoleak is present.

Diagnosis

Successful endovascular treatment of the patient's abdominal aortic aneurysm, with exclusion of the aneurysm, and no evidence of endoleak.

MR imaging has been evaluated in the follow-up of endografts, and has been demonstrated to be superior to CT for the detection of endoleak. Delayed images obtained as in the present case allowed the detection of even small amounts of endoleak.[1–3]

Note that the metallic artifact present does not significantly impair visualization of the lumen of the endovascular stent graft. In addition, the adjacent mural thrombus is clearly depicted. This stent graft was composed of nitinol, which produces very minimal artifact on MR imaging. Stent grafts composed of stainless steel, however, may produce extensive artifact and significantly limit the visualization of the aneurysm contents.

References

1. Weigel S, et al. Thoracic aortic stent graft: comparison of contrast-enhanced MR angiography and CT angiography in the follow-up: initial results. Eur Radiol. 2003;13(7):1628–1634.
2. Cejna M, et al. MR angiography vs CT angiography in the follow-up of nitinol stent grafts in endoluminally treated aortic aneurysms. Eur Radiol. 2002;12(10): 2443–2450.
3. Ersoy H, et al. Blood pool MR angiography of aortic stent-graft endoleak. AJR Am J Roentgenol. 2004;182(5):1181–1186.

Teaching File Case 144

12-year-old male with poor exercise tolerance

Category: Congenital

Findings

The short-axis images demonstrate normal left ventricular size and function. The right ventricle is within normal in appearance.

The 3-chamber view demonstrates abnormal turbulence arising within the left atrium. The 4-chamber view demonstrates the presence of a membrane traversing the left atrium. Subsequently obtained angiographic images demonstrate that the pulmonary venous confluence is separated from the remainder of the left atrial chamber by a thin membrane. This is the site of the turbulent flow.

The axial images demonstrate the presence of a left-sided superior vena cava, emptying into the coronary sinus. No right-sided superior vena cava is found.

The perfusion images demonstrate filling of the coronary sinus from a left arm injection.

Diagnosis

Cor triatriatum, with a persistent left superior vena cava and absence of the right superior vena cava.

Core triatriatum is a rare congenital abnormality in which there is failure of the normal developmental incorporation of the pulmonary venous confluence into the remainder of the sinus venosus portion of the left atrium as well as the primitive left atrium containing the left atrial appendage. As a result, a membrane is present in the left atrium separating the pulmonary venous confluence from the remainder of the left atrium. The degree of symptomatology and the age at presentation are dependent upon the size of the communication between the two left atrial chambers. The more restrictive the opening, the greater the degree of pulmonary venous obstruction, and the likelihood of an earlier clinical presentation increases. Most cases of cor triatriatum are identified during childhood. Untreated patients have a significant mortality risk.[1–3]

However, cor triatriatum can occasionally be unrecognized into adult life. In this instance, there usually no significant obstruction the left atrial inflow, or very mild obstruction.

Associated abnormalities include persistence of the left superior vena cava as noted in this instance. Atrial septal defect, patent foramen ovale, and patent ductus arteriosus are also frequently associated anomalies.

References

1. Bezante GP, et al. Cor triatriatum sinistrum and persistent left superior vena cava: an original association. Eur J Echocardiogr. 2002;3(2):162–165.
2. Sarikouch S, et al. Adult congenital heart disease: cor triatriatum dextrum. J Thorac Cardiovasc Surg. 2006;132(1):164–165.
3. Slight RD, et al. Cor-triatriatum sinister presenting in the adult as mitral stenosis: an analysis of factors which may be relevant in late presentation. Heart Lung Circ. 2005;14(1):8–12.

Teaching File Case 145

58-year-old female with chest pain and shortness of breath

Category: Mass

History

She also had an abnormal echocardiogram.

Findings

The left ventricle is normal in size and function.

Short-axis and 4-chamber views demonstrate a large mass originating in the right atrial free wall and extending into the right atrial cavity. This extends along the margin of the right atrial free wall to the posterior aspect of the right atrium as well. Pedunculated components are seen, which demonstrate mobility. A large mobile filling defect is seen to prolapse through the tricuspid valve and into the right ventricular chamber.

The lesion appears to transgress the wall of the right atrium, and extend into the pericardial space. On the 3-chamber view, the lesion can be seen to extend along the anterior margin of the aortic outflow tract.

The 4-chamber views also demonstrate an interatrial septal aneurysm.

Perfusion images demonstrate that the lesion demonstrates clear-cut enhancement. In addition, contrast is seen to outline the fossa ovalis, which is observed to bulge from right-to-left.

The fourth image series of the fourth row is a set of precontrast VIBE images (a fat-saturated T1-weighted gradient-echo sequence). These demonstrate that the lesion is high in signal on precontrast images, consistent with a significant component of hemorrhage within the lesion. The postcontrast images are seen in the next image, and demonstrate a significant region of enhancement within the mass as well as nonenhancing thrombus along the margins of the tumor.

Delayed-enhancement images with a long inversion time are seen in the first three images of the fifth row, and demonstrate that much of the lesion is low in signal intensity on these images. This indicates that there is likely abundant thrombus adherent to the large mass along the right atrial margin.

The morphologic images obtained in the axial sagittal and coronal planes demonstrate innumerable pulmonary metastatic lesions.

Diagnosis

Angiosarcoma arising along the right atrial free wall and extending along the epicardial surface. Abundant adherent thrombus is noted.

Angiosarcoma is the most common primary cardiac malignancy. It most commonly arises in the right atrium in an intramural location, but frequently extends to the epicardial surface and results in pericardial effusion. Often, a hemorrhagic component is seen, as noted in the present case.

Other primary cardiac malignancies include undifferentiated sarcoma, as well as osteosarcoma and other sarcomas. Many of these have a predilection for the left atrium, or for both atria in equal proportion. Rhabdomyosarcoma is notable for its frequent valvular involvement. It is the most common sarcoma of the heart in the pediatric age group. Nonsarcomatous primary malignancies are predominantly due to lymphoma.

Angiosarcomas have a slight male predominance, and usually arise in the fourth and fifth decades. Typically they are quite hypervascular and aggressive in appearance. The median life expectancy is approximately 6 months.[1–3]

The VIBE sequences are quite helpful in demonstrating the hemorrhagic nature of the lesion. The perfusion sequences are also helpful in demonstrating the vascular nature of the tumor. Delayed-enhancement imaging with a long inversion time is helpful in differentiating between the primary tumor and the adherent thrombus.

The morphologic images are helpful in documenting the extensive pulmonary metastatic disease.

References

1. Araoz PA, et al. CT and MR imaging of primary cardiac malignancies. Radiographics. 1999;19(6):1421–1434.
2. Best AK, Dobson RL, Ahmad AR. Best cases from the AFIP: cardiac angiosarcoma. Radiographics. 2003;23(Spec No):S141–S145.
3. Keenan N, et al. Angiosarcoma of the right atrium: A diagnostic dilemma. Int J Cardiol. 2005.

Teaching File Case 146

15-year-old male with a history of prior surgery and known congenital heart disease

Category: Congenital

Findings

Dextrocardia is apparent, with situs inversus also noted. Review of the orientation of the abdominal structures indicates that the liver is left-sided, and the spleen is right-sided. The viscero-atrial connections are concordant with this diagnosis, with a left-sided superior and inferior vena cava emptying into the morphologic right atrium which is located on the left. A right arch is noted, which is concordant with the patient's dextrocardia and situs inversus. The right arch has the expected branching pattern, with a left innominate seen as the first branch, followed by the right carotid and right subclavian arteries.

The left ventricular cavity is normal in size. There is no evidence of left ventricular hypertrophy. The interventricular septum is a normal appearance.

The right ventricle is normal in overall size, but demonstrates aneurysmal dilatation of its outflow tract. Slight depression of the right ventricular ejection fraction is noted, measured at 32%.

The aortic valve is normal in appearance. Absence of the pulmonic valve is apparent, with free pulmonic insufficiency noted. The regurgitant fraction is approximately 45%.

Also noted is pulmonary arterial stenosis at the division point of the main pulmonary artery into the right and left pulmonary arteries.

Delayed-enhancement images demonstrate enhancement of the right ventricular outflow tract, at the site of the prior surgery. The minimally dilated segment shows particular prominent hyper-enhancement.

Diagnosis

Situs inversus totalis. Post-op Tetralogy of Fallot, with absence of the pulmonary valve and extensive pulmonic insufficiency.[1]

Situs inversus totalis as seen in the present example has been associated with the immotile cilia syndrome, many of which will demonstrate the findings of Kartagener syndrome. At least 50% of patients with the immotile cilia syndrome will demonstrate situs inversus as seen in the present example.[2, 3]

In this disorder, the sides are completely reversed, resulting in the left lung demonstrating 3 lobes, and the right lung demonstrating 2 lobes. The bronchial branching pattern will reflect this abnormality.

In this instance, the mirror-image branching of the aorta as well as the L looping of the heart are concordant findings with the situs abnormality, and are normal for this disorder. In this circumstance, the Tetralogy of Fallot is an unrelated disorder.

The degree of segmental pulmonary stenosis can be assessed using the velocity-encoded images as demonstrated in the third row of the data set.[4]

Fibrosis of the right ventricular outflow tract associated with prior surgery has been demonstrated to show abnormal hyperenhancement on delayed-enhancement imaging, and correlates with impaired RV function in patients who have undergone prior patch annuloplasty for treatment of Tetralogy.[5]

References

1. Guit GL, et al. Levotransposition of the aorta: identification of segmental cardiac anatomy using MR imaging. Radiology. 1986;161(3):673–679.
2. Schidlow DV, Katz SM. Immotile cilia syndrome. N Engl J Med. 1983;308(10):595.
3. Yarnal JR, et al. The immotile cilia syndrome: explanation for many a clinical mystery. Postgrad Med. 1982;71(2):195–197, 200–102, 209–211 passim.
4. Norton KI, et al. Cardiac MR imaging assessment following tetralogy of fallot repair. Radiographics. 2006;26(1):197–211.
5. Babu-Narayan SV, et al. Ventricular fibrosis suggested by cardiovascular magnetic resonance in adults with repaired tetralogy of fallot and its relationship to adverse markers of clinical outcome. Circulation. 2006;113(3):405–413.

Teaching File Case 147

82-year-old male with acute chest pain

Category: Aorta

Findings

Static morphologic images demonstrate marked thickening of the wall of the ascending aorta, with atherosclerotic plaque apparent. Penetrating atherosclerotic ulcers are noted in multiple locations along the anterior margin of the ascending aorta. The volume rendered image displayed in the far right image of the top row demonstrates irregular outpouchings from the ascending aorta. No evidence of a dissection is seen.

Also evident was mild aortic stenosis along with mild aortic insufficiency. The overall left ventricular function was within normal limits. The right ventricle size and function are normal as well.

Diagnosis

Penetrating atherosclerotic ulcers.

Penetrating atherosclerotic ulcer, along with intramural hematoma and dissection represents one of the three causes of acute aortic syndromes.[1]

A penetrating atherosclerotic ulcer is one that extends beyond the intima, and into the media of the aorta. Continuity with the aortic lumen is noted in this circumstance. This can be accompanied by significant chest pain. The descending aorta is said to be more commonly involved than the ascending aorta. It is associated with a risk of rupture and pseudoaneurysm formation.[2]

This is distinct from an intramural hematoma, which represents a localized collection of blood within the wall of the aorta, not in continuity with the lumen. No flow is seen within an intramural hematoma. Many authorities have speculated these develop as a result of disruption of the vasa vasorum of the media of the aortic wall. They also have a propensity to progress to pseudoaneurysm formation, as well as the development of frank dissection. They may also proceed to rupture.[3]

Aortic dissection on the other hand represents a disruption of the intima, and often a portion of the media as well, with flow seen within a second false channel. They are classified according to the Stanford scheme, in which dissections involving the ascending aorta are termed type A dissection and those beginning in the descending thoracic aorta are termed type B dissections.[4]

References

1. Macura KJ, et al. Role of computed tomography and magnetic resonance imaging in assessment of acute aortic syndromes. Semin Ultrasound CT MR. 2003;24(4):232–254.
2. Eggebrecht H, et al. Penetrating atherosclerotic ulcer of the aorta: treatment by endovascular stent-graft placement. Curr Opin Cardiol. 2003;18(6):431–435.
3. Ganaha F, et al. Prognosis of aortic intramural hematoma with and without penetrating atherosclerotic ulcer: a clinical and radiological analysis. Circulation. 2002;106(3):342–348.
4. Krinsky G, Ribakove GH. Spontaneous progression of ascending aortic intramural hematoma to Stanford type A dissection fortuitously witnessed during an MR examination. J Comput Assist Tomogr. 1999;23(6):966–968.

Teaching File Case 148

20-year-old female with complex congenital heart disease, status–post reconstructive surgery

Category: Congenital

Findings

The left ventricle is mildly dilated, while the right ventricle is markedly hypoplastic. No outlet of the right ventricle is seen. The aorta arises normally from the morphologic left ventricle.

A large atrial septal defect is noted, allowing inferior vena caval blood to extend from the right atrium into the left atrium. The superior vena cava has been attached to the main pulmonary artery, with filling of only the left pulmonary artery apparent. The right pulmonary artery does not fill from the inferior vena caval flow or from the superior vena cava. The aortogram demonstrates changes consistent with a prior right-sided Blalock-Taussig shunt, which is now occluded, and very poor right lung blood flow is seen. Specifically, no discernible hilar pulmonary artery is seen on the right. Large collaterals are seen to arise from the aorta, as well as from the celiac axis in the abdomen, and filling of the pulmonary circuit on the right occurs via bronchial collaterals.

Note is also made of abnormal filling of sinusoidal vessels directly from the right coronary artery, which extend into the diminutive right ventricular cavity.

Diagnosis

This patient has pulmonary atresia with intact ventricular septum.

This resulted in marked hypoplasia of the right ventricle. Initially, pulmonary blood flow to the right lung was improved by performance of a Blalock-Taussig shunt. However, this subsequently became occluded. Construction of a Glenn anastomosis between the superior vena cava and the pulmonary artery was performed, but did not result in significant filling of the right pulmonary artery, but only of the left pulmonary artery. Currently her oxygenation is dependent upon this systemic venous to pulmonary arterial connection.

The inferior vena cava flow has been routed to the right atrium and subsequently to the left atrium via the septal defect. Thus, this patient is markedly cyanotic.[1]

This case illustrates the ability of MR imaging to visualize complex cardiovascular abnormalities.[2, 3] It allows depiction of surgically created shunts such as the Fontan and Blalock-Taussig shunts, as well as native great vessel relationships. By performing flow studies through the aorta and pulmonary artery, Qp/Qs ratios can be calculated. Quantification of function is also possible. Therefore, MR is the best means of non-invasively assessing complex congenital disease.

References

1. Agnoletti G, et al. Right to left shunt through interatrial septal defects in patients with congenital heart disease: results of interventional closure. Heart. 2006;92(6):827–831.
2. Powell AJ, et al. Accuracy of MRI evaluation of pulmonary blood supply in patients with complex pulmonary stenosis or atresia. Int J Card Imaging. 2000;16(3):169–174.
3. Geva T, et al. Gadolinium-enhanced 3-dimensional magnetic resonance angiography of pulmonary blood supply in patients with complex pulmonary stenosis or atresia: comparison with x-ray angiography. Circulation. 2002;106(4):473–478.

Teaching File Case 149

46-year-old female with a known systemic disorder

Category: Cardiomyopathy

Findings

The left ventricular cavity is moderately dilated, with a focal area of wall thinning and dyskinesia involving the inferolateral wall at the basal level. Review of the 4-chamber view demonstrates a focal area of aneurysmal outpouching in the inferolateral wall of the basal level extending to the mid-ventricular level. The anterior, septal, and inferior walls demonstrate normal contractility.

The right ventricle size and function are normal.

No significant valvular disorders are noted.

Delayed-enhancement imaging demonstrates transmural enhancement of the area of aneurysm formation at the inferolateral wall of the base. Patchy areas of abnormal enhancement are also seen in multiple foci involving the septum at the basal and mid-ventricular levels. Involvement of the lateral wall and the apical region is seen as well. Extensive enhancement of the aneurysmal segment is noted.

Diagnosis

Sarcoidosis, with aneurysm formation.

Coalescent sarcoid granulomas can result in extensive fibrosis and the formation of focal areas of aneurysm.[1] Basilar involvement predominates.

Patchy myocardial enhancement in the pattern described is characteristic of sarcoidosis, although it may be seen in other forms of myocarditis.[2–4]

Although ischemic disease is the most common cause of aneurysm formation, as can be seen in the present case, other etiologies are also possible. Given the focal patchy areas of abnormal delayed-enhancement seen elsewhere in a non- coronary artery disease pattern, alternative diagnoses should be considered.

Although Fabry disease can result in preferential involvement of the inferolateral basal wall, it is usually accompanied by concentric hypertrophy, which is not seen in the present case. In addition, it does not usually result in aneurysm formation.

References

1. Serra JJ, et al. Images in cardiovascular medicine. Cardiac sarcoidosis evaluated by delayed-enhanced magnetic resonance imaging. Circulation. 2003;107(20): e188–e189.
2. Smedema JP, et al. Cardiac involvement in patients with pulmonary sarcoidosis assessed at two university medical centers in the Netherlands. Chest. 2005;128(1):30–35.
3. Smedema JP, et al. Evaluation of the accuracy of gadolinium-enhanced cardiovascular magnetic resonance in the diagnosis of cardiac sarcoidosis. J Am Coll Cardiol. 2005;45(10):1683–1690.
4. Tadamura E, et al. Effectiveness of delayed-enhancement MRI for identification of cardiac sarcoidosis: comparison with radionuclide imaging. AJR Am J Roentgenol. 2005;185(1):110–115.

Teaching File Case 150

64-year-old female in for evaluation of chest pain

Category: Mass

Findings

Stress MR imaging is performed. The short-axis images in the upper demonstrate normal left ventricular size and function. The perfusion images in the second and third rows demonstrate no evidence of inducible ischemia.

The short-axis images through the inter-atrial septum demonstrate the presence of a sessile mass arising from the left atrial side of the fossa ovalis. Small field-of-view imaging is subsequently performed and demonstrates the finding quite well. In addition, a second small mass is seen at the orifice of the left upper lobe pulmonary vein.

Delayed-enhancement imaging shows no evidence of prior infarction. The lesion in question at the left atrial side of the fossa ovalis appears to demonstrate heterogeneous enhancement.

Diagnosis

Left atrial myxomas.

Secondary cardiac masses are estimated to be 20–40 times more common than primary cardiac masses. Of the primary cardiac masses, benign etiologies far outweigh malignant etiologies, and myxomas makes up of approximately 50% of cases.[1–3]

Myxomas are gelatinous tumors that most often arise in close proximity to the fossa ovalis. Approximately 80 to 85% originate in the left atrium, with approximately 10% originating in the right atrium or extending through the fossa ovalis. 5% or less arise within the ventricles. In addition, less than 5% are multiple as noted in this case. When multiple, syndrome association should be sought, including the Carney syndrome. This disorder is characterized by the presence of melanotic schwannomas, atrial myxomas, as well as breast fibroadenomas.

Myxomas demonstrate a heterogeneous enhancement pattern on delayed-enhancement images, and can usually be distinguished from thrombus, which demonstrates homogenous low signal intensity on inversion recovery images obtained with a long inversion time. Some confusion may occur in cases where thrombus coats a myxoma however, and detailed evaluation of the images is required.

References

1. Hoffmann U, et al. Usefulness of magnetic resonance imaging of cardiac and paracardiac masses. Am J Cardiol. 2003;92(7):890–895.
2. Araoz PA, et al. CT and MR imaging of benign primary cardiac neoplasms with echocardiographic correlation. Radiographics. 2000;20(5):1303–1319.
3. Wintersperger BJ, et al. Tumors of the cardiac valves: imaging findings in magnetic resonance imaging, electron beam computed tomography, and echocardiography. Eur Radiol. 2000;10(3):443–449.

Part III
Appendixes

This section is intended to serve as a practical resource and quick reference for day-to-day CMR scanning. Appendix A is a glossary that is presented first in the hope of rendering some clarity out of the "alphabet soup" of acronyms and abbreviations that permeates CMR. Basic technical issues, such as image acquisition planes, are covered in Appendix B. The majority of Appendix C is dedicated to a review of imaging modules and their constituent parts. Combinations of modules are what actually comprise most clinical cardiac MR exams are reviewed in Appendix D. Special emphasis is placed. They on protocols for evaluation of selected congenital heart defects, as patients with these lesions often present for CMR evaluation, but typically not in the sort of volume that would allow many centers to have developed great familiarity with specific protocol development. MR angiographic protocols are also presented, noting that wide variability between vendors in terms of scanner capabilities and sequences makes standardization difficult.

Appendix A
Acronyms

AI—Aortic insufficiency.
ARVD—Arrhythmogenic right ventricular dysplasia (also termed ARVCardiomyopathy).
AS—Aortic stenosis.
ASD—Atrial septal defect.
ASSET—General Electric proprietary version of parallel imaging.
CAD—Coronary artery disease.
CMR—Cardiovascular magnetic resonance.
DE-CMR—Delayed-enhancement CMR.
FIESTA—Proprietary term for SSFP sequence by General Electric.
FLASH—Fast low angle shot. A Siemens fast spoiled gradient echo sequence often used for T1 weighted rapid acquisitions such as angiography and perfusion sequences. Similar to GE -SPGR (spoiled gradient echo) and Philips-T1FFE (T1 weighted fast field echo).
FOV—Field-of-view.
FSE—Fast spin-echo.
Gd—Gadolinium.
GRE—Gradient echo (also called gradient recalled echo).
Half-Fourier imaging called ½ NEX by GE or half-scan by Philips.
HASTE—Siemens sequence. Half-Fourier acquistion turbo-spin echo. GE version=SSFSE-single-shot fast spin echo. Philips version=single-shot TSE.
HCM—Hypertrophic cardiomyopathy.
HE—Hyperenhancement.
HOCM—Hypertrophic obstructive cardiomyopathy.
IMH—Intramural hematoma.
IPAT—Integrated parallel acquisition technology. A parallel imaging technology used by Siemens. GE version=ASSET, Philips version= SENSE.
LGE—Late gadolinum enhancement. Synonymous with delayed-enhancement.
LV—Left ventricle.
LVOT—Left ventricular outflow tract.
MI—Myocardial infarction.
MIP—Maximum intensity projection.
MPR—Multiplanar reconstruction.
MR—Magnetic resonance.
MRA—Magnetic resonance angiogram.
PAD—Peripheral arterial disease.
PAU—Penetrating atherosclerotic ulcer.
PDA—Patent ductus arteriosus.
PET—Positron emission tomography.
Qp—Pulmonary blood flow.
Qs—Systemic blood flow.
RV—Right ventricle.
SPGR—Spoiled gradient echo. Also used by General Electric as the acronym for their fast T1W gradient echo sequence used for MRA.
RVOT—Right ventricular outflow tract.
SFOV—Small field-of-view. Often used to describe a specialized cine sequence used to image the valves.
SPECT—Single photon emission computed tomography. A commonly used nuclear medicine imaging technology.
SSFP—Steady state free precession.
STIR—Short tau inversion recovery. Often used to produce fat-suppressed T2 weighted images.

Tet—Tetralogy of Fallot.
TGA—Transposition of the great arteries.
True-FISP—True fast imaging with steady state free precession. A Siemens proprietary version of SSFP. GE version= FIESTA, Philips version= balanced FFE.
TR—Two potential meanings TR=Repetition time when referring to a specific sequence (eg. a T1 weighted sequence typically has a TR of 500ms or less and a short TE).
TR—can also refer to Temporal Resolution, usually when referring to a segmented acquisition (eg. a standard cine sequence should have a TR of <45ms).
TSE—Turbo spin-echo. Synonymous with FSE.
T1W—T1 weighted.
T2W—T2 weighted.
VEC—Velocity-encoded imaging.
VENC—Maximum velotcity value encoded by a velocity-encoded sequence. Values above this level will result in aliasing.
VIBE—Volumetric-interpolated breath hold exam. A Siemens proprietary name for a fat-saturated 3-D volumetric imaging study. Similar to the FAME sequence of General Electric.
VRT—Volume-rendered 3-D image.
VSD—Ventricular septal defect.

Appendix B
Cardiac Scan Planning

Step 1: Planning the 2-chamber scout view

Perform localizer scout imaging.

Using the axial scout image that shows the LV, plan a 2-chamber view by placing a line bisecting the apex and mitral valve plane.

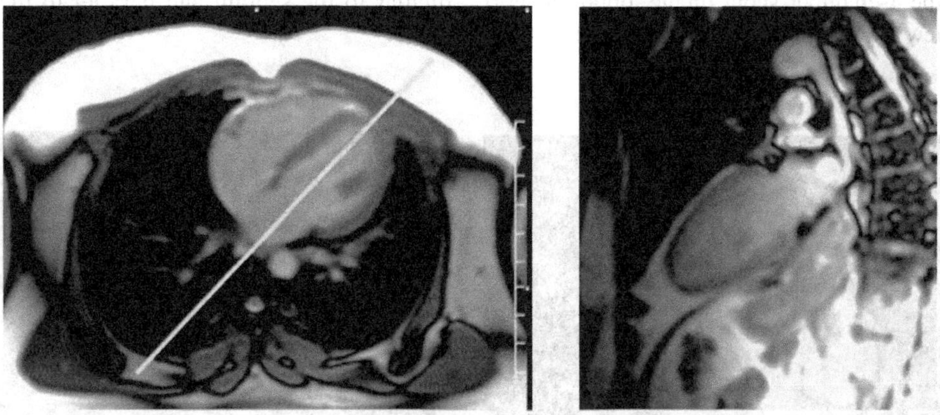

FIGURE B.1. The 2-chamber scout is planned from the axial scout. *(Left)* planning image; *(right)* resulting image

Step 2: Planning the 4-chamber scout view

From the 2-chamber scout, obtain the 4-chamber scout view by placing the imaging plane through the apex and left atrium.

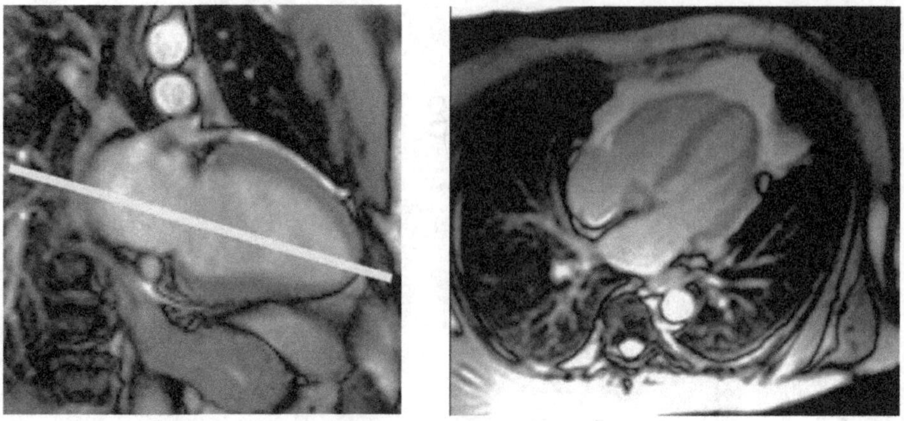

FIGURE B.2. The 4-chamber scout is planned from the 2-chamber scout. *(Left)* planning image; *(right)* resulting image

Step 3: Planning the short-axis scout view

From the 4-chamber scout image, obtain a short axis view by placing the imaging plane perpendicular to the septum and parallel to the mitral valve.

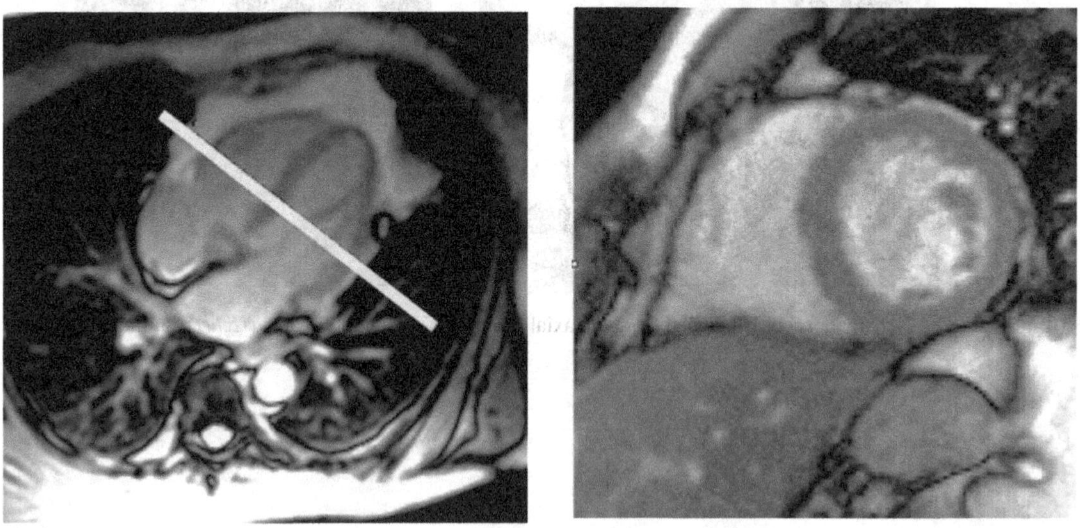

FIGURE B.3. The short-axis (SAX) scout is planned from the 4-chamber scout. *(Left)* planning image; *(right)* resulting image

Step 4: Planning the short-axis cine view

Open a standard cine sequence and using the low-resolution short-axis scout view, copy the image position. Check FOV, Phase, and the length of breath-hold. Make sure that breath-hold is reasonable. Adjust segments to keep temporal resolution <45 ms. Capture cycle, breath hold and run.

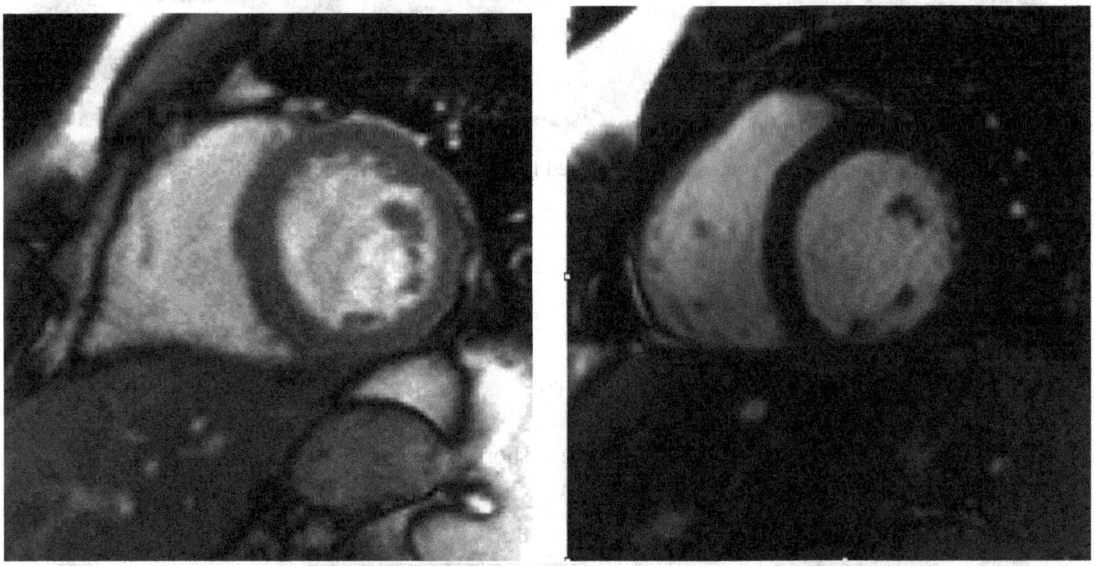

FIGURE B.4. The short-axis (SAX) cine is planned from the short-axis scout. *(Left)* planning image; *(right)* resulting image

---

Step 5: Acquiring the short-axis stack

Sequentially acquire images (6 mm with 4 mm gap or 8 mm with a 2 mm gap) at contiguous 1 cm intervals through the apex and back through the mitral valve.

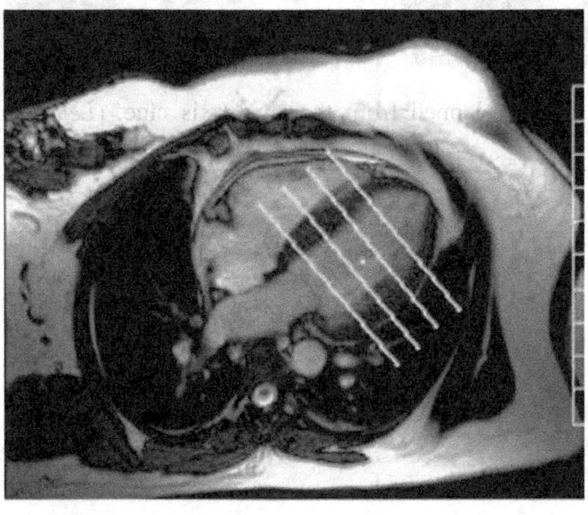

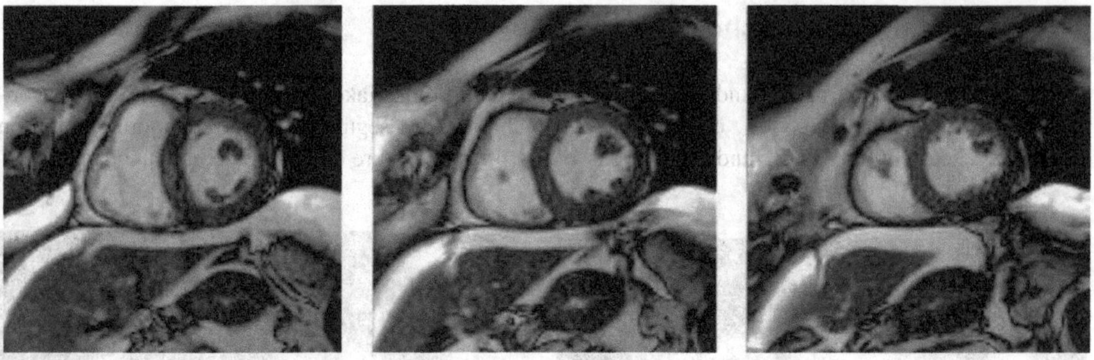

FIGURE B.5. The short-axis (SAX) cine stack is acquired from the base to the apex (not all views are shown)

Step 6: Planning the 3-chamber view

The 3-chamber view is acquired by placing a line through the mitral and aortic valves as seen on a short-axis view at the base of the heart.

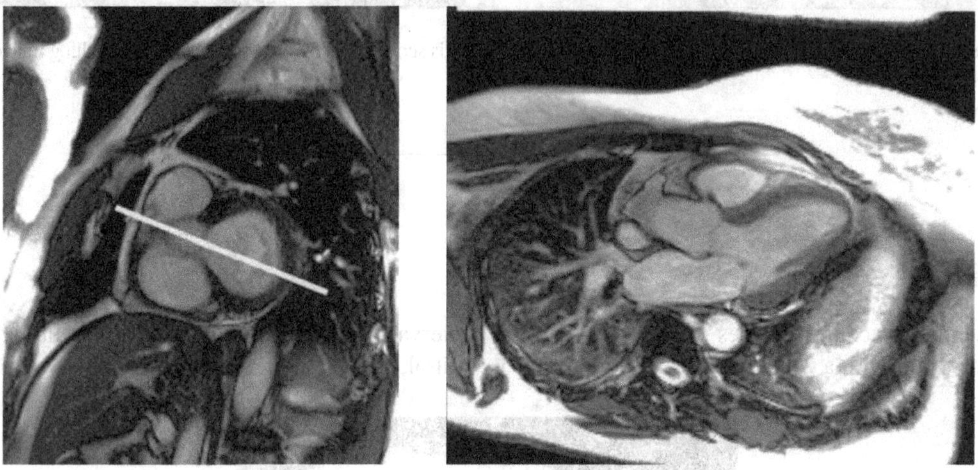

FIGURE B.6. The 3-chamber cine is planned from the short-axis cine. *(Left)* planning image; *(right)* resulting image

Step 7: Planning the 4-chamber cine view

The 4-chamber cine view can be planned from a short axis view by placing a line perpendicular to the inferior septum. In general, the line should traverse the acute margin of the RV free wall just above the diaphragmatic portion. Care should be taken to avoid the aortic valve.

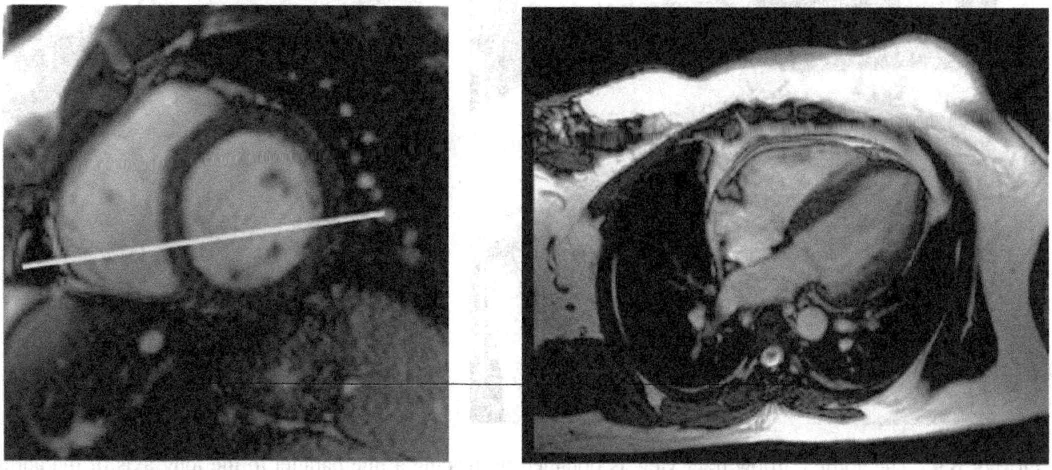

FIGURE B.7. The 4-chamber cine is planned from the short-axis cine. *(Left)* planning image; *(right)* resulting image

---

Step 8: Planning the 2-chamber cine view

Increase the overall FOV by approximately 10% prior to obtaining the 2-chamber view to prevent wrap artifact (alternatively only the FOV in the phase direction can be increased). This is planned using a short axis view by placing the imaging plane perpendicular to the anterior and inferior walls and parallel to the interventricular septum. (6 o'clock to 12 o'clock position in the figure below). The plane should also bisect the LV apex on the 4-chamber view.

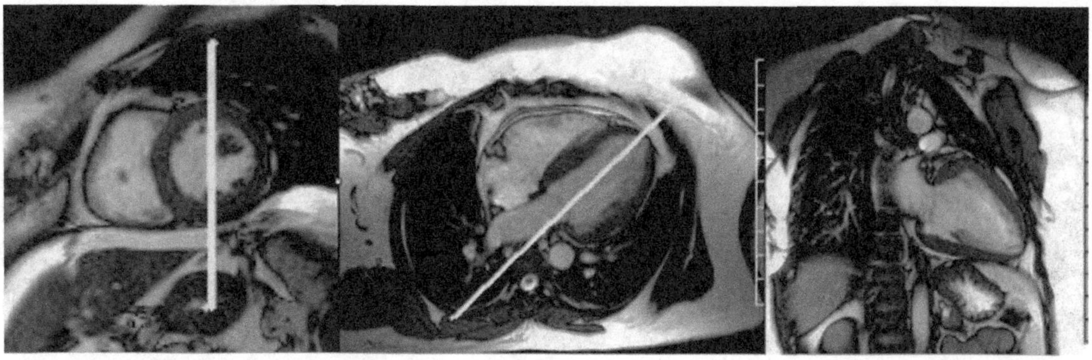

FIGURE B.8. The 2-chamber cine is planned from the short-axis and 4-chamber cines. *(Left)* planning image; *(middle)* planning image; *(right)* resulting image

Step 9: Planning the aortic outflow tract view

The aortic outflow view is obtained by placing the imaging plane through the aortic valve parallel to the long-axis of the proximal aorta on the 3-chamber view.

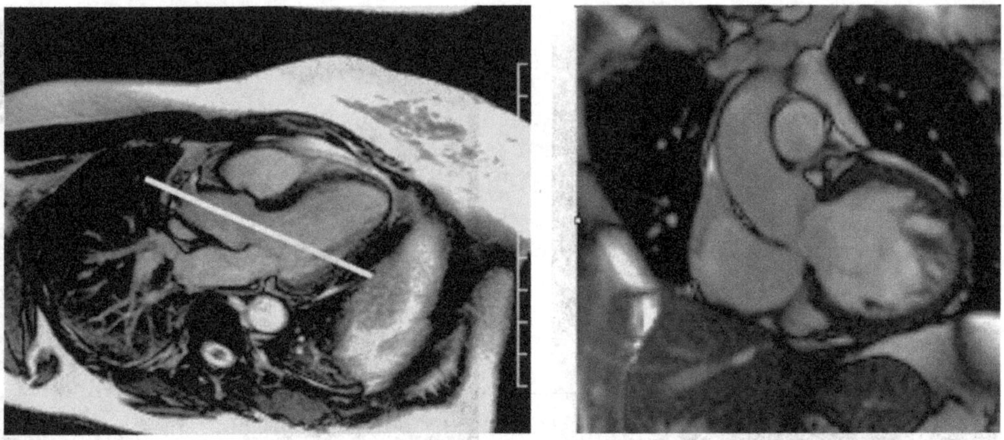

FIGURE B.9. The aortic outflow tract view is obtained by placing a line parallel to the long axis of the aorta and through the aortic valve. *(Left)* planning image; *(right)* resulting image

Step 10: Planning the aortic valve view

High-resolution imaging of the aortic valve is performed with a special cine through the valve plane. This small field-of-view cine of the aortic valve is acquired using the small FOV cine sequence by placing a perpendicular line across the aortic valve. Use both the 3-chamber and aortic outflow views to plan the acquisition.

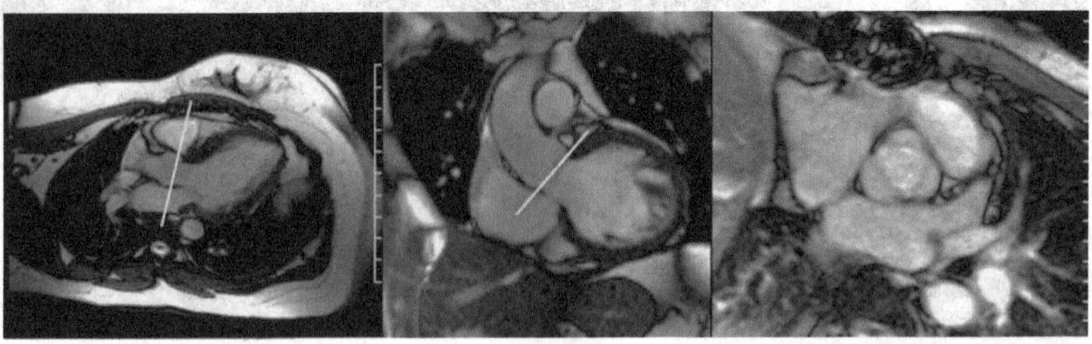

FIGURE B.10. Planning the aortic valve view. *(Left)* planning image; *(middle)* planning image; *(right)* resulting image

Appendix C
Cardiac Imaging Modules

LV Structure and Function

1. Scout imaging – axial, coronal, sagittal
2. (OPTIONAL) Axial (8–10 mm) set of steady state free precession (SSFP) or half Fourier single shot turbo spin echo (HASTE) through chest
3. 2-chamber (or vertical long-axis) and 4-chamber scout (or horizontal long-axis) images are obtained as per the scan-planning instructions. These are then used to plan the short-axis scout view. This is obtained perpendicular to the septum and approximately parallel to the mitral valve plane on the 4-chamber view.
4. The short-axis cine images are obtained using steady state free precession imaging from the mitral valve plane through the apex.
   a. Slice thickness 6–8 mm, at 1 cm contiguous intervals.
   b. Temporal resolution <45 msec between phases.
   c. Parallel imaging used as available.
5. SSFP cine images are also obtained using similar technical parameters in the 4-chamber, 2-chamber, and 3-chamber views as outlined in the scan planning section above.
6. Analysis
   a. The short axis images can be evaluated with computer aided analysis packages for planimetry of endocardial and epicardial borders at end-diastole and end-systole. Measurement of end-diasto lic and end-systolic volumes allows stroke-volume and ejection fraction calculation. Tracing of the epicardial contours allows determination of LV mass and regional wall thickening.
   b. Due to movement of the base of the heart towards the apex during systole, the 1 or 2 most basal slices may include only left atrium at end-systole. However, this slice at end-diastole will include some of the LV mass and volume, which will need to be measured for accuracy.

Delayed-Enhancement (Late Gadolinium Enhancement)

1. Imaging should be delayed approximately 10 minutes after gadolinium administration for the standard inversion recovery segmented GRE images. However, the single-shot inversion recovery SSFP images with a long inversion time (~ 600 ms) can be obtained earlier, at 2–5 minutes post contrast. These are used to evaluate for thrombus.
2. The high-resolution inversion recovery GRE images are obtained with a segmented acquisition during mid-diastole at the same slice positions and with the same slice thickness as the cine images.
3. Data (read-out) is acquired every other heart beat to allow recovery of magnetization before the next inversion pulse is applied. This may be adapted in cases of severe tachycardia (imaging at every third beat) or bradycardia (imaging at every heart beat).

4. The duration of readout during a heart beat should be less than 200 ms to adequately freeze motion during diastole. This period may need to be shortened in the setting of tachycardia.
5. The in-plane resolution should be ~1.2–1.8 mm. The inversion time should be adjusted to null the signal from normal myocardium. An inversion time scout series may be helpful in estimating the appropriate inversion time, but a few trial images are usually necessary to optimize image quality.
6. Phase-sensitive inversion recovery images may be a useful alternative, as a "fixed" TI (~300 ms) can be used.
7. Alternative/Optional.
   a. Inversion recovery SSFP single-shot imaging can be perf med as an acceptable alternative in patients with arrhythmias or difficulty with breath holding.
   b. 3-D IR sequences with parallel imaging are available and may be useful in selected patients.
8. Analysis
   a. Interpret visually using AHA 17-segment model.
   b. Estimate area (transmural extent) of hyperenhancement within each segment (0%, 1–25%, 26–50%, 51–75%, 76–100%).

First-Pass Perfusion

1. Perfusion imaging is performed using a heavily T1 weighted saturation-recovery GRE, GRE-EPI hybrid, or SSFP sequence. In general, GRE-EPI hybrid sequences are faster (better temporal resolution, more slices per heart beat, etc), and SSFP sequences seem to offer higher SNR, however, currently we favor simple GRE sequences (with parallel imaging acceleration) since they are the most robust and less prone to artifacts.
2. At least 3 short-axis images should be obtained every heart beat.
   a. Slice thickness 8 mm.
   b. Parallel imaging, 2-fold acceleration if available.
   c. In-plane resolution, at least 3.0 × 2.0 mm.
   d. Readout temporal resolution ~ 100 – 125 ms or shorter as available.
   e. A precontrast perfusion sequence is then obtained and evaluated for wrap artifact, and adjusted as needed.
   f. Contrast is given at a rate of 3–5 ml/sec followed by 30 ml saline flush at the same rate. An antecubital vein is preferred. The total dose of contrast is 0.05–0.1 mmol/kg/min.
   g. If real-time monitoring of the perfusion images is available, the patient is instructed to hold their breath when the contrast is visualized in the RV. If monitoring is not available, the patient should be instructed to breath hold beginning 5–6 seconds after the start of the contrast infusion. Images are obtained for 40–50 heart beats by which time contrast will have transited the LV myocardium.

Modification–Adenosine Stress-Rest Perfusion

1. Prior to scan initiation, two IV lines should be started; one for the administration of contrast and the other for the infusion of adenosine. Make sure that the blood pressure cuff will not interfere with contrast or adenosine infusion.
2. Following scout acquisitions, short-axis cine images are obtained from the mitral valve to the apex as described in the LV structure and function module.
3. A precontrast perfusion sequence is then obtained and evaluated for wrap artifact and adjusted as needed.
4. The patient may be moved partially out of the magnet for the initiation of the adenosine infusion. Adenosine is administered at a dose of 140ug/kg/min for at least 2 minutes, and the patient is then returned to the magnet while the infusion is continued.
5. Stress perfusion imaging is then performed as described in the first-pass perfusion module. Gadolinium contrast is given during the last minute of adenosine. The total adenosine infusion time is 3–4 minutes.
6. Rest Perfusion

a. Prior to acquiring the rest perfusion images there should be at least a 10 minute wait for contrast to washout from stress perfusion imaging. During this period stress images can be reviewed, cine imaging should be completed (e.g. long-axis views), valvular evaluation can be performed, etc.
b. The rest perfusion images are obtained in an identical fashion as for stress imaging (also same dose of contrast) without adenosine.
c. If stress images are completely normal, rest perfusion imaging can be skipped. Additional gadolinium, however, may need to be given for delayed enhancement imaging (for a total of 0.10 – 0.20 mmol/kg).

7. Delayed-enhancement imaging can be performed as described in the delayed-enhancement module; however, there should be at least a 5 minute delay after the second injection of gadolinium during rest imaging.
8. Analysis

   a. Visual interpretation is performed using the standard 17 segment AHA segment model (16-segment model can be used, leaving out apex).
   b. Side-by-side comparison of the cine, stress and rest perfusion, and DE-MR images at the same slice locations facilitates evaluation and is recommended.

Inflammation Imaging

T2-weighted imaging can be considered if myocardial inflammation is suspected. In general, this may be useful in the acute setting of myocardial disorders (e.g. acute MI, acute myocarditis, etc.) when edema may be present. Increased image intensity represents long T2 values, which may occur in the setting of reversible as well as irreversible myocardial injury.

1. Perform imaging prior to contrast administration.
2. For sufficient T2-weighting, TE should be at least 60 ms.
3. Consider imaging both with and without fat saturation.
4. Selected views are obtained usually based on abnormalities seen on cine imaging.
5. Slice thickness, 5–8 mm.
6. Currently, most often performed using a segmented fast spin-echo sequence with double inversion recovery preparation to produce a dark-blood image.

   a. Adjust readout to mid-diastole to minimize slow flow artifact and motion artifact, but keep in mind that the time to readout from the R-wave should be between 600–900 msec for the dark blood preparation to function well.
   b. Slice thickness of dark blood prep should be 2–3 fold greater than that for readout. Otherwise myocardium with good contractility (significant base-apex motion) may appear darker than hypokinetic regions. This effect can result in "bright" regions based on the amount of myocardium that experiences both the dark blood prep and the readout slice selection rather than because of tissue "edema".

7. "Bright-blood" T2-weighted imaging sequences are preferred since myocardial image intensities will be less dependent on myocardial motion and the presence of slow LV cavity blood flow.

Appendix D
Suggested Protocols

Protocols for Specific Disorders

Acute Myocardial Infarction

1. Cine imaging of the entire LV is performed as described earlier (LV structure and function module).
2. Optional–T2 weighted images (inflammation imaging module) can be obtained to aid in the differentiation of acute from chronic MI, and to possibly detect areas of ischemic injury. These can be obtained at selected locations.
3. Perfusion imaging is performed at rest to evaluate for microvascular disease and perfusion deficits (first-pass perfusion module).
4. Delayed enhancement imaging is then obtained after a delay of 10 minutes as described earlier. High inversion time (~600 ms) single-shot IR SSFP may be helpful in differentiating regions with microvascular obstruction (no-reflow zones) from viable myocardium, both of which can be dark in appearance. These can be obtained beginning at 5 minutes post-contrast and may be repeated after a 5–10 minute delay to differentiate between no-reflow zones and LV thrombus (no-reflow zones become smaller over time, whereas thrombus will remain the same size).

Chronic Ischemic Heart Disease and Viability Imaging

1. Cine imaging of the entire LV is performed as described earlier (LV structure and function module).

2. Optional - adenosine stress-rest perfusion imaging to comment on the presence or absence of ischemia.
3. Delayed-enhancement module.
4. Interpretation / Analysis

   a. Important to view the cine and DE-MR images side-by-side.
   b. The interpretation should use both the cine and DE-MR data. For example, "region is dysfunctional but viable".

Nonischemic LV Cardiomyopathies (Including Myocarditis)

1. Cine imaging of the entire LV is performed as described earlier (LV structure and function module).
2. Consider T2-weighted imaging (inflammation imaging module) in the acute setting when necrosis/edema may be present (e.g. acute myocarditis). These are obtained prior to contrast administration at selected slice locations usually based on cine imaging findings.
3. Delayed-enhancement module.
4. Analysis

   a. Examine the "pattern" of hyperenhancement and determine if the pattern is a "CAD" or "Non-CAD" pattern.
   b. If the pattern is a non-CAD pattern, attempt a more specific diagnosis using pattern recognition as described in Chapter 3.

5. Optional - adenosine stress-rest perfusion imaging (see stress protocols) to comment on the presence or absence of ischemia since a mixed cardiomyopathy may be present.
6. Optional–for hypertrophic cardiomyopathies – consider velocity flow imaging through LV outflow tract.

ARVC

1. Cine imaging of the entire LV and RV is performed as described earlier (LV structure and function module).
2. In addition, a stack of 4-chamber views covering the RV outflow tract should be acquired, along with an RV 2-chamber view. Evaluate for global RV enlargement and dysfunction, excessive trabeculation, and regional dyskinesia/ microaneurysm formation. These changes are often more apparent along the RV free wall and RV outflow tract.

   a. Higher temporal (<35 ms) and spatial resolution (near 1 mm in-plane, ≤5 mm slice thickness) than for normal cine imaging is desirable.
   b. Volumetric analysis of the LV and RV may be helpful.

3. Delayed enhancement module for identification of RV fibrosis (include additional RV views).

   a. Consider T1 nulling for RV (usually 30–40 ms shorter than normal).
   b. Consider performing delayed enhancement with fat-sat.

NOTE: CMR can add 1 major or 1 minor criterion (right ventricular enlargement, right ventricular wall motion abnormalities or aneurysms). A major finding is an easily visualized severe abnormality; a minor finding is a moderate abnormality, which may be less clear. Fat and delayed-enhancement are not used in the guidelines.

Valvular Disease

Patients with artificial valves can safely undergo CMR at 1.5 and 3 Tesla. The force exerted by the beating heart is many times higher than the force exerted by the magnetic field.

1. Cine imaging of the entire LV is performed as described earlier (LV structure and function module). The tricuspid valve is best seen on the 4-chamber view, while the mitral valve can be well seen on this view and the 3- and 2-chamber views. The aortic valve is seen on the 3-chamber view as well as on the basal short-axis, aortic outflow tract view (see scan planning section).

   a. Additional views (RV long axis, RV-outflow tract as needed).

2. Optional

   a. Valve morphology assessment with dedicated small field-of-view (SFOV) SSFP cine in the plane of the valve in question. Care must be taken to optimize angle of imaging and to take a full stack of images across the valve.
   b. Gradient echo imaging is often reported to be more sensitive than SSFP for milder degrees

of regurgitation; however, worse image quality may limit the utility of obtaining additional GRE cine views.

3. For measurements of flow/volume, phase-contrast imaging should avoid regions with turbulent high velocities (i.e. measure aortic flow distal to valve leaflet tips), otherwise flows are underestimated.
4. For measurements of peak velocity, phase-contrast imaging should be at the valve leaflet tips.
   a. The imaging plane should be perpendicular to the jet in at least 2 orthogonal planes.
   b. Adapt velocity encoding to actual velocity (using lowest velocity without aliasing).
   c. Use lowest TE possible.
   d. Use highest temporal resolution possible (i.e. the time for each cine phase should be as short as possible, preferably less than 40–50 ms)
5. Analysis
   a. Although many reports suggest normalizing velocities to reference in static tissue, we find that this may add as much error as remove it. Thus, we do not routinely perform this procedure. It is more important to use low gradient strengths, and to center the region of interest to the scanner isocenter.
   b. Single valve regurgitation can be measured by determining left and right ventricular stroke volume (other methods available).
   c. Mitral regurgitation can be measured by subtracting systolic aortic flow from the LV stroke volume.
   d. Multiple valve lesions can be assessed from comparison of the aortic and pulmonary diastolic regurgitant flow and the LV and RV stroke volumes.
   e. Cross-sectional aortic valve area (CSA) can be calculated using the continuity equation: $CSA_{AV} = CSA_{LVOT}$ * Velocity time integral$_{LVOT}$ / Velocity time integral$_{AV}$
   f. We generally measure aortic valve area by planimetry, keeping in mind that these measurements are usually somewhat larger (10–20%) than from the continuity equation because of a variety of reasons (peak systolic opening is greater than average systolic opening, actual orifice size is greater than effective orifice size, etc.).

Anomalous Coronary Artery Evaluation

1. LV structure and function module to look for wall motion abnormalities.
   a. Add repeat 4-chamber long axis with high temporal resolution sequence (≤ 20 ms per phase) to accurately determine quiescent period of RCA.
2. HASTE imaging in axial, sagittal, and coronal planes
3. Navigator-gated, 3-D T2-prepared free-breathing whole-heart MRA sequence:
   a. Axial slices spanning from just above the sino-tubular junction to the bottom of the heart.
   b. Slice thickness 1–1.5 mm; acquired spatial resolution in-plane < 1.0 mm.
   c. Slices – typically 50–80, as needed to encompass the entire heart.
   d. Parallel acquisition preferred
   e. Navigator placed over the right hemi-diaphragm.
   f. T2 prep time is 40–50 ms.
   g. Optional – image post gadolinium contrast administration to increase SNR. If imaging post contrast, T2 prep time can be increased.
4. Optional – breath-hold techniques if poor image quality, navigators unavailable, or of poor quality.

Congenital Heart Disease Protocols

VSD

1. Localizer scouts
2. Cine–stack of four chamber views (to locate the defect in the base-to-apex plane)
3. Cine–stack of short-axis views (to locate the defect in the antero-posterior plane)
4. VEC–through-plane images of the proximal aorta and pulmonary artery to measure flow

ASD

1. Localizer scouts
2. Cine–2-chamber and 4-chamber views
3. Cine–Stack of short-axis views from base to apex for assessment of LV and RV size and function

TABLE D.1. Sequences by exam type.

Sequence	Standard Exam	Stress/Rest Perfusion	Arrhythmia/ Uncooperative	Valve disorders	Mass	Pericardium
Localizer Scouts	X	X	X	X	X	X
Morphologic images (HASTE/SSFP)	Optional	Optional	Optional	Optional	X	X
CINE -stack of short-axis images, 2,3,4-chamber views	X	X		X	X	X
CINE -others				Small field of view of valves		
High-resolution DE (segmented)	matched to CINEs	matched to CINEs		X	X	X
Single-shot IR DE	Optional matched to CINEs	matched to CINEs	matched to CINEs	Optional matched to CINEs	X	X
Single-shot IR DE w long TI	Optional matched to CINEs		Optional matched to CINEs	Optional matched to CINEs	X	X
Perfusion		matched to SAX CINEs			Thru mass	
Velocity-encoded images				Thru valve, prox. aorta/ pulm. art.		
Real-time CINES			SAX, 2,3,4-chamber views			SAX with deep inspiration

4. Gadolinium (Gd)-enhanced 3-D cardiac magnetic angiography (MRA) to visualize pulmonary venous anatomy
5. VEC MRI sequences:
   a. "En face" view is particularly useful for quantification of secundum ASD severity and for visualization of ASD shape and location. The imaging plane is roughly parallel to the interatrial septum, but should be optimized to account for cardiac cycle interatrial septal motion and ASD flow direction (see chapter 4).
   b. Orthogonal in-plane views
   c. Perpendicular to the main pulmonary artery and ascending aorta to measure differential flow.

Tetralogy of Fallot

1. Localizer scouts.
2. Cine–2-chamber and 4-chamber views.
3. Cine– Stack of short-axis views from base to apex for assessment of LV and RV size and function.
4. Cine image parallel to the right ventricular outflow tract.
5. Gd-enhanced 3-D MRA.
6. VEC MRI sequences perpendicular to the main pulmonary artery, ascending aorta, AV valves and branch pulmonary arteries.
7. Post-gadolinium delayed-enhancement imaging to assess for myocardial fibrosis.
   a. Note that RV outflow tract patches usually hyperenhance.

Transposition of the Great Arteries

1. Localizer scouts.
2. Cine–stack of images in the axial plane with multiple contiguous slices from the level of the diaphragm to the level of the transverse arch to provide dynamic imaging of venous pathways, qualitative assessment of ventricular function, AV valve regurgitation, and great artery relationships.
3. Cine–Based on the previous sequence, multiple oblique coronal planes parallel to the superior and inferior vena cava pathways are obtained to image these pathways in long-axis.
4. Cine–Stack of short-axis views from base to apex for assessment of LV and RV size and function.
5. Gd-enhanced 3-D MRA.
6. VEC MRI sequences perpendicular to the main pulmonary artery, ascending aorta, AV valves and any further areas suspicious for obstruction.

7. Post-gadolinium delayed myocardial enhancement to assess for myocardial fibrosis.

Fontan Shunt Evaluation

1. Localizer scouts.
2. Cine–stack of axial images to cover the thorax.
3. Cine –2-chamber, 4-chamber, and short-axis stack to cover the heart.
4. Cine– images in the plane of the Fontan shunt.
5. Gd-enhanced 3-D MRA.
6. VEC MRI measurement perpendicular to the main and/or branch pulmonary arteries, ascending aorta, AV valves, and any other locations suspicious for obstruction.

Coarctation of the Aorta

1. Localizer scouts.
2. Cine–2-chamber, 4-chamber views.
3. Cine–stack of short-axis views for quantitative assessment of left ventricular dimensions, systolic function, mass and mass-to-volume ratio.
4. ine– images parallel to the left ventricular outflow tract and cross-section to aortic valve and root.
5. Cine images –in the long-axis view of the aortic arch (if high-velocity turbulent jets produce systolic signal voids on SSFP imaging, then cine gradient echo may be used; if there is artifact from previous endovascular stents then turbo spin echo is employed).
6. Gd-enhanced 3-D MRA.
7. ECG-gated VEC MRI measurement in the ascending aorta and the descending aorta distal to the coarctation.

Sequences for Evaluation of Congenital Heart Disease.

TABLE D.2. Congenital heart disease protocols.

Sequence/ Lesion	VSD	ASD	Tetralogy	TGV	Fontan	Coarctation
Localizer Scouts	X	X	X	X	X	X
Morphologic images (HASTE/SSFP)	X	X	X	X	X	X
CINE -stack of short-axis images, 2,3,4-chamber views	X	X	X	X	X	X
CINE -others	Stack of 4-chamber views	Optional -Stack of 4-chamber views	In plane of RVOT/ pulmonic valve	Stack of axials thru chest and in plane of SVC/IVC	In plane of shunt	Candy-cane view of aorta, hi-res of aortic valve
High-resolution DE (segmented)			X -to evaluate RVOT, septal HE			
Single-shot IR DE			X (if unable to do hi-res)			
Perfusion	optional	optional		optional		
Velocity-encoded images	Thru prox. PA/ Ao for Qp/Qs	Thru prox. PA/ Ao for Qp/Qs. Also in the plane of the atrial septum and orthogonal to it	Perpendicular to the main pulmonary artery, ascending aorta, AV valves and branch pulmonary arteries.	Perpendicular to the main pulmonary artery, ascending aorta, AV valves and any obstructions.	Perpendicular to the main pulmonary artery, ascending aorta, AV valves and any obstructions.	Transaxial to aorta proximal, distal, and at the coarc for flow and gradients
MR Angiogram		To evaluate pulmonary veins	To evaluate pulmonary artery, aorta, and collaterals	To evaluate pulmonary artery, aorta, and collaterals	To evaluate shunt	To evaluate aorta

Magnetic Resonance Angiography Protocols

Thoracic

1. Three plane localizer scout images.
2. Stack of axial morphologic images –Half-Fourier single-shot TSE (HASTE) and/or SSFP (to cover entire thorax).
3. Axial T1-weighted TSE through aorta (for intramural hematoma, dissection) or pre-contrast fat-suppressed 3-D volumetric T1 weighted acquisition (VIBE)
4. SSFP cine imaging in oblique sagittal plane parallel to the long axis of the aorta ("candy-cane view"), using 3-point scan planning if available. SFOV imaging of the aortic valve is also performed.
5. Pre-contrast angiogram using thin-section 3-D T1-weighted gradient echo MRA sequence. Check for coverage, wrap artifact, and adjust as needed.
6. Contrast timing

   a. Option 1 -Axial test bolus at level of the mid-thoracic aorta. 2cc injection of Gd-chelate, followed by 30cc saline. Administer at the same rate that will be used for the angiogram. Determine time to peak contrast enhancement following injection. Calculate trigger time from the observed circulation time using the formula –Start time = Circulation time+ (injection duration/2) - (scan duration/2).
   b. Option 2 – "Fluoroscopic" monitoring of the contrast passage (Care bolus) can be used to trigger the scan, with monitoring of the contrast in the same plane as the planned angiogram. In this case, elliptic centric k-space acquisition should be used.
   c. Option 3 – Rapid multiphase 3-D acquisitions without timing sequences

7. 3-D contrast enhanced MRA (0.1–0.2mmol/kg Gd-based contrast) (optional – ECG-gated acquisition). These are exactly matched to the pre-contrast images so that subtraction images can be obtained. These can be pre-programmed in advance.

   a. Use spatial resolution at least 1.5mm.
   b. Parallel acquisition if available.
   c. At least 2 acquisitions after contrast injection.

8. Optional - axial T1 weighted gradient-echo post contrast for aortitis, or VIBE sequence. DE-MRI can also be obtained.
9. Analysis - MPR-Reconstruction, MIP and thin slab MIP images are reviewed interactively at a dedicated workstation, along with the source images.

Pulmonary Veins

1. LV structure and function module (if pre-ablation).
2. After a non-contrast mask acquisition, breath-hold nongated contrast-enhanced MRA performed in the modified coronal projection encompassing the pulmonary veins and left atrium (greater anterior coverage if breathholding permits) (optional – optimize oblique projections, ECG-gated acquisition), following an initial non-contrast planning exam.

   a. Gd-chelate (0.2mmol/kg) injected at 2–3cc/sec.
   b. Slice thickness 1–2mm; acquired spatial resolution in-plane 1–1.5mm.
   c. Slices – typically 60–80, as needed to encompass the left atrium and pulmonary veins.
   d. Parallel acquisition used as available, using 2-fold acceleration.
   e. 2 volumetric acquisitions – each breathhold typically no longer than 15–18 seconds.

3. Optional – In cases of suspected stenosis, through-plane phase contrast flow studies can be acquired through each pulmonary vein.
4. Analysis

Contrast-enhanced MRA evaluated qualitatively by scrolling through the source images. The number and position of pulmonary veins is accounted for noting common trunks, accessory veins, and evidence for stenosis or thrombosis. A 3-D workstation is used for MPR analysis to calculate major and minor axes, and cross sectional area of each pulmonary vein ostium. Compare pre- and post-ablation images side by side.

Abdominal

1. 3-plane localizer images.
2. HASTE (Half-Fourier single shot TSE) images are obtained in the sagittal, coronal and axial planes.

3. SSFP stack of axial images, without breath holding
4. Axial 3-D T1-weighted fat-suppressed gradient-echo sequence (Volumetric interpolated breath-hold exam– VIBE).
5. Contrast timing –May be performed using a timing bolus run, or "fluoroscopic" monitoring (Care bolus).
6. 3-D contrast enhanced MRA (0.1–0.2 mmol/kg Gd-based contrast)
   a. Use spatial resolution of at least 1.5 mm; 1 mm isotropic images preferable.
   b. Parallel acquisition if available.
   c. At least 3 acquisitions after contrast injection (arterial, early venous, late venous phases).
7. Re-run the axial 3-D T1-weighted fat-suppressed gradient-echo sequence (Volumetric interpolated breath-hold exam– VIBE).
8. Analysis - MPR-Reconstruction, MIP and thin slab MIP images are reviewed interactively at a dedicated workstation, along with the source images.

Peripheral Moving-Table

1. Dedicated phased-array peripheral vascular coils are preferred, although other coil configurations can be used. Optional–venous compression cuffs (placed on the thighs, and inflated to 50 mm Hg) may be used to slow the contrast passage and decrease venous opacification.
2. 3-plane vessel scouting is performed at all three (or four if necessary) stations with time-of-flight MRA or SSFP localizer sequences.
3. Pre-contrast 3-D gradient echo MRA sequences are obtained for later subtractions.
4. Contrast timing
   a. Option 1 – Axial test bolus at level of distal abdominal aorta. 2cc injection of Gd-chelate, followed by 30 cc saline. Determine time to peak contrast enhancement following injection. Use the same flow rate as will be used for the scan.
   b. Option 2 – "Flouroscopic" monitoring (Care bolus) to time start of scan
5. Stepping-table, contrast-enhanced MRA performed in the coronal projection from the mid abdominal aorta to the feet.
   a. Gd-chelate injected at 1.4cc/sec × 20cc, followed by 0.4cc/sec for 20cc followed by saline flush. This biphasic injection is used to minimize venous contamination.
   b. Slice thickness 1–1.5 mm; acquired spatial resolution in-plane 0.8–1.5 mm.
   c. Slices – typically 60–80, as needed to accommodate vessels of interest.
   d. Volumes obtained of Abdomen/pelvis and thighs may be coarser spatial resolution (larger vessels), while those of the legs preferably are sub-millimeter spatial resolution. The former acquisitions typically require 15–20 seconds, while the leg acquisition may take 45–60 seconds for increased spatial resolution. Elliptical centric k-space acquisition is advantageous for the legs. If available, time-resolved acquisitions are preferred for the legs (see the following detailed MRA protocol).
   e. Parallel acquisition recommended (multichannel surface coil needed)
   f. The contrast-enhanced acquisitions are obtained with the same parameters as the pre-contrast acquisitions and image subtractions are then performed. These can be programmed in advance for in-line subtraction and MIP creation.
6. Analysis
   a. MIP and MPR reconstructions are performed in the orthogonal views for each station. Contrast-enhanced MRA at each station is evaluated qualitatively by scrolling through the coronal slices. The presence, number, and degree of stenoses are evaluated qualitatively.

Alternative: dual injection protocol (Hybrid techniques)

1. An initial angiogram is performed at the calf level. This can be done in one of two ways:
   a) A high-resolution sequence can be obtained at the lower leg level using a pre-contrast mask MRA dataset followed by a timing bolus. 15cc of contrast are then administered at 1cc/sec, with 30 cc saline flush at the same rate. 2 postcontrast datasets are acquired, and then standard moving-table imaging of the abdomen-pelvis and upper-leg stations is

performed as above using a second contrast injection.

b) OR, an initial time-resolved acquisition can be obtained at the calf station either using TRICKS (GE) or by modifying the sequence parameters to shorten the imaging time (see below; the changes result in slightly lower spatial resolution). Following an initial mask acquisition, 8cc of contrast are administered at 1cc/sec with a 30cc saline chaser given at the same rate. Multiple datasets are then obtained, and coronal MIP images are created using in-line subtraction. The standard moving-table peripheral MRA can then be obtained.

See the specific example below of a peripheral MRA protocol with time-resolved imaging as used in this Teaching File.

Sample Peripheral Protocol with Time-Resolved Imaging

Protocol Steps:

Siemens Avanto with time-resolved sequence

1. Patient placed in magnet feet first, and centered at midabdomen
2. Abdomen True-FISP Scout localizers (3 planes)–20sec
3. Table moves 375mm (pt <5′10″) or 420mm (pt>5′10″) –2 sec
4. Upper leg 3 plane scout– 20sec
5. Table moves (see above)–2sec
6. Lower leg 3 plane scout–20sec
7. Lower leg non-contrast mask image for time-resolved sequence –8.5 sec
8. Contrast indicator clicked ON
9. Contrast injected at 1cc/sec for 8cc total, with 25cc flush at 1cc/sec
10. Time-resolved dynamic acquisition started at same time—programmed in advance for 10–15 repetitions, and for in-line subtraction and coronal MIPs –90–130 sec
11. Contrast indicator clicked OFF (VERY IMPORTANT-Later subtractions depend on this)
12. 3-D standard angio non-contrast acquisition at lower leg (26 sec)
13. Table moves to upper leg station –2sec
14. 3-D standard angio non-contrast acquisition –21sec
15. Table moves to abd/pelvis station –2sec
16. 3-D standard angio non-contrast acquisition –15sec
17. Contrast indicator clicked ON (VERY IMPORTANT)
18. CARE-Bolus acquisition (in coronal plane centered on aorta) started
19. Contrast injected at 1.4cc/sec for 18cc, then at .4cc/sec for remainder with flush at .4cc/sec
20. 3-D angio dataset of abdomen/pelvis post-contrast acquisition triggered when contrast seen in abdominal aorta –15sec. (in-line subtraction from pre-contrast mask pre-programmed, along with SAG and COR MIPs)
21. Table moves to upper leg level –2sec
22. Upper leg 3-D post-contrast angio dataset obtained –21 sec (with in-line subtraction, MIPs pre-programmed)
23. Table moves to lower leg station –2 sec
24. Lower leg 3-D angio dataset acquired ×2 –26 sec each (sub/MIPs etc pre-programmed)
25. Additional VIBE post-contrast sequences at abdomen, femorals, popliteals prn.

NOTE: For venous studies following arterial studies, simply re-run the sequence in reverse order—wait approximately 30 seconds and re-acquire the lower leg, then the upper leg, then the abdomen/pelvis

TABLE D.3. Siemens avanto sequences for protocol above.

Sequence	Localizer Coronal	Localizer Sagittal	Localizer Transverse
TR(msec)	3	3	3
TE(msec)	1.5	1.5	1.5
Flip Angle(degrees)	64	64	64
Slice thickness(mm)	8	8	8
Number of slices	15	18	20
Field-of-view(mm)	500 ×500	500 ×500	500 ×500
Matrix(lines)	256 × 180	256 × 180	256 × 180
Averages	1	1	1
Acceleration factor	0	0	0
Bandwidth(Hz/pixel)	900	900	900
Scan duration(sec)	23	23	23

TABLE D.4. 3-D angio sequence with time-resolved imaging.

	Abdomen/pelvis	Thigh	Calf	Calf time-resolved
TR(msec)	2.9	3.51	3.51	2.91
TE(msec)	1.1	1.25	1.25	1.07
Flip Angle(degrees)	20	25	25	30
Slice thickness(mm)	1.4	1.4	1.2	1.3
Number of slices	88	80	104	60
Field-of-view(mm)	500 × 375	500 ×406	500 × 406	500 × 400
Matrix(lines)	384 × 245	512 × 291	512 × 291	448 × 186
Spatial resolution(mm)	1.4 × 1.3 × 1.4	1.4 × 1.0 × 1.4	1.4 × 1.0 × 1.2	1.9 × 1.1 × 1.3
Averages	1	1	1	1
Acceleration factor	2	2	2	2
Bandwidth(Hz/pixel)	500	360	360	470
Scan duration(sec)	15	21	26	8.5
k-space acquisition	linear	linear	centric	centric

Index

9781848000896